COMMERCIALIZATION SECRETS FOR

SCIENTISTS AND ENGINEERS

COMMERCIALIZATION SECRETS FOR

SCIENTISTS

AND

ENGINEERS

MICHAEL SZYCHER, Ph.D.

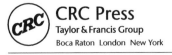

CRC Press
Taylor & Francis Group
Boca Raton London New York

CRC Press is an imprint of the
Taylor & Francis Group, an **informa** business

CRC Press
Taylor & Francis Group
6000 Broken Sound Parkway NW, Suite 300
Boca Raton, FL 33487-2742

© 2017 by Taylor & Francis Group, LLC
CRC Press is an imprint of Taylor & Francis Group, an Informa business

No claim to original U.S. Government works

Printed on acid-free paper
Version Date: 20161115

International Standard Book Number-13: 978-1-4987-3060-0 (Paperback)

Library of Congress Cataloging-in-Publication Data

Names: Szycher, M. (Michael), author.
Title: Commercialization secrets for scientists and engineers / Michael Szycher.
Description: Boca Raton : CRC Press, 2017.
Identifiers: LCCN 2016049768| ISBN 9781498730600 (paperback : acid-free paper) |
    ISBN 9781498730617 (ebook)
Subjects: LCSH: Technology transfer. | Research, Industrial. | New business enterprises. |
    Science--Vocational guidance. | Engineering--Vocational guidance.
Classification: LCC T174.3 .S99 2017 | DDC 658--dc23
LC record available at https://lccn.loc.gov/2016049768

Visit the Taylor & Francis Web site at
http://www.taylorandfrancis.com

and the CRC Press Web site at
http://www.crcpress.com

Printed and bound in the United States of America by
Edwards Brothers Malloy on sustainably sourced paper

This book is dedicated to my wife, Laurie; my son, Mark and his wife, Rachel;

my son, Scott and his wife, Diane; and my wonderful grandchildren,

Arielle and Jason.

Contents

Section II   Classical Initial Decisions

Section III Product Launch

Section IV Pathways to Profitability

List of Abbreviations

3Fs	Friends, family, and fools
4Cs	Consumer, cost, communication, and convenience
4Ps	Product, price, promotion, and place
ACA	Affordable Healthcare Act
AOR	Authorized Organization Representative
ARRA	American Recovery and Reinvestment Act
B2B	Business to Business
BRIC	Brazil, Russia, India, and China
BTC	Beta Test Coordinator
CCR	Central Contractor Registry
CDC	Certified Development Company
CDRH	Center for Devices and Radiological Health
CEO	Chief executive officer
CER	Comparative effectiveness research
CFR	Code of Federal Regulations
cGMP	Current good manufacturing practice
CI	Competitive intelligence
CMO	Contract Manufacturing Organization
CMS	Centers for Medicare and Medicaid Services
CPI	Consumer Price Index
CRO	Contract Research Organization
DoD	Department of Defense
DUNS	Data Universal Numbering System
E-Biz POC	E-Business point of contact
EGC	Emerging growth company
EHR	Electronic health record
EIN	Employer identification number
eRA	Electronic Research Administration
EU	European Union
FDA	Food and Drug Administration
GDP	Gross domestic product
GE	General Electric
GPO	Group purchasing organization
GUI	Graphical user interface
HHS	Department of Health and Human Services
HIT	Health information technologies
IDE	Investigation Device Exemption
IND	Investigational New Drug
IP	Intellectual property
IPO	Initial public offering

JV	Joint venture
KISS	Keep it simple, stupid
KM	Knowledge management
KPI	Key performance indicator
M&A	Mergers and acquisitions
MCPI	Medical Consumer Price Index
MRI	Magnetic resonance imaging
NAICS	North American Industry Classification System
NB	Notified body
NDA	New drug application
NIH	National Institutes of Health
NBA	National Bankers Association
NSF	National Science Foundation
OECD	Organisation for Economic Co-Operation and Development
ONC	Office of the National Coordinator for Health Information Technology
OOPD	Office of Orphan Products Development
PI	Principal investigator
PMDL	Pharmaceutical and Medical Device Law
PMA	Premarket approval
PMN	Premarket notification
R&D	Research and development
ROI	Return on investment
SBA	Small Business Administration
SBIC	Small Business Investment Company
SCORE	Service Corps of Retired Executives
SIA	Strategic international alliance
SME	Small and medium-sized enterprise
SO	Signing official
STTR	Small business technology transfer
SWOT	Strengths, Weaknesses, Opportunities, and Threats
VC	Venture capital
VHRD	Virtual human resource development

Section I

Development on a Shoestring

1

Risk Is a Four-Letter Word

Do you have a solution to a problem, or do you have a solution looking for a problem?

1.1 Introduction

Commercialization is profiting from innovation through the sale of or incorporation of a specific technology, for example, high-temperature superconductivity, into products, processes, or services. Commercialization emphasizes activities including product/process development, manufacturing, and marketing, as well as any supporting research. Commercialization, not innovation or invention *per se*, is primarily driven by firms' expectations of securing a competitive advantage in the marketplace [1]. Innovation delivers the benefits of a new method, idea, product, or procedure to customers or clients, whereas commercialization monetizes innovative ideas. For most start-ups, commercializing innovative ideas allows founders and shareholders to reap the financial benefits.

Commercializing a knowledge-based product or service requires a realistic, methodical approach combined with a great deal of perseverance. In this book, we use the terms *technology commercialization* and *technology transfer* as (1) transforming research into practical applications with commercial potential, (2) seeking patent protection for those innovations, and (3) licensing to industry participants via contractual agreements. Commercialization includes extensive market research, competitive analysis, value proposition development, and business plan development.

This book is intended to serve as a high-level guide to key questions and critical issues that will confront you, the founding entrepreneur, as you begin your quest to commercialize your knowledge-based innovations emanating from your laboratory.

1.1.1 Invention and Innovation

Invention and *innovation* are commonly used in overlapping ways to refer to developing new technology and incorporating it into new products, processes, and services. Confusion often arises from subtle differences in the meaning of each term; hence, for our purposes, these two terms will be defined as follows:

Invention: devising or fabricating a novel device, process, or service. Invention is the conception of a new product, process, or service, but not putting it into use. Although inventions can be protected by patents, many are not, and most patents are never exploited commercially.

Innovation: the development and application of a new product, process, or service, and assumes novelty in the device or in its application. Thus, innovation encompasses either using an existing product in a new application or developing a new device for an existing application. Innovation includes activities that support dissemination and application of an invention, such as scientific, technical, and market research; product, process, or service development; and manufacturing and marketing.

1.2 Commercializing Knowledge-Based Products

Developing, distributing, and commercializing knowledge-based, scientific, and advanced high-technology products reflect a growing worldwide trend toward high-technology industries, including wireless communications, information technology, pharmaceuticals, life sciences, nanotechnology, and education. Commercializing knowledge-based products is a complex undertaking—Figure 1.1 depicts the process of going "from your brain to your bank account."

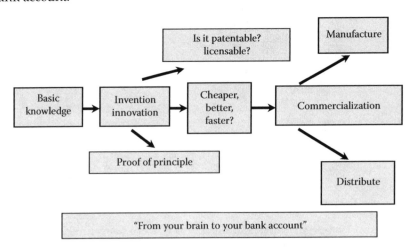

FIGURE 1.1
Commercialization of knowledge-based technology.

TABLE 1.1

Famous Solutions for Common Problems

Product Name	Description	Problem ("Need")
Ronco power spray guns	Gun that washes cars in less than 5 min	Waxing/washing cars simultaneously
Chop-O-Matic	Kitchen appliance to quickly cut onions, potatoes, etc.	Teary eyes Time-consuming tasks
Dial-O-Matic	Slice a potato so thin you can read a newspaper	Cutting food ultrathin
Veg-O-Matic	Slices, dices, and juliennes to perfection	Lower kitchen skills for specialized recipes
Feather-touch knife	So sharp it can shave the eyebrows off a NJ mosquito	Incredibly sharp table knives
Ginsu knife	So sharp it can cut a cow in half. And that's no bull	Ruggedly sharp large knives

Source: Modified from Popeil, R. *The Salesman of the Century.* Delacorte Press, New York, 1995.

Ron Popeil, the so-called Salesman of the Century, became famous for mass marketing household products on television. Although Table 1.1 lists consumer products, notice that each item is targeted toward solving a specific problem, that is, the "need."

Although you begin your quest as the great specialist with a vision for an innovative product and its associated need, you must become the great generalist and communicator once you have started your company and hired your team (as seen in Figure 1.2). In addition, you must familiarize

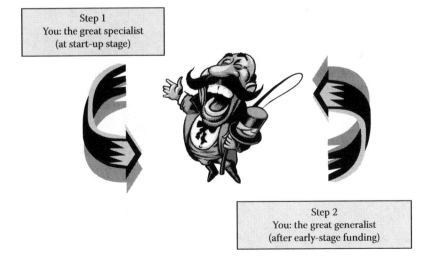

FIGURE 1.2
The great secret.

yourself with a myriad of specialties including manufacturing, marketing and sales, legal, accounting, finance, and human relations, as shown in Figure 1.2.

1.2.1 Establishing Your Communications Platform

Furthermore, much like Ron Popeil, you must become your company's greatest communicator (i.e., salesman). Who better than you to lead your team to commercial success and its attendant financial rewards (as shown in Figure 1.3)?

In a start-up company, your ability to communicate is the heart and soul of attaining fair value. While a business plan is essential, your emotion and deep commitment to the enterprise's success cannot be conveyed to a potential investor from a business plan or a PowerPoint slide deck. Your communication skills will instill confidence and trust, thereby adding needed credibility to everything written down on paper.

Positioning within the marketplace and communicating value to both investors and customers are critical. Irrespective of whether your company is a start-up or a more mature endeavor, you can achieve these goals in four sequential steps [2]:

Step 1. Develop your investment proposition

Step 2. Identify and target your investor and customer audience

Step 3. Develop your communications platform

Step 4. Maintain constant communications with the marketplace

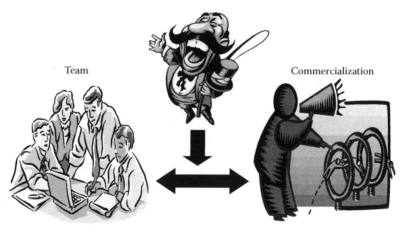

FIGURE 1.3
You: the great communicator.

1.3 Risk in a Start-Up Environment

The word *risk* is derived from the Latin *riscare*, "to dare" or "run into danger." Risk is omni-present and involves many disciplines including probability, statistics, psychology, and history. In entrepreneurial terms, *risk* is uncertainty around financial and operating results. In a start-up environment, risk is the possibility of losing a portion of the invested capital, at best delivering less-than-projected results, and at worst threatening the viability of the new enterprise.

Peter Drucker, the management guru, identified four business risks [3,4]:

1. Risk inherent to the business
2. Risk one can afford to take
3. Risk one cannot afford to take
4. Risk one cannot afford not to take

Start-ups face unique risks, and the reality is that only certain innovations may be suitable for the creation of a start-up company. Along with the invention team, management should analyze several factors to determine whether a start-up is the most appropriate path to commercialization.

1. **Demand:** Potential for the core technology to provide a solid platform for multiple markets or product opportunities
2. **Competition:** Identification of other companies that address similar needs or offer similar solutions
3. **Licensing:** Likelihood of interest from existing companies in licensing your technology
4. **Early-Stage Funding:** Availability of capital to build and grow your business, together with the interest, capabilities, and track record of likely investors
5. **Commitment:** Level of commitment and personal involvement of the inventors
6. **Support:** Presence of a true business champion for both your technology and your new venture

Most successful knowledge-based businesses are started by people who already have several years of relevant technical experience. A profound understanding of the technology involved, of customer behavior, and of market dynamics are critical to grow an innovative idea into the minimal level of sales to become financially viable (also known as breakeven or escape sales velocity).

For example, before founding Intel, Gordon Moore and Robert Royce already had several years' experience at Fairchild Semiconductors. Conversely,

TABLE 1.2

Examples of Crucial Start-Up Risks

Within the Organization (Internal)	In the Marketplace (External)
Key executive/managerial positions cannot be filled	Sales are only 50% of prediction
A key member of staff, such as the head of R&D, leaves abruptly	Inability to obtain patent protection
Prototype delays	Costs spiral out of control
Failure to obtain regulatory approvals	Distributor partner breaches agreement

TABLE 1.3

Your Risk Mitigation Table

Risk Category	Issues to be Answered by Team
1. Technological	Does the new technology really work?
2. Financial	Can you raise enough capital?
3. Market	Is the market size large enough?
4. Regulatory	Can you meet FDA, EPA, OSHA, ISO, SEC, IRS, etc. regulations?
5. Operational	Is adequate management in place?
6. Force majeure	Are you prepared for natural disasters, fire, floods, hurricanes, etc.? Can you afford adequate business insurance?

there are examples (albeit fewer) of revolutionary concepts that have been invested and commercialized by visionaries with no experience whatsoever. Steve Jobs and Steve Wozniak quit their university studies to found Apple, and Fred Smith developed FedEx's concept of "on-time delivery" while still a graduate student in business school. Table 1.2 presents four crucial internal and external risks to consider when deciding whether or not to start a company.

As a start-up founder, your most important goal is to mitigate business risks. Develop a "risk mitigation table" and work to minimize each risk's likelihood and impact. Generally, for knowledge-based entrepreneurial companies, there are six major sources of risk, as shown in Table 1.3.

1.4 Your Innovation and Opportunity Recognition

Were you aware that Thomas Edison did NOT invent the light bulb? Not only did 22 inventors have the idea before Edison did, but 22 researchers actually invented incandescent electric lamps before Edison did. Edison did not steal their ideas, but instead improved on their idea by first understanding the market. He realized that a lower-priced and longer-lasting light bulb was necessary if light bulbs were to enter mainstream use, so he and his dream team created the incandescent light bulb, and the rest is history. The

1. Unique selling proposition. "Unique" defined from the customer's viewpoint, not R&D or design departments. Superiority is derived from design, features, attributes, specification, and positioning.
2. Strong market orientation that prevails throughout the entire new product project.
3. Pre-development strategy that includes market and technical studies, market research, business analysis, prototype production, etc.
4. Unambiguous and early product definition. Including target market definition, concept and benefits, positioning strategy, product failures, and prioritized attributes.
5. Clearly specified budgets (including materials, capital equipment, and staff).

FIGURE 1.4
Top five reasons for new product successes.

moral of the story is that (s)he who had the idea first doesn't necessarily win. In fact, if your idea is so good, there is a good chance that many others have thought of it before you. The winner takes the idea to market first (first mover advantage), continues development based on customer feedback, and then commercializes and scales the business to achieve escape velocity.

Your innovative idea must appeal to potential investors. You must develop a roadmap, not an advertising leaflet or a technical description, which answers the following two questions: (1) What is the customer benefit? (2) What market problem "pain" does your idea alleviate?

Commercial success is generated from satisfied customers, not from amazing products. Customers buy a product to satisfy a need or to solve a problem—perhaps by reducing effort, increasing pleasure, enhancing their self-image, and so on. Thus, the first characteristic of a successful business idea is that it clearly articulates the need it will satisfy or problem it will solve, and whether it will be delivered as a product or as a service. Marketing specialists often refer to a product or service's distinctiveness as its "Unique Selling Proposition." Figure 1.4 summarizes the top five reasons for new product successes.

1.5 What Is the Level of Market Pain?

What market problem are you trying to solve? A business idea only has real economic value if people want your product or service and are willing to pay for it at a price that is profitable to you. Furthermore, a successful business idea has a clearly identifiable market need and a target customer group(s).

How will it make money for you and your investors? Most products generate revenue directly from sales. In some cases, however, the "revenue mechanism"

- Meets a screaming market need
- Highly innovative or disruptive
- Unique product/service
- Focused to mitigate risks
- Promises high long-term profitability

FIGURE 1.5
The five characteristics of a killer idea.

can be more complicated: for example, the product is given away free of charge to the consumer but is paid for by advertisers. Last, a successful business idea clearly articulates how and when money will be made.

To merit the consideration of professional investors, any business idea must meet the "five killer criteria" shown in Figure 1.5. Although investors live with the risk of losing their money, they will limit this risk as much as possible, so a single issue may halt their pursuing a business idea.

1.6 Presenting Your Business Idea

The way you present your business idea to an investor will be the acid test of your efforts. Investors will notice and show interest based on content and your professional qualifications. Remember that most venture capitalists, whose time is limited, receive up to 40 business ideas *every week*.

Therefore, your first goal is clarity. Investors will typically not have familiarity with your product's technology or the jargon of your trade, and are unlikely to take the time to understand confusing terms or concepts. Your second goal is conciseness of content and expression. If an investor shows interest, there will be ample opportunity at a later time for detailed descriptions and exhaustive financial calculations.

Developing business ideas is only one aspect of starting a business. Your ideas must be screened and evaluated to determine those that warrant further investigation. Should your product or service be deployed by an existing company, or should a new company be launched?

Entrepreneurs must provide compelling answers to questions such as

- What is the size of the market served by this product?
- Are there competitive products already in this market?
- How does your product compare to and differentiates from competing products?
- Who are your current competitors?

Many concepts may be feasible under the right conditions, and the feasibility tests listed in Table 1.4 will help you determine those conditions.

TABLE 1.4

Assessing Your Business Risks and Market Pain

	Strong	Weak
Your industry		
What are the demographics, trends, patterns of change, and life cycle stage of your selected industry?		
Are there low or high barriers to entry? If so, what are they?		
What is the development status of your innovative technology?		
What are typical profit margins in your industry?		
What is the status of your target industry? Expanding? Contracting?		
Your target market		
Is there a market large enough to make your concept feasible and worth the time and effort to create a new product/service?		
Customers		
What are the current and expected demographics of your target market?		
What is your customer profile? Who is your customer?		
Have you contacted some of your largest customers?		
Who are your competitors and how do you differentiate yourself?		
Product/service		
What are the features and benefits of the product or service?		
What are the product development tasks and what is the timeline for completion?		
Is there potential for intellectual property rights (copyrights, patents, etc.)		
How is your product or service differentiated from others in the market?		
Finance		
What are your start-up capital requirements?		
What are your working capital requirements?		
What are your fixed cost requirements?		
How long will it take to achieve positive cash flow?		
What is the break-even point for your start-up business?		
Distribution channels		
What are potential distribution channels and which customers will be served by them?		
Are there ways to innovate in the distribution channel?		
Your start-up team		
Can an appropriate start-up team be put together to execute your concept?		
What executive and technical expertise does your team possess?		
What are the team gaps and how do you plan to fill them?		

Note: Entrepreneurs are willing to work 80 hours a week to avoid working 40 hours a week.

1.7 Sizing Your Intended Market

Technology entrepreneurs face a unique problem of sizing their intended market since they typically develop their business from a research and development (R&D) perspective, often ignoring the intricacies of new or emerging markets. It is difficult to determine the rate at which a new technology will be accepted and the rate at which your innovation may replace existing approaches to solving the same problem.

The rate of market acceptance depends on factors such as

- New legislation and enforcement of existing legislation
- Number of competitors
- Approval from governmental entities (if required)
- Product pricing
- Training required to use the technology
- Capital invested in alternative approaches
- Other synergistic technologies

Factors that affect the rate at which an emerging market adopts your technology create financial risk, and investors are often reluctant to provide significant financing while the market risk is high. Instead, they wait until preliminary customer acceptance is demonstrated before making significant investments. As such, targeting a very large intended market is crucial to attracting investors.

The *market buildup method* is commonly used to size your intended market. Market buildup is a market forecasting technique that involves identifying the set of potential buyers within a particular market and learning their product preferences or choices. Forecasting demand in an emerging market provides companies with a sense of whether the product or service would attract a sufficiently large number of buyers to be financially viable.

Your emerging market demand is the total product volume (1) as a function of a customer group, (2) in a geographical area, (3) during a particular period, (4) in a specified marketing environment, and (5) under a defined marketing program.

1.8 Before You Start...

A good idea does not necessarily result in a good product. And a good product does not necessarily result in a successful company. The first

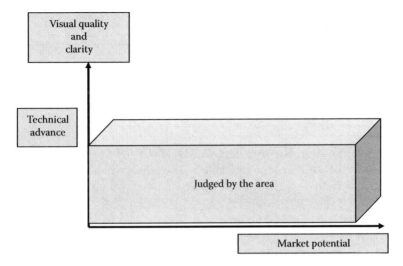

FIGURE 1.6
Presenting your ideas convincingly.

milestone in starting a high-growth company is to develop a convincing product that solves a market problem. To do so, you must consider your idea from the investor's perspective, that is, to clearly and concisely demonstrate how customers benefit from your idea, how you will deliver the product or service and in which markets, and how and when money will be made. Last, you must present your idea in a convincing fashion, as shown in Figure 1.6.

In general, most entrepreneurs are "technology driven," whereas investors are "market driven." While technology driven focuses on the scientific or technical merits of the idea, market driven is the profit potential versus the financial risks of the start-up organization. Thus, there is a clear dichotomy between entrepreneurial and investment cultures, with the former focused on cutting-edge innovations and the latter focused on market needs. The entrepreneur must bridge this cultural gap by ensuring that his or her technology addresses a "crying market need."

1.8.1 Your Business Planning and Commercialization Channels

Many technology entrepreneurs view business planning as a necessary evil, an admission "ticket" to the commercialization game, but business planning is actually the business counterpart of scientific theory construction, and is the process by which "conjecture is turned into certitude" and "intuition is replaced by facts" [5]. Business planning is the precursor of commercialization, and your business plan and commercialization channels must be clearly communicated to all your stakeholders. There are three broad channels for commercializing your technology:

1. Selling or assigning ownership of the technology to an existing company
2. Licensing the technology to an existing company
3. Starting a new company

Choosing the right channel is critical. Key variables to making this decision include the nature of the technology itself, the industry it will be applied to, and the objectives of the inventor. Many will consider starting a new company for the following reasons:

- Market potential for the opportunity is worth the added risk.
- Maximizing the value of the technology.
- Desire to work with an experienced business person who can lead the company.
- Existing contacts to create a business team and access to other support and resources.
- Prior attempts to license the technology have been unsuccessful.

1.8.2 Key Initial Considerations

Creating a successful new company is difficult, and success is often heavily influenced by factors outside your control. The stark reality is that a very large proportion of start-ups fail. Although creating a new company to commercialize your technology holds the highest risk, it can also lead to the highest reward. Following are items to consider when deciding whether to start a new company:

1. Is your invention a disruptive technology? If not, how would it be categorized?
2. How soon can a commercial product come to market?
3. What is the level of risk associated with this start-up?
4. Does the technology have clear applications and a definable market?
5. Who owns the intellectual property?
6. What will be your role in the new company: full-time employee, advisory board member, executive, or consultant?
7. What are the goals for the company? Is it to grow the company and position it for an acquisition or a possible initial public offering? Or, is it to build a small, yet sustainable business?

8. Will capital from private investment companies be needed? If so, will the company eventually be sold or go public? Private investors rely on these exit strategies to get a return on their investments.

9. What is the current valuation of the company? Valuations are based on several factors, including stage of development, proof-of-concept lab data, whether there is a working prototype, if there are any paying customers.

10. Have you spoken to potential customers? Valuable information includes what customers care most about, needs most critical to address, current solutions (if any) to their problems, and how much they are willing to expend on a solution.

Finally, the following legal steps are necessary before you start:

- Select the legal form for the business (sole proprietorship, corporation, partnership, or Limited Liability Company).
- Apply for federal and state employer tax identification numbers (if needed).
- Obtain the proper licenses that apply to your business.
- Apply for workers' compensation and other insurance through private insurance carriers.
- Register a trade name if applicable.
- Apply for any trade name registration, registration, trademarks, copyrights, or patents necessary to protect your assets.
- Engage and consult qualified advisors in law and taxes as needed.

Legal counsel may greatly enhance the decision-making process when starting a company. An attorney with experience in small business entity formation and equity considerations can be a reliable and trusted advisor.

1.9 After You Start...

Firms may encounter difficulties bringing new technology to market at any of several points during the commercialization process. Often, the most difficult stage is converting a prototype into a salable product. In the pharmaceutical industry, for example, a new drug must undergo costly and time-consuming clinical trials with no guarantee of a successful outcome. In electronics, scaling up production using state-of-the-art manufacturing facilities can cost in excess of several hundred million dollars with significant uncertainty as to the time required to achieve full-scale production with acceptable yields.

Small firms face daunting financial constraints in the cost-prohibitive stages of commercialization. Because venture capital and contributions from wealthy individuals (often called angels) are rarely sufficient to these commitments, small firms frequently ally with partners that provide the necessary working capital. As compensation for contributing working capital, these partners may demand patent licenses, equity, and/ or other forms of remuneration. Such arrangements are more likely to succeed when the small firm and its partner(s) are in the same line of business. For instance, several large pharmaceutical companies have provided support to small biotechnology firms in return for a license to the new drug. Large companies, by contrast, can manufacture and market a new drug through existing distribution channels with no need to establish a partnership [1].

As shown in Figure 1.7, inadequate capitalization is the most prevalent cause of new product failures, but there are others to consider.

The following legal steps are necessary after you start:

- File returns for both state and federal taxes.
- Comply with all state and federal requirements for withholding and payment of payroll taxes on behalf of employees (if any).
- Comply with all state/federal sales and use tax regulations, as applicable.
- Pay local property taxes, as applicable.
- Obtain a US Employee Identification Number, if needed (IRS Form SS-4).
- Protect the intellectual property that is the foundation of the new company.

1. Inadequate capitalization—biggest reason small companies fail
2. Target market—large enough to be profitable
3. Poor product quality/performance—product does not meet customer needs
4. Insignificant differentiation—product is not a major improvement on competitive offerings
5. Poor execution of marketing mix—wrong price, wrong distribution, wrong product launch

FIGURE 1.7
Top five reasons for new product failures.

Also, continue to refine and practice your 1-min "elevator pitch," and network with other entrepreneurs and representatives in the industry.

1.9.1 Your Product Pipeline

Investors are attracted to innovative discoveries that could lead to multiple products or product lines (so-called platform technologies). A platform technology is a technology that could lead to multiple additional products and is the basis of a product pipeline. Investors often ask, "Is it a product or a company?" Single product ideas ("one-pony shows") are viewed as inherently more risky.

A new enterprise can certainly be formed around a single product, but the enterprise will be less attractive to institutional investors unless the product represents a huge, untapped market opportunity.

Determining a company's initial product is often very difficult—especially for platform technologies with many different applications. In some cases, the inventor might want to consider licensing the platform technology for further development to an established company, rather than creating a start-up with multiple products.

1.10 How to Think Like an Executive

To become a successful executive, you will require traits to operate, influence, and lead a commercialization team. This book will assist you in

- Identifying your knowledge boundaries—and how to expand your horizons
- Preparing for uncertainty and the unexpected
- Focusing on results, not activities
- Hiring people smarter than you
- Becoming the great communicator
- Demonstrating your ability to not only invent but also lead

Successful innovation and commercialization of your product depend on more than a strong scientific and technological base. Commercialization is based on reasoned judgments about future profitability from investments in product design and development, manufacturing, marketing, sales, and distribution. Figure 1.8 presents the commercialization process from an executive perspective, that is, by focusing on major milestones.

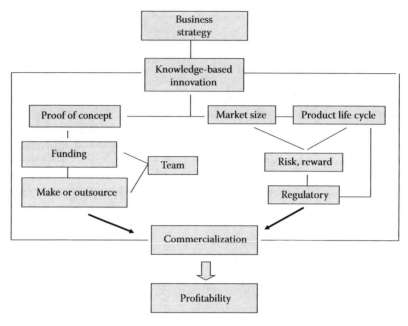

FIGURE 1.8
Commercialization from an executive's perspective.

1.11 Five Pillars of Small Businesses Success

Some 40 million businesses are started each year, yet a paltry 350,000 break out of the pack, grow, and ultimately become profitable. So how can a small business owner overcome common pitfalls and achieve success? Whether you're already in business or preparing to start a business, it takes hard work, tenacity, and drive. Here are the five pillars that make a small business successful [6].

1. **People**

    For your small business to succeed, you need a fantastic team. Surround yourself with people who are much smarter than you and who complement your knowledge and skills. Your company can accomplish amazing things with leadership, and a team that is inspired is hardworking and believes in the mission. Success in business requires passion about a problem that fills a crying need in the marketplace.

2. **Plan**

    Just about everyone in the business world agrees that having a plan is important. A business plan is akin to a PhD thesis, but in contrast to a thesis, a business plan may start slow and then grow over time. Your business plan must answer three key questions:

- Who are your target customers?
- What problems are you trying to solve for them?
- What are the most effective marketing and promotional strategies?

3. **Process**

Dr. W. Edwards Deming, the father of Statistical Quality Control said, "85 percent of the reasons for failure to meet customer expectations are related to deficiencies in systems and processes … rather than the employee." It's crucial that you have a full and clear understanding of your company's processes and have the right systems in place.

As a start-up, implementation is everything—you must assign responsibilities and accountability, set goals, and track performance.

4. **Product**

Does your product solve a problem? Does the product exist yet? Is there something in the marketplace that your product addresses in a different way? Is there a true demand for your product?

5. **Profit**

Profitability is the ultimate measure of business success, so a critical component of running a successful business is understanding your company's finances. "If you want to be successful in business, you need to become proficient at handling certain numbers. You need to be able to read and understand your financial dashboard" [7].

In summary, starting and running a successful business can be a fulfilling and rewarding experience. As a small business owner, you should never stop learning, innovating, planning, and growing. Leaders spend 5% of their time on the problem and 95% of their time on the solution.

References

1. Office of Technology Assessment, 1995.
2. Corbin, J. *Investor Relations: The Art of Communicating Value.* Aspatore, Inc., 2004.
3. Drucker, P.F. *Innovations and Entrepreneurship*, HarperBusiness, reissue edition, 2006.
4. Drucker, P.F. *Managing for Results*, HarperBusiness, reissue edition, 2006.
5. Servo, J.C. *Business Planning for Scientists and Engineers.* Fourth Edition, p. 5. Dawinbreaker, 2005.
6. Carbajo, M. https://www.sba.gov/blogs/5-pillars-small-businesses-success.
7. Fotopulos, D. *Accounting for the Numberphobic: A Survival Guide for Small Business Owners.* AMA, New York, 2015.

2

The Innovation Imperative

When a great executive meets up with a bad business, it is usually the business whose reputation remains intact.

Warren Buffett

2.1 Introduction

Innovation is a buzzword that means many different things to different people, so defining terms is in order. **Innovation**, derived from the Latin *innovatio*, to renew or to change, is the application of knowledge in a novel way for economic benefit. **Innovation activities** are all scientific, technological, organizational, financial, and commercial steps undertaken to implement an innovation, but may also include research and development (R&D) not directly related to a particular innovation.

"Innovation is the ability to see change as opportunity, not a threat," as Steve Jobs famously quipped. The minimum requirement for an innovation is that the product, process, marketing, method, or organizational method must be new (or significantly improved) to the firm [1]. Innovation can thus be viewed as three distinct activities, as seen in the following:

1. The acquisition of new knowledge through leading-edge research
2. The application of new knowledge to create products and services
3. The introduction of advanced-technology products and services into the marketplace

The process starts with an invention, and then progresses to innovation, and finally to commercialization, as discussed in the subsequent paragraphs.

2.2 Invention, Innovation, and Commercialization

Invention is the creation of new products or processes through new knowledge or from a combination of existing knowledge. **Innovation** is the initial

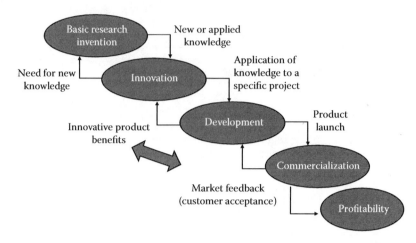

FIGURE 2.1
The five recognized steps from invention to profitability.

commercialization of invention by producing or selling a new product, service, or process. As discussed in Chapter 1, **commercialization** is the process of turning the invention, concept, or innovation into a product or service that can be sold in the marketplace.

Most technological innovation consists of certain predictable incremental steps in knowledge-based industries. Generally, there are five recognized steps from basic research innovation to profitability as graphically shown in Figure 2.1.

Innovation encompasses an **entire process** from opportunity identification, ideation, or invention to development, prototyping, production marketing, and sales. Conversely, entrepreneurship is focused solely on commercialization [2].

2.2.1 Types of Innovation

According to Professor Clayton M. Christensen of Harvard Business School in his book, *The Innovator's Dilemma* [3], innovations are either (1) sustaining or (2) disruptive, as shown in Figure 2.2.

1. **Sustaining**
   - Continuous
   - Discontinuous
2. **Disruptive**
   - Improve products in an unexpected fashion
   - Lower price
   - Enabling technologies

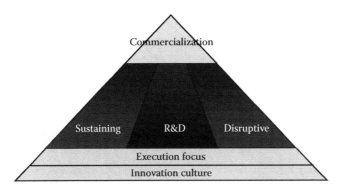

FIGURE 2.2
Ideal types of start-up innovations.

Sustaining innovations improve the performance attributes that are most valued by mainstream customers when choosing a product. For example, the data storage capacity of a USB flash drive increased from 8 MB in 2000 to 8 GB by 2007. The two types of sustaining innovation are *incremental innovation* and *radical innovation*. **Incremental innovation** is created during the ordinary course of business by companies producing and selling established products. Most of the time, an innovator is an employee of the company and often has a personal interest (e.g., a bonus or a promotion) as motivation [4]. Incremental innovation frequently occurs within large established organizations and is typically performed by "intrapreneurs."

Radical innovation creates new value and entirely new competencies within an industry. Importantly, radical innovation may lead to abandoning an existing practice or product. For example, the introduction of minimally invasive coronary stents has nearly eliminated the practice of open-heart procedures for coronary artery bypass surgeries.

Sometimes, though, performance improvements progress beyond market demand for such improvements. In their efforts to provide better products than their competitors, companies may "overshoot" the consumers' appreciation or willingness to pay for improved performance or technological sophistication.

Disruptive innovations, sometimes referred to as breakthrough innovations, destroy the competencies of incumbent firms in an industry. Breakthrough innovations are generally considered "out-of-the-blue" solutions that cannot be compared to any existing practices or techniques. These innovations employ enabling technologies (a technology that can be applied to drive radical change) and create new markets. Most breakthroughs are developed by R&D groups that often have not thought specifically about a particular commercial market application.

Conventional wisdom says "listen to the market," but breakthroughs often come from research laboratories, universities, or other entities that do not have ready touchpoints with customers. These technologies are introduced to the marketplace with the expectation they will be adopted by the consumer [5]. Some examples of disruptive innovations include digitized medical records, super-strong glass that keeps mobile device screens from breaking, and mobile payments via smartphones.

2.2.2 Disruptive Technologies

Clayton M. Christensen and Joseph Bower coined the term *disruptive technologies* in their 1995 article "Disruptive Technologies: Catching the Wave" [6]. Currently, "disruptive" is used in business and technology literature to describe innovations that improve a product or service in ways that the market does not expect, typically by lowering price or orienting toward a different set of consumers.

Disruptive innovations create a new (and unexpected) market by applying a different set of values. This is summarized in Table 2.1.

2.2.2.1 Disruptive High-Tech Innovations

The brisk pace of technology innovations—including mobile devices and apps, social networking, and the cloud—heralds unprecedented opportunities for start-ups in the dynamic high-tech field. Innovations are transforming a variety of sectors in unforeseen ways in this "connected" era. Leaders such as Amazon, Facebook, Google, and Microsoft are joined by upstarts from many countries in the world.

2.2.2.2 Porter's Model

Published in 1980, Michael E. Porter's *Competitive Strategy: Techniques for Analyzing Industries and Competitors* lays out a model called "Five Forces," which has since become a widely used and recognized tool for analyzing industrial structure, competition, and the strategic options of players. In the

TABLE 2.1

Disruptive Technology Examples

Old Technology	New Technology
Slide rules	Handheld calculators
Chemical photography	Digital photography
Movie theaters	VCR rentals
Vinyl records	CDs
Typewriters	Computer word processors
Open-chest coronary bypass surgery	Catheter-based coronary stents
Exploratory gastro-enteric surgery	Capsule endoscopy (pill that you swallow and transmits continuous images via telemetry)

context of disruptive technologies. Porter's Five Forces model can be used to determine to what extent and in what ways a disruptive trend has unfolded (ex-post) or is likely to manifest its impact (ex-ante) [7].

The model is based on the insight that a successful corporate strategy might seize the opportunities and guard against the threats of the organization's external environment. Porter identifies five competitive forces (bargaining power of suppliers, threat of new entrants, bargaining power of buyers, threat of substitute products, and rivalry among competitors; see Table 2.2) that shape every industry and every market, and focuses on the activities and influences of a company's main external actors (customers, suppliers, existing competitors, and new entrants) and on the characteristics of the goods or services that are bought and sold. These forces determine the intensity of competition and hence the profitability and attractiveness of an industry. The objective of corporate strategy should be to modify these competitive forces in a way that improves the competitive position of the organization by influencing or exploiting particular characteristics of its industry.

An innovation is classified as "disruptive" (or at least as having disruptive potential) if it has or may have a **major impact on at least one** of the five competitive forces. For example, one disruptive impact of the Internet in consumer markets is the significant increase in transparency of prices across sellers, thus increasing the bargaining power of consumers. In media markets, the Internet has become a substitute for classified advertising in newspapers. Table 2.2 provides some examples to illustrate how new technologies or other innovations (also including changes in the regulatory framework,

TABLE 2.2

Disruptive Innovations and Their Impact on Competition (Porter's "Five-Forces" Framework)

Competitive Force	Disruptive Innovation Examples
Rivalry in the market	Internet: sales of used cars are increasingly initiated on specialized Internet platforms
Threat of new entrants	Digital photography enabled electronics companies to enter the camera market
	Online intermediaries taking commission from existing service providers (e.g., hotel reservation services, best price finders)
	Online retailers competing with conventional retail stores
Bargaining power of customers	Internet has increased price transparency in consumer goods
	Changes in the regulatory framework/liberalization of markets, allowing customers to select providers (utilities, telecoms)
Bargaining power of suppliers	Electronic components requiring rare earth elements (dependence on raw material providers)
	Substitution of products/services
	Internet: substation of classified advertising
	Computers replacing typewriting machines

which can also be framed as a disruptive innovation) have had impacts on their respective competitive forces.

2.2.3 Classifications of Innovations

Every year, *BusinessWeek* publishes its popular "50 Most Innovative Companies" [8]. *BusinessWeek* classifies Apple as a product innovator, Google as a customer experience innovator, and IBM as a process innovator. These classifications can help us answer questions such as, "What are we innovating around?" and "How many levers are we turning?" [9]. According to this classification scheme, there are four types of innovation:

- **Process innovation:** Process innovation updates internal business processes to improve efficiency. For example, a hypothetical coffee shop called Coffee Express uses a new and faster machine to make cappuccino for customers. Toyota is considered the role model of process innovation through continuous improvement ("kaizen").

- **Product/offering innovation:** Product/offering innovation provides a new product or service to existing customers. For example, 3M began offering Post-It® Notes to customers of its existing office supply lineup.

- **Customer experience innovation:** Customer experience innovation involves improving the customer's shopping experience, which might include enhancing the visual appeal of a retail location or enhancing the website to provide additional product information of recommendations for complementary products. Visual merchandizing is an example from the retail industry.

- **Business model innovation:** Business model innovation is a reconfiguration of one or more of the following: target customer base, degree of insourcing or outsourcing production or inputs to the production process, or product pricing model.

In established organizations, each type of innovation happens in a different department. For example, the delivery or product departments drive process innovation, while new product development, business development, or portfolio management departments develop product/offering innovations. Brand managers are typically responsible for customer experience innovations, and business model innovations are developed within strategy departments.

2.2.4 Oslo Classification of Innovations

The Organisation for Economic Co-operation and Development of the European Union published "Proposed Guidelines for Collecting and Interpreting Technological Innovation Data," known as the Oslo Manual.

According to the Oslo Manual [10], innovations can be divided into the following four distinct classes:

1. **Product innovation:** introduction of a new product or significant improvements to an existing product related to its inherent characteristics or intended uses. Product innovation includes advancements in technical specifications, components/materials, incorporated software, user friendliness, or other functional characteristics. Product innovations can utilize new knowledge or technologies or can be based on new uses or combinations of existing knowledge or technologies.

2. **Process innovation:** implementation of a new or significantly improved production or delivery method, including significant changes in techniques, equipment, or software. A process innovation can be designed to decrease unit costs of production or delivery, to increase quality, or to produce or deliver new or significantly improved products.

3. **Marketing innovation:** implementation of a new marketing method involving significant changes in product design or packaging, product placement, promotion, or pricing. Marketing innovations are aimed at better addressing customer needs, opening up new markets or newly positioning a firm's product on the market, with the objective of increasing the firm's sales.

4. **Organizational innovation:** implementation of a new organizational method in the firm's business practices, workplace organization, or external relations. Organizational innovations can be designed to increase a firm's performance by reducing administrative or transaction costs, improving workplace satisfaction (and thus labor productivity), gaining access to nontradable assets (such as noncodified external knowledge), or reducing costs of supplies.

In a start-up organization, the entrepreneur and the team must decide which innovation classification best fits their organizational goals.

2.2.5 An Innovation Culture

An **innovation culture** is focused on (1) discovering hidden opportunities and (2) commercially exploiting proprietary technologies. Harvard business strategy guru Gary Hamel stated that "pursuing incremental improvements while rivals re-invent the industry is like fiddling while Rome burns" [11].

Developing a culture of innovation is one of the key drivers of success—or failure—of a start-up organization. A good, well-aligned culture can propel a start-up to success, but the wrong culture will stifle its ability to adapt to a fast-changing world. So how do you evaluate your corporate culture? And what steps can you take to create a strong corporate culture that will best support your organization's activities? As founder, you must decide what type of organization culture to establish.

Organizational culture is the collective behavior of people in an organization and the meanings that the people attach to their actions. Culture includes organization values, visions, norms, working language, systems, symbols, beliefs, and habits. It is also the pattern of such collective behaviors and assumptions taught to new organizational members as a way of teaching these new members to perceive, think, and feel. Organizational culture affects the way people and groups interact with each other, with clients, and with stakeholders [12].

Deal and Kennedy [13] defined organizational culture as *the way things get done around here* and created a model of culture based on four different types of organizations. Each organizational type quickly defines the feedback received by the organization, the way members are rewarded, and the acceptable level of risks:

1. **Work hard, play hard**
   - Rapid feedback/reward and low risk
   - Stress from quantity of work expected rather than uncertainty
   - High-speed action coupled with high-speed recreation
   - Examples: restaurants, software companies, and ladies' shoe manufacturers

2. **Tough-guy macho**
   - Rapid feedback/reward and high risk
   - Stress from high risk and potential loss/gain of reward
   - Focus on the present rather than the longer term
   - Examples: police, surgeons, politicians, and sports figures

3. **Process culture**
   - Slow feedback/reward and low risk
   - Low stress, plodding work, comfort, and security
   - Stress from internal politics and stupidity of the system
   - Bureaucracies and other means to maintain status quo
   - Focus on security of the past extending into the future
   - Examples: banks, insurance companies, teaching hospitals, and universities

4. **You-bet-your-company culture**
   - Slow feedback/reward and high risk
   - Stress from high risk and delay before knowing if actions have paid off

- Focus on executing business plans and strategies
- Examples: aircraft manufacturers, oil companies, and start-ups

2.2.6 Mechanisms of Innovation

Technology can enable and drive innovation, but to truly capitalize on technology's potential and unleash an organization's creative energy, technology know-how must be combined with business and marketing insights. Entrepreneurs should view consistent business and technology integration as crucial to innovation. Some mechanisms of innovation include the following:

- Novelty in product or service (differentiation; offering something no one else does)
- Novelty in process (offering products in a new way)
- Complexity (offer something that others find difficult to master)
- Timing (first mover advantage, fast follower)
- Add/extend competitive factors (e.g., price, quality, choice)
- Robust design (contribute a technology platform on which other variations can build)
- Reconfiguring the parts (building more effective business networks)

2.2.7 Most Iconic Failure-to-Innovate

What's wrong with this picture? In 2002, Kodak, defeated by the digital photography revolution, filed for Chapter 11 bankruptcy *despite* the early invention of a digital camera by a Kodak engineer, Steven Sasson, in 1975 [14]. Sadly, the digital camera was only one of countless technological innovations that Kodak failed to successfully commercialize.

Immensely successful companies can become myopic and product oriented instead of focusing on consumers' needs. Kodak's story of failure has roots firmly planted in its successes, which made the company stagnant and resistant to change. Its insular corporate culture led executives to believe that its strength was in its brand and marketing, and the company tragically underestimated the threat of an innovative technology such as digital photography [15].

Kodak's history shows that innovation alone is insufficient; companies must also have a clear business strategy that can adapt to changing times. Without such a strategy, disruptive innovations can sink a company's fortunes—even when the innovations are their own.

It wasn't always that way at Kodak. When Kodak's founder George Eastman [16] first began using his patented emulsion-coating machine to mass produce dry plates for photography in 1880, he was the one being disruptive. For more than a century thereafter, Kodak dominated the world of film and popular photography. In 1976, Kodak commanded 90% of film sales and 85% of camera sales in the United States [17], surpassing $10 billion in sales in 1981.

In 2015, the digital photography market—cameras, lenses, printers, and complementary products—was valued at more than $70 billion. Photography services account for several hundred billion more in revenues, and opportunities for providing these services digitally have become big business [18].

Just 25 years ago, very few people foresaw the opportunity for digital photography, and even fewer could have predicted digital photography's impact on related markets. Even fewer would have predicted the rise of the microstock photography market and the proliferation of and growth in Internet photo-sharing sites. While perhaps the impact on the photo processing market could have been predicted, most were surprised by how rapidly digital photography has displaced film. When digital cameras were introduced, customizing merchandise with personal photographs was in its infancy, with few firms offering customized products to customers who mailed in photographs.

Before the advent of the digital camera, photography-related markets included cameras, interchangeable lenses, film, film processing equipment, photo printers, scanners, and some storage products. However, the introduction of the digital camera disrupted all these markets. Overall, these markets are substantially larger than in the past since a far greater number of people who are involved with digital photography (e.g., using smartphones) than ever used traditional silver halide photography.

2.3 What Gets Measured Gets Attention… and What Gets Attention Gets Done

The sad truth is that 80%–90% of all innovations fail to produce the desired financial results [19]. Why? Following are the 10 most common reasons for innovation failures:

- Failure to meet needs of the market
- Poor launch timing
- Negative market conditions
- Ineffective or inconsistent branding
- Technical or design problems
- Overestimation of market size
- Poor positioning and segmentation

- Inadequate or nonexistent distribution
- Inappropriate metrics to measure success
- Insufficient differentiation from existing products

In today's business world, innovation is the mantra of success. For start-ups, the big winners are those that match new, marketable ideas with customers' needs before anyone else can. It takes flexibility, creativity, and exceptional planning. But measuring innovation is tricky, since such metrics are a combination of art and science. We throw around terms such as *creativity, breakthroughs, sustaining innovation,* and *disruptive innovation,* without any sense of how to shape, track, and measure the innovation process.

Why don't more companies measure innovation? Because innovation is a nebulous term, definitions differ, and expectations vary [20]. Following are some ways to think about developing metrics.

1. **Garbage in, garbage out. Nothing in, nothing out.**

   If you believe in the age old adage "garbage in, garbage out," then the scope of the problem becomes painfully poignant. Nothing in, nothing out. If you don't measure innovation, how do you know if you are getting it? You don't know, at least not in any systematic way.

   The most innovative organizations carefully consider what goes *into* the innovation process, but also consider what should come *out* of it. They focus on different types of measurements and include both quantitative aspects of the business (e.g., financial results, number of new products brought to market) and qualitative elements (e.g., leadership behaviors).

2. **Articulate the end game: Define the outputs.**

   Many companies zero in on the basics of the financial bottom line—top line revenue and overall profitability—when gauging success. Many also focus on their "net promoter score" (a customer loyalty metric) [21]. These high-altitude metrics are indeed important, but they have limited value when measuring—and driving—innovation. Why? Because these metrics are difficult to interpret within the context of innovation and organizational initiatives, and thus do not inspire action around clearly identifiable operating goals.

3. **Fuel the innovation engine: Identify the inputs.**

   Innovation also involves setting specific goals around ways of *fueling* innovation—things you do internally to help you hit your targets [22].

4. **Create your own metrics.**

   GE (General Electric) takes a customized approach. Over the past decade, employees have filed more than 20,000 patents, many of which have paved the way for the company to assume a leadership position in sustainable energy development and the "industrial Internet." GE's emphasis on protecting intellectual property runs deep in the company's culture and started when GE's founder established its R&D function in the early 1900s. GE has viewed patents as an essential "input" to innovation and has developed metrics around patent awards.

2.3.1 Key Performance Indicators

What are the primary challenges faced by start-ups to measuring innovation effectively? According to the research firm Arthur D. Little [23], there are three challenges: (1) use of key performance indicators (KPIs), (2) benchmarking, and (3) deployment.

2.3.1.1 Use of KPIs

First, innovation performance is difficult to measure and interpret. Most companies have some form of KPI system to show performance and help manage innovation. However, few companies believe that their KPIs are the right ones; nearly 72% of companies rate their innovation performance indicators as weak.

Next, many companies are unable to systematically obtain credible data for peer companies or even from their own organization, resulting in unending internal debates over data robustness and credibility. Ultimately, these debates engender a gradual loss of confidence in their KPI system altogether.

Furthermore, companies face difficulties interpreting when employing metrics such as market share, gross margins, or time to market. Although these metrics are computationally straightforward, they are less than helpful in differentiating between cause and effect. For example, if your average time to market is 14 months, should your market share decrease because your execution is simply too slow compared to competitors', or should your market share increase since you are only considering incremental low-return innovations?

2.3.1.2 Benchmarking

Even useful KPIs are challenging to translate into meaningful improvements. Where KPIs are measured and interpreted, companies struggle with setting shared priorities for improvement. For example, an R&D manager may correctly conclude from benchmarks that the company should innovate more in partnership with its suppliers, but may have trouble finding common ground with a procurement officer who has to meet yearly savings targets. And even when there is a consensus about priority improvements, are you focusing on what matters most for the company as a whole?

2.3.1.3 Deployment

Incidental improvements rarely mature into a system and culture of continuous improvement. Regularly changing priorities (and KPIs) often hinder companies in tracking innovation performance and trends over time, and demonstrating the success of the implemented improvement actions. Senior leadership support for actions can also be lost because the business case is rarely proven, often despite improvements in innovation performance.

2.4 What Gets Rewarded Gets Done Even Faster

Advancements in science and technology directly or indirectly create the overwhelming majority of newly created jobs. Furthermore, at least half of US GDP (gross domestic product) growth in recent decades has been attributed to technological innovation.

Manufacturing in the United States plays an outsized role in supporting and driving American innovation, and increasingly our ability to manufacture undergirds our future abilities to innovate and to create high-paying jobs [24].

- Manufacturing represents 12% of US GDP but contributes 60% of US R&D employees, 75% of US private sector R&D, and most patents issued in the United States [25].

- US manufacturers develop innovations at more than twice the rate of their counterparts in service industries and other US economic sectors. Thirty percent of US manufacturers reported an innovation between 2010 and 2014 compared to only 13% for nonmanufacturing businesses [26]. High-tech manufacturers report even higher rates of product and process innovation.

- For many technologies, the capabilities gained in production are intertwined with new learning and knowledge-based activities of research, development, and design. The iterative innovation cycle between engineering and production on the shop floor is responsible for a range of breakthrough technologies and has prompted many firms to reconnect production with development and design [27].

- Manufacturing output has increased 30% since the end of the 2009 recession, growing at roughly twice the pace of the economy overall. The years 2009 to 2015 mark the longest period since 1965 during which manufacturing outpaced overall US economic output [28].

- Since February 2010, the United States has added 725,000 manufacturing jobs, expanding employment in this sector at the most rapid pace in nearly two decades [29]. Manufacturing also supports millions of additional jobs throughout its supply chain and in local communities [30].

- Global executives in every industry and geography ranked the US #1 destination for business investment because of its highly productive workforce, sizeable and transparent markets, low-cost energy, and historic lead in innovation [31].

- The United States' renewed competitiveness in manufacturing is luring production back onto its shores. Nearly 54% of US-based manufacturers surveyed have returned manufacturing to the United States, a phenomenon known as reshoring.

However, not all industries were born equal regarding product or process innovations. There are wide disparities among industries in average percentages of companies reporting at least one innovation in a given year. For example, the electrical appliances industry reports 53% per year while all other industries average 13%. Manufacturers of communications equipment, aircraft and spacecraft, pharmaceuticals, and computers report rates of innovation at least double the US manufacturing sector average [32]. Additional statistics on innovation across industries are shown in Figure 2.3.

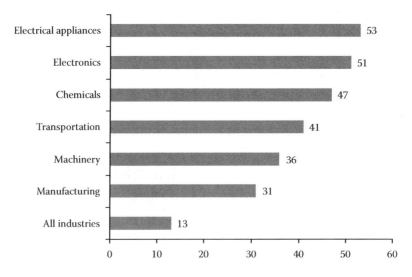

FIGURE 2.3
Companies introducing a new product or process innovation (2008–2010, in percentage). (From National Science Foundation, National Center for Science and Engineering Statistics. *Science and Engineering Indicators.* Arlington, VA (NSB 14-01), February 2014.)

TABLE 2.3

Core Competencies of Innovation

Behavior Patterns	Knowledge, Skills, and Abilities
1. Creativity	• Generating ideas • Critical thinking • Synthesis/reorganization • Creative problem solving
2. Enterprising	• Identifying problems • Seeking improvement • Gathering information • Independent thinking • Technological savvy
3. Integrating perspectives	• Openness to ideas • Research orientation • Collaboration • Engaging in non-work-related interests
4. Forecasting	• Perceiving systems • Evaluating long-term consequences • Visioning • Managing the future
5. Managing change	• Sensitivity to situations • Challenging the status quo • Intelligent risk taking • Reinforcing change

2.5 Your Innovation Core Competencies

To build a culture of innovation, founders must foster and develop "innovation competencies." Innovation competencies are a group of behavior patterns that result from a critical mass of knowledge, skills, and abilities, combined with motivation and persistence. These competencies form a necessary basis for exceptional executive performance [33].

Table 2.3 presents five core competencies necessary to support a culture of innovation.

2.6 Five Discovery Skills of Innovative Leaders

In the *Innovator's DNA*, Christensen et al. list five behaviors (discovery skills) that characterize innovative leaders [34]:

1. Associational thinking
2. Questioning

3. Observing
4. Networking
5. Experimenting

Christensen denotes these attributes as "discovery skills," all of which focus on identifying new opportunities as a critical element of the front end of the innovation process.

In addition to these important idea-generating qualities, other skills are equally important to navigate the entire innovation process given its inherently high level of ambiguity and uncertainty. Accordingly, the five personal leadership competencies essential for success in today's environment are as follows:

1. **A Leapfrogging Mind-Set.** Leading disruptive innovation requires a mind-set focused on *leapfrogging*, that is, creating or doing something radically new or different that produces significant progress. Leaders with an unyielding commitment to creating breakthroughs secure an advantage by focusing all efforts on adding value to the market.

2. **Boundary Pushing.** Pushing boundaries occurs on both the personal level and the strategic level. Leaders who live abroad, work across different functions, and surround themselves with diverse team members continually expand their mind-sets and creative problem-solving abilities. At the strategic level, leaders continually push the limits of their teams, organizations, and partners.

3. **Data-Intuition Integration.** Most leaders demand hard data when making important decisions, but in times of disruption, robust data rarely exist. Leaders must use whatever information they can obtain from any and all sources inside and outside the organization—but then be comfortable using their intuition and experience to fill the gaps.

4. **Adaptive Planning.** Leading disruptive innovation requires managing incredible levels of uncertainty. Adaptive planning creates a feedback loop between action and outcomes, whereby the organizations continually examine results to successively modify and optimize assumptions and approaches. Outcomes, both positive and adverse, provide insights to more effectively calibrate to the needs of the market.

5. **Savoring Surprise.** Disruptive innovation is laden with surprise— unexpected technological advancements, competitive moves, customer feedback, political and regulatory shifts, and other unforeseen events. Most companies strive to avoid surprises, but leaders who

recognize that surprises are inevitable (and natural in business, and life) are better able to actually use surprise as a strategic tool. These leaders are more agile and more likely to capitalize on the unforeseen or unexpected.

To summarize, leaders who want to make a significant difference for themselves and their organizations need to embrace new skills in today's increasingly disruptive competitive environment. While new behaviors are important, so are new mind-sets. Leading disruptive innovation requires a new set of assumptions, many of which require humility, that is, the recognition that we do not (and cannot) have all the answers, and that disruptive innovation is all about finding clarity while embracing uncertainty.

Innovation does not necessarily proceed linearly from basic scientific research to product development; instead, it is an iterative process of both matching market needs to technological capabilities and conducting research to fill gaps in knowledge. Such iterations occur in all phases of the innovation process, including product conception, product design, manufacturing, and marketing. Commercial success depends as much on establishing and protecting a proprietary advantage in the marketplace as on generating scientific and technical advances [35].

2.7 The Process of Innovation

The process of innovation varies dramatically across industries and product lines. In some industries such as pharmaceuticals, innovation depends heavily on scientific breakthroughs, while in others (e.g., electronics), innovation is driven by product and process design. In addition, innovation takes on different characteristics throughout product and industry life cycles. Nascent industries exhibit high levels of product innovation as firms settle on the primary characteristics and architectures of their new offerings; later phases are characterized more by process innovation, as firms improve manufacturing for existing product lines.

Technological innovation is developing and utilizing new products and processes, and demands novelty in the product/process/service and/or application. Innovation therefore includes not only development of entirely new products, processes, and services that create new applications but also development of new products, processes, and services for use in existing applications. Examples include integrated circuits replacing vacuum tubes in electronic applications and manufacturers of flat panel displays adapted semiconductor manufacturing equipment to their needs.

Innovation is more than just invention—innovation must lead to new products, processes, and services that are not obvious to someone skilled in the field and that represent clear departures from prior practice. Innovation requires an invention entering the ordinary course of business in an industry. Many inventions are never put into practice; some cannot meet users' cost or performance requirements, while others lack technologically feasibility.

2.8 Innovation in Different Industries

No single model accurately depicts the process of innovation; innovation occurs differently in different industries and in product lines as firms develop products and processes that meet market needs. In the pharmaceutical industry, for example, innovation is closely coupled to scientific discoveries and follows a fairly linear pathway through manufacturing and marketing. Nonetheless, firms often commence activities with longer lead times earlier than when these activities would otherwise be undertaken, for example, constructing manufacturing facilities while the drug is undergoing clinical trials.

Many obstacles impede the innovation process in pharmaceuticals. For example, existing products are often protected by strong patent protection, markets are quite easily identified and quantified, and third-party payment systems (e.g., insurance companies, health maintenance organizations) relax some cost constraints on new products.

In contrast, innovation in the semiconductor industry is driven primarily from new product design and improvements in manufacturing technology rather than from advances in basic science. Commercial success in the semiconductor industry is more elusive, as product life cycles tend to be short (typically not longer than 3 years) and consumers are highly sensitive to cost.

The aircraft industry's innovation is highly concentrated in a few producers that act as integrators of components from a broad range of suppliers. Furthermore, aircraft product cycles are several decades long, and manufacturers work closely with users to define product specifications and costs.

As the aforementioned examples suggest, innovators face different obstacles in developing and marketing new products, processes, and services, and must proceed through a different set of steps to successfully bring a new invention to market. Not only do differences in industry structure and the nature of markets impose different constraints on the innovation process, but science, technology, and innovation in different industries are linked in different ways. Innovators follow many different pathways through the innovation process, and facilitating innovation and the commercialization of emerging technologies necessarily takes different forms.

2.9 Creating Your Own Innovation Culture

Innovative technology is the cornerstone of value creation, enabling the previously impossible. Start-up entrepreneurs must develop their own "innovation culture" that is capable of achieving success. Research has identified the 10 most desirable characteristics in the innovator-leader, as follows:

1. Initiative
2. Assertiveness
3. Achievement
4. Efficiency
5. High quality
6. Systematic planning
7. Monitoring
8. Commitment
9. Relationships
10. Creativity

A culture of innovation can be the start-up's primary source of competitive advantage, but to create this culture, you cannot merely hold a couple of meetings and pay lip service. You must execute. Some companies, such as Apple, are always innovating popular products, while most others are merely spectators in a contact sport. Innovation gives start-ups their strength, staying power, and value.

The most successful start-ups strike the optimal balance between breakthrough innovations and incremental innovations. Admittedly, when one thinks of innovation, *bold* as opposed to *incremental* more readily comes to mind. Bold conjures up a mental image of people in white coats bent over laboratory benches conducting scientifically or technologically challenging research. Ultimately, the balance between incremental and breakthrough innovations depends on the growth objectives of the start-up. The company will need to pursue a greater percentage of breakthrough innovations to achieve a higher targeted growth rate, provided finances permit. Incremental innovations, meanwhile, protect the market share of pipeline products and complement the breakthrough innovation portfolio.

Ultimately, the portfolio balance between incremental and breakthrough innovations will depend on your growth objectives. The higher your targeted growth rate, the higher the percentage of breakthrough innovations you will need to pursue, risk appetite permitting. Incremental innovations, meanwhile, help protect market share and margins of existing products and services and in that way complement your company's breakthrough innovation. This is visually summarized in Figure 2.4.

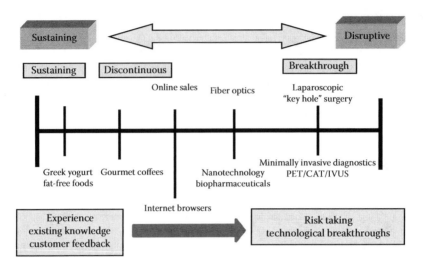

FIGURE 2.4
The innovation continuum.

Innovative start-ups command a price premium in the financial markets. The price premium may be observed in initial valuation or may become apparent during subsequent financing rounds.

References

1. Tiwari, R. Defining Innovation. February 2002, http://www.global-innovation.net.
2. Solow, R. Heavy Thinker, *Review of Prophet of Innovation: Joseph Schumpeter and Creative Destruction*, by Thomas K. McCraw. The New Republic, May 21, 2007.
3. Christensen, C. The innovator's dilemma, *Harvard Business Review*, 1997.
4. Wikipedia, http://en.wikipedia.org/wiki/Innovation.
5. Wikipedia, http://www.go4funding.com/Articles/Types-Of-Innovations.aspx.
6. Christensen, C.M. and Bower, J.L. Disruptive technologies: Catching the wave, *Harvard Business Review*, January–February 1995.
7. INNO-Grips—Global Review of Innovation Policy Studies. http://www.proinno-europe.eu/innogrips2.
8. http://www.businessweek.com/magazine/toc/10_17/B4175innovative_companies.htm
9. Catalign Innovation Consulting, http://www.catalign.in/2009/11/4-types-of-innovations-businessweek.html.
10. Oslo Manual: Guidelines for Collecting and Interpreting Innovation Data, 3rd Edition, October 2005.
11. Hamel, G. Strategy as revolution. *Harvard Business Review*, July–August 1996.

12. Wikipedia, http://en.wikipedia.org/wiki/Organizational_culture.
13. Deal, T.E. and Kennedy A.A. *Corporate Cultures*, Perseus Book Publishing LLC, HarperCollins Publishing, New York, 1982.
14. What's wrong with this picture? Kodak's 30-year slide into bankruptcy, http://knowledge.wharton.upenn.edu/article/whats-wrong-with-this-picture -kodaks-30-year-slide-into-bankruptcy/.
15. http://www.forbes.com/sites/avidan/2012/01/23/kodak-failed-by-asking-the -wrong-marketing-question/
16. http://en.m.wikipedia.org/wiki/Eastman_Kodak
17. Kılıç, E., Hatem, M., Lofty, R., with the collaboration of O. Amat, Barcelona School of Management, Universitat Pompeu Fabra, 2013. Eastman Kodak Co., http://www.econ.upf.edu/docs/case_studies/61en.pdf.
18. Digital Photography: Global MarketsPR Newswire, http://s.tt/1d19c.
19. Andreoli, S. http://www.forbes.com/sites/steveandriole/2015/02/20/why-inno vation-almost-always-fails/.
20. Kaplan, S. http://www.fastcodesign.com/3031788/how-to-measure-innovation -to-get-real-results.
21. http://en.wikipedia.org/wiki/Net_Promoter
22. http://www.quintiles.com/~/media/library/fact%20sheets/re-ignite-product -development-and-sales-data-insights.pdf
23. Kolk, M., Kyte, P, van Oene, F., and Jacobs, J. Innovation: Measuring it to man-age it. Arthur D. Little, Prism/1/2012, http://www.adlittle.com/downloads /tx_adlprism/Prism_01-12_Innovation.pdf.
24. Making in America: U.S. manufacturing entrepreneurship and innovation. June 2014, http://www.whitehouse.gov/sites/default/files/docs/manufacturing _and_innovation_report.pdf.
25. Bureau of Economic Analysis, Department of Commerce.
26. National Science Foundation, Science and Engineering Indicators.
27. MIT Production in the Innovation Economy Commission. *Production in the Innovation Economy*, 2013.
28. Bureau of Economic Analysis, Department of Commerce, NIPA tables.
29. Bureau of Labor Statistics, Department of Labor, Current Employment Statistics Survey.
30. McKinsey Global Institute. *Manufacturing the Future*, November 2012.
31. AT Kearney. Foreign Direct Investment Confidence Index, 2014.
32. National Science Foundation, National Center for Science and Engineering Statistics. Science and Engineering Indicators, 2014.
33. Innovation Competency Model, http://www.innovationinpractice.com/inno vation_in_practice/2011/04/innovation-competency-model.html.
34. Dyer J., Gregersen, H., and Christensen H.W. The Innovator's DNA: Mastering the Five Skills of Disruptive Innovators. *Harvard Business School Publishing, July 19, 2011.*
35. U.S. Congress Office of Technology Assessment. *Innovation and Commerciali-zation of Emerging Technology*, OTA-BP-ITC-165. US Government Printing Office, Washington, DC, September 1995.

3

Development on a Shoestring
(Bootstrapping)

A Rolex does not keep time any better than a Timex.

3.1 Introduction

Start-ups are not a small version of a large company. A start-up is a temporary organization designed to search for a repeatable and scalable business model ... that someday aspires to grow up to become a real company! A start-up is an organization dedicated to innovation under conditions of extreme financial constraints. Large companies have the luxury of allocating budgets to new products and can weather market uncertainties.

So where do start-ups get their initial financial resources? The answer is many start-ups are financed on a "shoestring" or "bootstrapping" basis. **Shoestringing** or **bootstrapping** is the *internal generation* of initial financing, using primarily your own personal resources, and sometimes complemented by various forms of equity investments or loans from family, friends, and relatives.

Bootstrapping is entrepreneurship in its purest form. It is the transformation of inventive value into financial capital. The overwhelming majority of entrepreneurial companies are financed through this "highly creative" process, as well as formal sources of private equity [1]. Interestingly, academic research has suggested that bootstrapping techniques can minimize risk because of the absence of outside venture capital (VC) investors [2]. When everybody says "no"—from the banker to the private investor—the tough small business owners turn to themselves ... they raise money from within by bootstrapping [3].

Because bootstrappers have no choice except to be resourceful, they may have an ironic advantage over other individuals who hail from more resource-rich environments in terms of developing their managerial and entrepreneurial skill sets. To a certain extent, being deprived of resources forces the entrepreneur to find other inventive ways to make do (or make do without) [4].

Entrepreneurial bootstrapping is more celebrated, studied, and desirable than ever before. Business school students flock to courses on entrepreneurship. Managers, fearful of losing their perch on the corporate ladder, yearn to step off on their own. Policymakers pin their hopes for job creation and economic growth on start-ups rather than on the once-preeminent corporate giants.

3.2 Cutting Corners and Pinching Pennies

Of course, not every entrepreneur bootstraps. The legendary Mitch Kapor raised nearly $5 million of VC in 1982 (a small fortune in those days), enabling Lotus to launch the 1–2–3 spreadsheet. Lotus 1–2–3 was the software industry's most successful advertising campaign. Significant initial capital is indeed a must in industries such as biotechnology or supercomputers where tens of millions of dollars have to be spent on research and development before any revenue is realized. Bootstrapping follows a predictable two-stage sequence, as depicted in Figure 3.1.

Many start-ups rely on bootstrapping, which is easier said than done. History shows that successful bootstrappers follow these principles:

- Place great emphasis on critical prelaunch preparations. Conduct enormous amounts of research: library research, bookstore research, Internet research, and especially field research (the nonscholarly translation of field research: network, network, network, with prospective

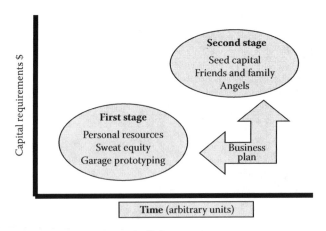

FIGURE 3.1
Stages of bootstrapping financing.

• Establish low administrative salaries from
  the start. You can always go up.
• Remember: every dollar spent on
  administration takes a dollar away from
  producing sales.
• Overhead or profits: your choice.
• Do not overhire: make everyone multitask.

FIGURE 3.2
Overhead bootstrapping.

suppliers, customers, advisory board members, and other potential
friends of the business).

• Crawl before you walk. Learn to barter. Think outside the box—like
  the editor who trades her proofreading services in exchange for an
  ad for her business in a local trade publication.

• Forget appearances. A Taj Majal–style headquarters will only serve
  you after you are successful, not before. Start your business out of
  your home.

• Negotiate terms carefully. Negotiate terms for purchases from vendors and sales to customers. When possible, arrange the purchase–
  sales sequence in a way that customers finance the purchase of
  inventory through prepayment terms.

• Advertise a product that could be produced, if response to the ad
  justifies its production.

• Develop business communications and media skills. Be worthy of
  media attention (i.e., be newsworthy) as a result of a unique product,
  company history, team, or even aspiration.

• Be extra careful of your overhead expenses, as summarized in
  Figure 3.2.

3.3 Bootstrapping Start-Ups via Sweat Equity

An early-stage technology company will almost certainly need some kind
of financial support to successfully get started. The key problem is that most
institutional funding organizations (e.g., banks and most conventional investors) will be accustomed to investing in very different propositions. Table 3.1
summarizes the different investing propositions between institutions and
start-ups.

While you may get some support from the bank, you will almost certainly
have to put up some sort of personal security against the loan. Be very wary

TABLE 3.1

Investing Propositions versus Start-Up Characteristics

Banks and Some Investors Prefer These Characteristics	Technology Start-Up Business Have These Characteristics
• Stable cash flow forecasts	• Fluctuating cash needs
• Business track record	• Business inexperience
• Steady growth forecasts	• High growth rate
• An easy-to-understand market	• New markets/complicated technology
• High fixed asset ratio	• Low fixed assets ratio

of this; remember that setting up a business and commercializing research is extremely high risk. If you are unable to pay off your debts, the banks will collect on their security.

At first, most entrepreneurs spend their own money, technical resources, and time in the yet-to-be formed company. At this point, the company is in the "dream" or "idea" stage and the entrepreneur is accumulating "sweat equity."

According to Investopedia, sweat equity "is the contribution to an innovative project or startup enterprise in the form of effort and toil." Sweat equity is the ownership interest, or increase in value, that is created as a direct result of hard work by the owner(s) and is the preferred mode of building equity for cash-strapped entrepreneurs in their start-up ventures, since they may be unable to contribute much financial capital to their enterprise. In the context of real estate, sweat equity refers to value-enhancing improvements made by homeowners themselves to their properties. The term is probably derived from the fact that such equity is considered to be generated from the "sweat of one's brow" [5].

For example, consider an entrepreneur who spends a year in her start-up. After a year of developing the business and getting it off the ground, she sells a 25% stake to an angel investor for $500,000. The sale gives the business a valuation of $2 million (i.e., $500,000/0.25), of which the entrepreneur's share (sweat equity) is $1.5 million.

Bootstrapping diminishes your dependence on banks and other forms of financing. Some typical examples are as follows:

- Negotiating extended terms with vendors
- Negotiating advance payments from customers
- Working from home until the business is established
- Keeping inventories at a minimum
- Leasing equipment (usually from the manufacturer)

3.3.1 Bootstrapping Best Practices

Lahm and Little [6], in their excellent study entitled "Bootstrapping Business Start-ups: A Review of Current Business Practices," identified and discussed two methods that broadly address bootstrapping. These two methods include the acquisition and control of resources (both tangible and intangible) and the efficient uses of those resources to finance the enterprise for growth. These authors provide a list of 13 practical suggestions for bootstrapping business start-ups, as shown below:

1. Start-up entrepreneurs with little capital should be advised to strongly consider a business model that entails compensation before the delivery of a product or service (e.g., consulting, mail order, or niche-oriented Internet businesses that do not require a glitzy website).

2. An emphasis on prelaunch preparations, perhaps several years in advance, may be wise.

3. More education and training are needed for would-be entrepreneurs such that they are more familiar with traditional sources of capital and nontraditional sources. Bootstrapping should be a course unto itself in university-level entrepreneurship programs.

4. Stockpile nonperishable business assets over a long period. Businesses that have resulted from a hobby often start out with many of the necessary tools, contacts, sources, and skills on the part of the owner to be well equipped from their inception.

5. Conduct enormous amounts of research: library research, bookstore research, Internet research, and especially field research (the non-scholarly translation of field research: network, network, network, with prospective suppliers, customers, advisory board members, and other potential friends of the business).

6. Consider an agency or brokerage-type business: connect a party who needs to sell with a party who needs to buy.

7. Get quotes. Provide a vendor with a general idea of a needed end result for a manufactured product (or a service) and ask for design specifications, pricing, projected delivery schedules, and terms (be sincere as a prospective customer).

8. Negotiate terms carefully. Negotiate terms for purchases from vendors and sales to customers. When possible, arrange the purchase–sales sequence in a way that customers finance the purchase of inventory through prepayment terms.

9. Choose a location wisely. Consider the "image" needs of the business, but also seek economic development dollars (or stakeholders) and co-location opportunities in neighbors with synergistic potential. Do not choose a location because it is close to home and convenient for the owner. It must be convenient for the customer, for the logistical needs of the business, and in a nurturing environment.

10. Advertise a product that could be produced, if response to the ad justifies its production.

11. Develop business communications and media skills. Be worthy of media attention (i.e., be newsworthy) as a result of a unique product, company history, team, or even aspiration.

12. Be generous. People are willing to follow a leader who understands their needs and fulfills those needs.

13. Sell in volume at wholesale, rather than one unit at a time.

3.3.2 Savings, Investments, and Salable Assets

This is always the preferred place to start. Theoretically, all you are doing is transferring your assets from one investment (your savings account) to another (your new business). But understand that you are increasing your risk by a quantum leap, although you are also increasing your opportunity for future rewards.

3.3.3 Your Family and Friends Network

Beyond sweat equity, most tech start-ups raise their first capital from friends and family. Friends and family financings are always the easiest to complete, often taking less than 2 months from start to finish. Friends and family rounds usually raise $25,000 to $150,000 in total [7].

Friends and family investors share the following characteristics:

- They do not need to be "Not accredited"
- May be "unsophisticated" in finance
- Invest their own capital
- Investing in a friend (you), not necessarily in the business
- Passive investors (do not demand board seats or managerial posts)

3.3.4 Life Insurance

If you own life insurance policies with a cash value, you probably shouldn't, because term life insurance is a far better deal. Consider cashing in such policies and putting that money to far better use—your business. Remember, however, that you may owe some income tax on accumulated interest (in excess of the premiums you paid) from your life insurance policy.

Ask yourself whether you really need life insurance at all. If you have no financial dependents, you won't need it to replace your income if you pass away. If you do need life insurance, however, secure good term life coverage before you cancel or cash in your current policy. Otherwise, your dependents will be in trouble if you pass away after you have canceled your current policy but before you have secured new coverage.

3.3.5 Credit Cards

Credit cards provide expensive money, perhaps, but easy money as well. No personal guarantees here, no bankers looking over your shoulder; just sign your name and get on with the business at hand. In the increasingly competitive credit-card market, interest rates on some cards are around 10%, so be sure to shop around rather than simply accumulating a balance on whatever platinum-hued card currently happens to be in your wallet or pitched through an ad, and when you carry a balance from month to month, always make your credit-card payments on time unless you enjoy paying even higher interest rates—in many cases upward of 20%.

3.3.6 Home Equity

Proceed with extreme care when borrowing against home equity. A misstep could cost you the roof over your family's head. Do not even consider this option until you have thoroughly reviewed your overall personal financial situation.

3.3.7 Financing with a Business Plan

Lenders and professional investors read a business plan as much to find out about the preparer as to understand the business. They look for thoroughness, professionalism, and attention to detail in the plan, in addition to the presentation of a credible scenario for running a successful business. After all, thoroughness, professionalism, and attention to detail are the same traits they want to see in the person responsible for managing the money they invest in or lend to the business. What better early indication of these characteristics than your business plan?

The sophisticated investor has learned from experience—horses don't win races; jockeys do. The jockey is you, the business owner, and the business plan is the first official indication of the kind of race your horse is going to run.

Business plans take a lot of time and focus to prepare well and are not to be confused with an afternoon jaunt at the beach. Similar to successfully locating the right financing and finding the right mentor, developing a successful business plan separates the potential doers from the dreamers.

By and large, only the truly committed take the trouble to prepare a business plan. You find some exceptions, of course; some potential small business owners have enough of their act together to carry a good business plan in their head, and, yes, some of those business owners have gone on to achieve great success. But these same business owners may have accomplished even greater success and avoided some early mistakes if they had taken the time to record and refine their ideas in a tangible business plan. The depth of your early commitment to writing a business plan directly correlates to your chances for success, and a well-thought-out business plan demonstrates your depth of commitment to end up at the helm of a successful small business.

Occasionally, investors will fund a start-up business strictly on the basis of a compelling business plan. In this case, the investors will be putting all their trust in you, the entrepreneur, to execute the business plan as presented.

3.3.8 Fundraising Importance of Patents

Patents enable entrepreneurs to acquire financial capital under the most favorable terms in earlier founding rounds [8]. Firms having larger patent portfolios enjoy a greater likelihood of sourcing initial capital, and of achieving liquidity through an initial public offering. Given the lengthy government certification process, it provides an early reliable "due diligence" signal for investors by which the quality of their investment can be better quantified [9].

Given the fundraising importance of patent protection, the entrepreneur/investor must guard against making innocent mistakes that may prevent their ability to obtain a patent. An inventor has 1 year from the date of "first public disclosure" of the invention to file a patent application in the US Patent Office. **First public disclosures** are many, and surprisingly they include the following:

- Disclosures at presentations and poster sessions
- Prior public uses or demonstrations
- Prior conversations with potential partners
- Prior publications or interviews
- Prior sales of prototypes at beta sites

Also, keep in mind that if the US application is filed after the public disclosure, the inventor is not able to file for patent protection in many countries. There is only a 6-month "grace" period in Japan, Korea, and Russia There is a 1-year grace period in Canada, Australia, and Mexico.

Also understand that the loss of foreign patent rights greatly diminishes the financial value of intellectual property in the eyes of investors. For that reason, and for your maximum protection, consider filing a patent application before embarking on any public disclosure.

- Is the patent in a subject area that is earning significant profits?
- Are there currently patent litigation cases in process in the subject area?

- Does the invention allow for reduced costs or increased performance?
- Are there any competitors that could directly benefit from your invention?
- Are there blocking or dominating patents in this area?
- Do you have freedom to operate?
- Do you have an inventorship/ownership policy in place?

In summary, a patent can help your company be more "investable." Fundamentally, investors will analyze the risks and potential rewards of a single investment. Owning one or more patents can reduce the risk of the company by strengthening the competitive advantage and providing an additional marketable asset.

3.4 Outsourcing for Your Capital Needs

Outsourcing institutions—banks, the Small Business Administration (SBA), Small Business Investment Companies (SBICs), angel investors, and venture capitalists—are *not* primary resources for start-up capital.

This is because most of these outsourcers are looking for either significant collateral and operating history (banks and the SBA) or a business in an industry with uncommon opportunities for return on investment (venture capitalists). Meanwhile, angels are the most versatile of the outsourcing resources, but they're also the most difficult to find. We discuss each of these resources in this section [10].

Outsourcers, with the possible exception of SBICs, have a well-deserved role in the financing world; that role just doesn't happen to be at the start-up stage. After your business has matured and has a track record, the outsourcers may become a part of the financing game for your business.

The first thing to discover when considering which outsourcer to use is whether they're loaning you money (banks, SBA, and others) or investing their money (venture capitalists, some angels, and the like). Or, stated another way, will they be creditors or will they be part owners?

Outsourcing resources fall into two general categories: banks and nonbanks. Most banks don't make start-up loans to small business owners unless an owner's collateral is such that it will cover 100% of the loan. Examples of such collateral include real estate (including home equity) and stocks and bonds.

A bank's primary role in the small business lending arena is funding growth, for example, financing the expansion of a small business that has a track record. Most banks can offer a wide variety of creative loan packages designed to finance the existing small business. These loans include the financing possibilities discussed in the subsequent sections.

3.4.1 Asset-Based Financing

Asset-based financing is a general term describing the situation whereby a lender accepts as collateral the assets of a company in exchange for a loan. Most asset-based loans are collateralized against either *accounts receivable* (money owed by customers for products or services sold but not yet paid for), inventory, or equipment. Accounts receivable is the favorite of the three because it can be converted into cash more quickly (theoretically within 30 days, if these are terms you are offering). Banks advance funds only on a percentage of receivables or inventory, the typical percentages being 75% of receivables and 50%, or less, of inventory.

For example, using these percentages, if your business has $30,000 in receivables due from customers and $50,000 in inventory, the bank may loan you 75% of $30,000 (which is equal to $22,500) and 50% of $50,000 (which is equal to $25,000). The total of the two ($47,500) would then be available for you to use as working capital. These percentages vary based on the industry and the quality of the receivables and the inventory.

3.4.2 Banking on Banks

The old joke goes: "A bank will always loan you money, as soon as you prove you don't need it." Contrary to the popular opinion that bankers enjoy turning down prospective borrowers, bankers are in business to lend money. Every time bankers sit down in front of a prospective borrower, they hope that what they're about to see is a deal that will work. After all, *no loans* means no investment income for the bank, and no investment income means no marble columns—and without marble columns, what would hold up their gold-inlaid ceilings?

Make no mistake about it, banks are in business to lend money and make profits, which banks do by playing the spread—charging you more to use their money than they're paying somebody else (namely, depositors) to get it.

Banks tend to shy away from small companies experiencing rapid sales growth, a temporary decline, or a seasonal slump. In addition, firms that are already highly leveraged (a high debt-to-equity ratio) will usually have a hard time getting more bank funding.

Banks rely on four key requirements to lend you money. These key requirements are summarized in Figure 3.3.

If you have decided to seek a bank loan, the following terms are generally required to qualify:

- A written business plan or loan proposal
- Investment of your own money (usually 10% to 30% of the loan amount)

- You know your business and your market niche
- Credible forecast covering the load period
- You will be able to repay the loan:
  – Risks are minimized
  – Financial ratios are conservative and attainable
  – Hard assets are available as collateral
  – Personal loan guarantee
- Current revenues

FIGURE 3.3
What bankers want to see.

- Enough assets to collateralize the loan (usually one to two times the loan)
- Good character and personal credit
- Personal guarantee (your personal assets will be at risk)
- Obtaining a loan for 100% of capital needs is usually not possible
- Lenders usually require borrowers to have some personal or other source of cash to cover at least 25% or more of the total need
- Loans usually must be for business equipment, inventories, and operating expenses. Loans to cover loss of income are not available

3.4.3 Line of Credit

A line of credit involves the bank's setting aside designated funds for the business to draw against the ebb and flow of cash as needs dictate. As line-of-credit funds are used, the credit line is reduced; conversely, when payments are made, the line is replenished.

An advantage of line-of-credit financing is that no interest is accrued unless the funds are actually used. Ironically, the best time to arrange for your business's line of credit is when your business is doing well and you need the money the least. Why? Because that's when getting approval from the banker for the line of credit will be easiest, and you'll qualify for the best loan terms.

Don't make the mistake of overlooking a line of credit just because you don't presently need money. (Remember, a "line" doesn't cost anything if you don't draw against it.) Establish your credit line when things are going well. Sooner or later, if you're like most small businesses, you'll need the cash.

3.4.4 Letter of Credit

A **letter of credit** is a guarantee from the bank that a specific obligation of the business will be honored. Letters of credit are most often used to buy products unseen from overseas vendors. The bank generates its income in these situations by charging fees for making the guarantee.

3.5 Getting Money from Nonbanks

Banks don't have a lock on the small business lending market. Investment brokerage firms and major business conglomerates are also important players in the small business lending market. Most nonbank lenders find their niche by specializing in a specific category of loan, such as leasing or asset-based financing.

Leasing companies (where you can lease your business's equipment or furniture and fixtures), for example, are the most common nonbank financing resource, with 25% of small businesses availing themselves of some sort of leasing financing. *Leasing* is basically a rental—you pay a monthly fee for the use of an item, and at the end of the lease term, you return the item to the company that leased it to you. A compilation of nonbank resources follows in this section.

3.5.1 The Small Business Administration

An SBA loan is a loan made by a local lender (bank or nonbank) that is, in turn, guaranteed by a federal agency called the Small Business Administration (SBA). The SBA provides its backup guarantee as an inducement for banks to make loans that otherwise may be too risky from a banker's perspective.

Only in rare cases does the SBA actually provide the money itself. SBA loans usually provide longer repayment terms and lower down-payment requirements than conventional bank loans. They're available to most for-profit small businesses that don't exceed the SBA's parameters on size (which can vary depending on the industry). SBA loans can be used for a number of reasons, including (in infrequent cases) start-up monies if you have sufficient collateral in long-term assets.

Getting an SBA loan is not easy; to the contrary, the agency is extremely selective about whom it approves. Consider the primary criteria the SBA looks for when considering guaranteeing a loan:

- The owner must have invested at least 30% of the required capital and must be willing to guarantee the balance of the loan.
- The owner must be active in the management of the business.
- All principals must have a clean credit history.
- The business must project adequate cash flow to pay off the loan, and the debt/net worth ratio must fall within the SBA's approved guidelines.
- The SBA does not lend money. It provides guarantees to a bank that if a person does not repay a loan, the SBA will pay a major percentage of the loan back to the bank.

- All banks can make SBA-guaranteed loans but most have restrictions on what types of loans they are willing to make.
- The SBA only wants to guarantee loans to people who are likely to repay the loan.
- All SBA loans are made to individuals for a business. The individual is personally liable to repay the loan.

SBA loans have a reputation for being cumbersome and subject to enormous red tape. This reputation had been deserved in years past, but technology has made inroads everywhere, even in the government. The SBA's LowDoc Program (short for "low documentation"), for loans under $100,000, promises to process loan requests in less than 48 h and requires the borrower to fill out only a one-page application form. Other documentation you can be expected to furnish when applying for an SBA loan in excess of $100,000 includes (1) a personal financial statement, (2) 3 years of tax returns, and (3) 3 years of financial projections (Pro Forma Statements).

The SBA offers a wide variety of educational materials and seminars for both current and aspiring small business owners. It also provides financial assistance through loans and loan-guarantee programs. In recent years, these programs have become significantly more user-friendly, and today, the SBA is an excellent resource for the capital-seeking small business owner who has trouble attracting funding through the conventional private-sector sources.

The SBA, however, does not have any grant programs to start a business. Beware of the common myth that there is a lot of "free government grant money" for start-ups.

To find a local bank or nonbank institution that works with the SBA, look in the Yellow Pages for SBA Approved Lending Sources or call the SBA at 800-827-5722. If you're on the Internet, see www.sba.gov for more information about SBA loans that may work for you.

3.5.2 Small Business Investment Companies

SBICs are privately owned, quasi–venture capital firms organized under the auspices of the SBA. SBICs either lend money to, or invest money in, small businesses primarily within their local area. Categorized as *Federal Licensees* (meaning the federal government has given the SBIC its stamp of approval), SBICs either fund start-ups or provide operating funds with which to expand existing businesses. Through their relationship with the SBA, they're also able to offer particularly favorable terms and conditions to *disadvantaged businesses* (businesses owned by women and minorities).

Hundreds of SBICs operate around the country. To find out more about them, call the SBA at 800-827-5722, check out the SBA's website (www.sba .gov), or contact a nearby Small Business Development Center.

3.5.3 Certified Development Companies

Another program of the SBA, the Certified Development Company (CDC) program (also known as the 504 Loan Program), provides long-term (10- and 20-year) fixed-rate loans for small businesses. This program focuses on financing fixed assets, such as real estate (land and buildings). CDCs work with a local lender; typical financing may include 50% from the local lender, 40% from the CDC, and 10% down from the small business being helped. The asset being purchased acts as its own internal collateral. Several hundred CDCs exist nationwide. For the CDC nearest you, call the SBA at 800-827-5722 or visit the SBA's website (www.sba.gov) and inquire about the 504 Loan Program.

3.5.4 Your State's Economic Development Department

Many states have an Economic Development Department (sometimes a stand-alone governmental agency, possibly housed within the state's Department of Commerce) that offers a variety of loan programs to statewide businesses. The programs offered are usually modeled after SBA loans but can often offer better terms and conditions than the SBA, especially for those businesses that employ many employees. Such state departments will also generally offer *microloan* programs designed to assist small business start-ups.

3.5.5 Minority Funding Resources

The resources for low-income and minority funding (which, in many cases, is defined to include women-owned businesses) are many. Look to the following for starters:

a. The National Bankers Association (NBA) in Washington, DC, represents minority-owned banks that target loans to minority-owned businesses. For the nearest member bank in your area, call the NBA at 202-588-5432 or visit its website at www.natianalbankers.org.

b. Most states have an agency that provides one-stop assistance on financial services for small businesses. Check the library or the phone book for such an agency in your state and then ask about state-operated minority funding resources.

c. At the federal level, the SBA can help direct callers to local organizations that can, in turn, help locate low-income and minority funding opportunities. Call the SBA at 800-827-5722 for the resource nearest you or surf its website at www.sba.gov.

d. The U.S. Commerce Department's Minority Business Development Agency funds Business Development Centers nationwide whose function is, in part, to help minority-owned start-up businesses. Call 888-324-1551 for more information or visit its website at www. mbda .gov.

3.5.6 Exploring Your Ownership Options

In theory, all businesses have three ownership options:

- Privately held, with the founder being the only shareholder
- Privately held, sharing ownership with partners or other shareholders
- Publicly held, meaning that shares in your company are available to the investing public via the stock market

In reality, of course, most businesses only have the first two of these options—going for it alone or having partners or minority shareholders. Few businesses have the management, resources, and appeal needed to go public, either at the start-up stage or in the course of the business's growth.

There is no right or wrong answer as to which of the three options you should use, but there is a right or wrong way to determine which works best for you. At the heart of making that decision is … you guessed it… you! You are the primary ingredient that will determine which of the three options will work best for your business. Your criteria to use in making this decision should include the kind of person you are, the way you communicate, the way you delegate, and the manner in which you work with people.

The kind of business you intend to start also can be a factor. If, for example, you intend to start a high-tech manufacturing business, you may find that the key employees you want will demand some ownership as part of their compensation packages. On the other hand, if you intend to go into the consulting business, sole ownership is the likely ticket for you.

3.5.7 Service Corps of Retired Executives

The Service Corps of Retired Executives (SCORE) has helped create more than 56,000 new businesses and allowed more than 107,000 businesses increase revenue.

Federally funded, SCORE consists of more than 10,000 volunteers in hundreds of cities across the United States who provide free counseling, mentoring, and advice to prospective or existing small businesses. SCORE volunteers provide the specific advice and resources you need through customized, one-on-one or team mentoring.

SCORE, an excellent concept to be sure, can be a tad on the hit-or-miss side, however, because the majority of SCORE's volunteers are ex–large-company employees. Thus, not all of them have known what it's like to have been there as their own small business takes off. If you happen to be assigned to the right volunteer, however, SCORE can be the best deal in town—occasionally even providing you with a much needed mentor. SCORE is definitely a service worth trying, especially to pose online questions to counselors or to contact the office nearest you (website at www.score.org, or call 800-634-0245).

3.5.8 Consider Looking for a Partner with Deep Pockets

This is one of the most overlooked sources of money. Many small businesses resist this approach because they want to own 100% of the business. However, it is better to own 50% of a growing successful business than 100% of a business that never gets off the ground. Funding sources can come from any one of these "other" deep pocket sources:

- A specialized supplier
- A strategic partner
- A venture capitalist
- A private equity dealer
- A private offering
- A private investor
- An "angel" investor

3.5.9 Finding a Guarantor or Loan Co-Borrower

This works well when a family member or close friend is reluctant to give you cash up front but they think you have a good idea for a business and a good chance to succeed. They may be willing to either guarantee a loan or co-sign for a loan. Before going out looking for money, remember three tips described below:

1. **When you need a loan, establish a personal relationship.** Loans are about trust, and trust starts with familiarity. Invite your lender to your place of business. Impress the lender with your product samples or services. Take advantage of their experience and contacts by asking for help on nonbanking issues. Ask him to join your informal business advisory board. You may even learn more about your business from your lender.

2. **Know your numbers cold.** Every business loan has terms and conditions. Be sure you understand them. Learn about a balance sheet, a profit and loss statement, and cash flow projections.

3. **Sweeten the deal.** What lenders want even more than your loan are new customers. Ask about the lender's other products and services. If you are pleased with the lender's products and services, refer family

and friends to do business with the lender company, but whatever you do

- Don't fool yourself. Know your weaknesses.
- Know your financial break-even point. If you are bad with numbers, hire a good bookkeeper or accountant.
- Do not bankrupt your business because you are too proud to admit that you need help.
- Know what you should say when you meet with a lender.
- Thoroughly describe your background, experience, and education.
- Stick to the facts. Be truthful with the lender. Confidence in your ability and integrity is very important.
- State exactly how much money you require. Never ask "how much can I get?"
- Outline what you plan to do with the money. Using the cash to replace lost income is not a valid reason for a loan.
- Define how the business will generate the cash flow required to pay back the bank loan.
- Tell the lender how much of your own money you are investing in the business. Most lenders require your share to be 25%–30%, which includes investments you have already made.
- Bottom line, "When in doubt, tell the truth."

3.5.10 Small Business Investment Company

Congress created the SBIC program in 1958 to fill the gap between the availability of VC and the needs of small businesses in start-up and growth situations. SBICs, licensed and regulated by the SBA, are privately owned and managed investment firms that use their own capital, plus funds borrowed at favorable rates with an SBA guarantee, to make VC investments in small businesses. Virtually all SBICs are profit-motivated businesses.

They provide equity capital, long-term loans, debt-equity investments, and management assistance to qualifying small businesses. The only small businesses that cannot qualify for SBIC assistance are other SBICs, finance and investment companies, finance-type leasing companies, companies with less than one-half of their assets and operations in the United States, passive or casual businesses (those not engaged in regular and continuous business operation), and companies that will use the proceeds to acquire farm land.

There are two types of SBICs—regular SBICs and specialized SBICs, also known as 301(d) SBICs. Specialized SBICs invest in small businesses owned by entrepreneurs who are socially or economically disadvantaged. The SBIC Program makes funding available to all types of manufacturing and service industries. The cost of money on SBIC loans and debt securities issued by small concerns is regulated by the SBA in the interest of the small business concerns and is limited to the applicable state regulations governing such loans and debt securities, or by SBA regulations, whichever is lower.

Loans made to and debt securities purchased from small concerns should have minimum terms of 5 years. Many investment companies seek out small businesses with new products or services because of the strong growth potential of such firms. Some SBICs specialize in the field in which their management has special knowledge or competency. Most, however, consider a wide variety of investment opportunities. Information on local SBICs can be obtained by contacting the Small Business Answer Desk at 1-800-U-ASK-SBA or by visiting the SBA Home Page on the Internet at http://www.sbaonline .sba.gov. Contact: U.S. Small Business Administration Office of Financial Assistance 409 Third Street, SW, Washington, DC, 20416.

3.6 Controlling Your Initial Start-Up Expenses

There's a fine line between starting your business on a shoestring and watching it fail because of a lack of resources. You don't want to invest lavishly at first, yet you want to look professional in the eyes of your potential customers. The paradox and the challenge are to maintain the image of a solid, successful company without letting your expenses lead to uncompetitive pricing and failure [11].

The trick is to determine the point at which your business runs both effectively and efficiently. This is a key issue for any start-up that can determine whether you'll be able to survive. The good news is, if you master the art of trimming expenses early in the game, you'll develop good habits that'll serve you well as your company grows.

The first thing to do is cut your initial budget to the bare minimum. Chances are your business will start slow, so doing things for a dime that would otherwise cost a dollar is a great discipline. Here are some tips to keep early costs under control.

3.6.1 Four Tips for Reducing Your Start-Up Costs

One of the biggest concerns for new entrepreneurs is start-up costs. Even if you are not renting an office or laboratory space for your business, there are still other bills to be paid before you start seeing a profit. While most business owners plan for these expenses, many don't anticipate just how many extra costs they'll encounter along the way. If you're starting a business on a budget, follow the four tips shown in Table 3.2 to minimize your expenses and maximize your bottom line [12].

TABLE 3.2

Minimize Your Expenses and Maximize Your Bottom Line

Tips	How Best to Proceed
1. Create a realistic budget	..... and stick to it "come hell or high water"
2. Be flexible	When you developed your business plan, you probably also had a vision of the things you wanted for your business: all the latest equipment, a full-time staff, and your own private office. Every entrepreneur hopes that they will be able to make these business dreams come true, but the reality is that you'll sometimes have to sacrifice them to keep your company running.
3. Go inexpensive, but not cheap	Many small business owners who spend a lot of money up front on services like marketing and Web design end up regretting it in the long run. There are countless cost-effective tools available for small business owners who want to save money by taking care of their own branding and website development. However, "free" isn't always the right answer.
4. Evaluate and reevaluate	If you've followed all of these steps to save money in the early stages of your start-up, the best way to continue saving as your business grows is to continually revisit and revise your budget. Seek financial advice from accountants and fellow small business owners and then go over your expenses and try to cut back where you can.

3.6.2 Controlling Labor Costs

Controlling labor costs is probably the most formidable challenge you will face. Don't learn the hard way, for example, that turnover wreaks havoc on your profits. When it's time to hire, do it carefully and intelligently, and if an employee's performance is not up to your standards, do not be too quick to fire him or her. Work with the individual to improve job performance.

While competitive compensation is essential to attracting good people, it doesn't have to all be in the form of salary. Remember the tip about turning your fixed costs into variable ones? It works in compensation as well. Supplement a small salary with the potential for healthy bonuses based on your company's earnings.

Give your employees perks, such as flexible work hours. Train them adequately for their responsibilities, and take the time to give them timely feedback and direction. Be passionate about your company and about your employees.

Refrain from hiring too much staff and expanding too quickly. With each new employee, there will be associated expenses that you may not be ready to underwrite. A better choice might be to outsource noncore competencies. You may outsource functions such as payroll, accounts payable, accounts receivables, periodic financial statements, taxes, legal, advertising, and so on [13].

3.6.3 Controlling Your Sales Performance

You have only three ways to increase your business's financial performance:

- Increasing sales (in which case, those increased sales may or may not have a positive impact on profitability)
- Increasing prices (in which case, the entire amount of the increase will have a positive impact on profitability, assuming that you don't lose customers because of the price increase)
- Decreasing expenses (in which case, the entire decrease will have a positive impact on profitability, assuming that you don't lose business because the expense reduction has a negative impact on your product or service quality)

In other words, you'll find a one-to-one leverage factor at work on your bottom-line profits when you increase prices or cut expenses. This is why the successful small business owner always looks to the expense and pricing categories first when in a profitability crunch: Results can be instantaneous, and the impact is usually dollar on dollar.

Whether starting a new company or running an existing one, you must always remember that controlling expenses is a cultural issue, and cultural issues begin at the top. This means that many of your employees are going to emulate you. If you have overstuffed chairs in your office and idle secretaries in your foyer, your employees are likewise going to demonstrate a penchant for spending unnecessary money. We're talking about the old practice of leading by example.

Whenever we walk into a business's lobby or reception area and we're greeted by the gurgle of cascading waterfalls and the sight of bronze sculptures, we're reminded again of Sam Walton and Wal-Mart. Linoleum floors and metal desks were the order of the day at Wal-Mart's frugal corporate headquarters in Bentonville, Arkansas. No wonder they could underprice and outperform such longtime competitors such as Sears, Montgomery Ward, and J.C. Penney, whose overhead included the cost of maintaining plush corporate offices in the towering skyscrapers of Chicago and Dallas.

3.6.4 Controlling Fixed and Variable Expenses

Two kinds of expenses need controlling: fixed and variable. *Fixed expenses* don't fluctuate with sales; they're usually negotiated in the start-up stage and then left to their own devices until the original negotiations lapse and it's time to renegotiate them. Such periods may be anywhere from 1 year to 5 years.

Effective control of these fixed expenses, which include such categories as insurance, rent, and equipment leases, requires the small business owner's skillful negotiation, because after they're established, renegotiation time probably won't come around for a while. That cost is then fixed, and you can do little about it.

Variable expenses are those expenses that fluctuate with sales—as sales go up, variable expenses go up as well (and vice versa). You can delegate the determination of the prices to be paid for variable expenses, as long as you remember that the responsibility for controlling them, in the early stages of a business anyway, should always rest with you (the owner). You should approve all purchase orders and sign all checks that relate to variable expenses.

As your company grows, you may choose to delegate the responsibility for controlling expenses to other responsible individuals inside the company, or you may still choose to maintain control by signing the checks and questioning the invoices that support those checks.

A key to controlling expenses is keeping your employees cost-conscious: If the employees know that you or other key managers are cost-conscious and will question unreasonable or unnecessary expenses, then they, too, will be motivated to contain them. Incentives are also an often-used tool for cutting costs—give your employees a reason (bonus, perks, recognition) to look for unnecessary costs, and they're sure to find them.

Always be aware that the 80–20 rule is alive and well when it comes to managing your expenses. In this case, the 80–20 rule says that 80% of your wasted expense dollars can be found in 20% of your expense categories. For businesses that have a number of employees, the wages and salary account is usually the largest expense category and, thus, the most often abused.

We don't mean to say that expenses shouldn't be challenged in every category. Quick and easy dollars can usually be found by rooting around in such expense accounts as utilities, travel, insurance, and, of course, the compost heap of them all, the "miscellaneous" expense account.

Effective expense control isn't only a profitability issue; it is also an important element for controlling cash flow. Because lack of cash is usually the number one warning signal of a small business's impending failure, how better to begin building a solid foundation than by controlling your company's expenses?

3.6.5 Controlling Your Budgeting Process

Start-up businesses of all sizes need accurate budgets to help balance financial accounts and create business goals. You can design a weekly, monthly, quarterly, or annual budget. A start-up business should develop at least one general budget that captures projected expenses and sales revenues. Without a solid budget, a new business might spend more than it earns and become insolvent [14].

One critical mistake many start-up entrepreneurs make is underestimating the budgeting process [15]. The traditional budgeting process proceeds as follows:

- Set goals that will enable you to grow.
- Break the goals down so that there is clear ownership and accountability for each goal by a specific team.
- Refine goals into measurable targets.
- Figure out how many new people are required to hit the targets.
- Estimate the cost of the effort.
- Benchmark against the industry.
- Make global optimizations.
- Execute.

This all sounds very mechanical and automatic, but your budget is your roadmap for the future. Do it right the first time around!

3.6.6 The Golden Rule

For many small businesses, the cost of getting started and keeping the business going for the first few months is quite high while income is unusually low. Budgeting for those initial costs will tell you how much capital you will need to have available to you upfront before it is sensible to start spending it all. The budgeting rule is not only to have a reasonably reliable figure but also to know how you came up with it for your budgeting process [16].

Budgeting (also known as *forecasting*) is the periodic (usually annual) review of past financial information with the purpose of forecasting future financial conditions. If you've completed your business plan, you, in effect, prepared your first budget when you forecasted your profit and loss statement for the upcoming year.

The only difference in preparing a budget for your ongoing business is that you'll now enjoy the advantage of having yesterday's figures to work with. The process of budgeting is one that should apply not only to your business but also to your personal finances, especially if you have trouble saving money.

In your small business, you have two ways to budget expenses from year to year. The first—the easy way—is to assume a percentage increase for each expense category, both variable and fixed. For example, say that you decide that your telephone expense (a variable expense) will increase by 5% next year, your rent (a fixed expense) will remain the same, and your advertising and promotion (a variable expense) will increase by 10%. Whoosh! A few multiplications later, and you have budgeted these expenses for the course of a year.

3.6.6.1 Zero-Based Budgeting

Zero-based budgeting, on the other hand, makes the assumption that last year's expenses were zero and begins the budgeting process from that point. For example, the zero-based formula assumes that your supplies' expense account begins at zero; thus, you must first determine who consumed what supplies last year, who will be consuming them this year, and how much will be consumed. Then, you must determine what price you'll pay for this year's supplies.

In this manner, zero-based budgeting forces you to annually manage your consumption at the same time that you're annually reviewing your costs. The effect of zero-based budgeting is that you'll no longer include prior years' mistakes in the current year's budgets. For example, when budgeting telephone expenses for the year, instead of increasing it by a flat percentage, zero-based budgeting demands that you make sure that your prior year's bill was the lowest it could be. This assumption forces you to determine who's using your phones for what kind of activity and also to reprice your rates with telephone carriers. Instead of forecasting a 5% increase, you may well end up projecting a 5% decrease. The zero-based method also assumes that you'll check out prices with vendors other than those that you're presently using.

Far too many small businesses don't budget expenses at all. Furthermore, of those small business owners who do, few use zero-based budgeting, despite its many advantages. Not budgeting is truly one of the most expensive mistakes you can make as a small business owner. Sure, zero-based budgeting may take more of your time, but it can pay big dividends in controlling your bottom-line profitability.

Remember that cash is king. The most critical piece is your cash flow management. You need a system that will give you an accurate picture of your bank account balance right now, as well as at various points in the future. Will you make payroll on the 30th? Will you make rent on the first? When in the next 2 months should you buy those fancy 3D printers or expensive analytical equipment [17]?

3.7 Minimizing Start-Up Risk with Part-Time Ventures

Some people believe that starting your own business is the riskiest of all small business options. However, if you're starting a business that specifically uses your skills and expertise, the risk may not be nearly as great as you think.

Besides, risk is relative: Those who are employed by someone else are taking a risk, too—a risk that their employer will continue to offer them the opportunity to remain employed.

One way to minimize the risk of starting a full-time business is to work into a part-time one. Suppose for a moment that you're a computer trouble-shooter at a large company and making $75,000 per year. You're consider-ing establishing your own computer consulting service and would be happy making a comparable amount of money. If you find through your research that others performing the services you intend to provide are charging $80 per hour, you'll need to actually spend about 20 h/week consulting (assum-ing that you work 50 weeks per year).

Because you can run your consulting business from your home (which can generate small tax breaks) and you can do it without purchasing costly new equipment, your expenses should be minimal. (Note: We have ignored your employer's benefits here, which, of course, have value, too.) Rather than leaving your day job and diving into your new business without the safety of a regular paycheck, you have the option of starting to moonlight as a con-sultant. Over the course of a year or two, if you can average 10 h/week of consulting, you're halfway to your goal.

Then, after you leave your job and can focus all your energies on your business, getting to 20 h/week of billable work won't be such a stretch. Many businesses, by virtue of leveraging their owner's existing skills and expertise, can be started with low start-up costs. You can begin building the framework of your company using *sweat equity* (the time and energy you invest in your business, as opposed to the capital) in the early, part-time years. As long as you know your competition and can offer your customers a valued service at a reasonable cost, the principal risk with your time business is that you will not do a good job marketing what you have to offer.

3.7.1 Buying an Existing Business

In the event that you do not have a specific idea for a business you want to start, but you have exhibited considerable business management skills, consider buying an established business. Although buying someone else's business can, in some cases, be riskier than starting your own, at least you know exactly what you're getting into right from the start. The good news, however, is that you often don't have to waste time and energy creating an infrastructure—it's already in place, which allows you, the buyer, to dive right into the business, without having to waste time on the peripherals.

Buying an existing business often requires that you invest more money at the outset, in the form of a down payment to buy the business. Thus, if you don't have the ability to run the business and it performs poorly, you have a lot more to lose financially.

3.7.2 Evaluating Buying a Business

In the American legal system, an accused is presumed innocent until proven guilty beyond a reasonable doubt. When you're purchasing a business, however, you should assume, until proven otherwise, that the selling business owner is guilty of making the business appear better than reality.

We don't want to sound cynical, but more than a few owners out there try to make their businesses look more profitable, more financially healthy, and more desirable than they really are. The reason is quite simple: Business sellers generally seek to maximize the price their business will command. Thus, don't trust only your gut when evaluating a business, because you could be fooled.

Buying a business can be tricky because the business brokerage market rarely favors the buyer. The following list presents some of the obstacles you're likely to encounter when buying a business:

- The necessary confidentiality of transactions: You can't publicly investigate a lot of the background information.
- Few listings: A paucity of businesses for sale means that the seller is in control. For good businesses that are fairly priced, there are usually plenty of potential buyers waiting in the wings.
- Unpublished prices of previous sales: There are no benchmarks. No templates to follow.
- Emotional circumstances surrounding the sale: People can get more emotional about selling their business than they do about selling real estate. Blood, sweat, retirement, and, yes, egos, are involved. Emotions run high, on both sides.

Buying a business is a long, detail-ridden, and stressful procedure. Don't rush it; be sure to cover your bases. We hit all the key points of consideration in this chapter.

3.7.3 Kicking Their Tires

Before you make an offer to buy a small business, you're going to want to do some digging into the company to minimize your chances of mistakenly buying a problematic business or overpaying for a good business. This process is known as *due diligence,* and it is every bit as important as hiring an attorney or signing the purchase agreement.

Smart buyers build plenty of contingencies into a purchase offer for a small business, just as they do when buying a home or other real estate. If your financing doesn't come through or you find some dirty laundry in the business (and you're not buying a laundromat), contingencies allow you to back out of the deal legally. However, knowing that you'll draft all purchase offers with plenty of contingencies shouldn't encourage you to make a purchase offer casually. Making an offer and doing the necessary research and homework are costly, in both time and money.

Before making an offer for a business, you'll want reasonably clear answers to the important due diligence questions discussed in the following sections.

3.7.4 Due Diligence on Owners and Key Employees

A business is usually only as good or bad as the owners and key employees running it. Ethical, business-savvy owners and key employees generally run successful businesses worthy of buying. Unscrupulous, marginally competent, or incompetent business owners and key employees are indicative of businesses that you should avoid.

Just as you wouldn't (we hope) hire employees without reviewing their resumes, interviewing them, and checking employment references, you shouldn't make an offer to buy a business until you do similar homework on the owners and key employees of the business for sale. Here's a short list of information we suggest gathering as well as suggestions on how to find it:

Business background: Request and review the owner's and key employees' resumes, remembering that some people may fabricate or puff up information on that piece of paper. Are the backgrounds impressive and filled with relevant business experience? Just as you should do when hiring an employee, check resumes to make sure that the information they provide is correct. Glaring omissions or inaccuracies send a strong negative message as to the kind of people you're dealing with.

Personal reputations in the business community: The geographic and work/professional communities to which we belong are quite small. Any business that has been up and running for a number of years has had interactions with many people and other companies.

Take the time to talk to others who may have had experience dealing with the business for sale (vendors, Chamber of Commerce, Better Business Bureau, and so on) and ask them their thoughts on the company's owners and key employees. Of course, we shouldn't need to remind you that you can't always accept the statements of others at face value. You have to consider the merits, or lack thereof, of the source.

Credit history: If you were a banker, we hope you wouldn't lend money to anyone without first assessing their credit risk. At a minimum, you should review the seller's credit history to see how successful they've been at paying off, on time, money they've borrowed. Even though you won't be lending money to the business seller you're speaking with, we recommend that you check his credit records. A problematic credit record could uncover business problems the owner had that he may be less than forthcoming in revealing. The major agencies that compile and sell personal credit histories and small business information are Experian (www.experian.com), Equifax (www.equifax.com), Transunion (www.transunion.com), and Dun & Bradstreet (800-234-3867; www.dnb.com).

Key customers: The people who can usually give you the best indication of the value of a business for sale are its current customers. Through your own research on the business or from the current owner, get a list of the company's top 5 to 10 customers and ask them the following questions:

- In general, how is the company perceived by its customers?
- Does it deliver on time?
- How do its products or services compare to its competitors' offerings?
- Does it have a culture of integrity?
- What does the company do best?
- What does it need to improve?

Key employees: If the employees of the business for sale are aware of the prospects of the impending sale, be sure to interview them and get their insider's take on the condition of the business. You also want to know whether they intend to remain as employees under the new ownership.

3.7.5 Why Is the Owner Selling?

After you locate a potentially attractive business for sale, the serious work begins. First, try to discover the reason the owner is selling. Small business owners may be selling for a reason that shouldn't matter to you (they've reached the age and financial status where they simply want to retire), or they may be selling for reasons that should matter to you (the business is a never-ending headache to run, it isn't very profitable, or competition is changing the competitive landscape).

If an owner wants to sell for some negative reason, that shouldn't necessarily sour you on buying the business. If the business has a low level of profitability, it isn't necessarily a lemon—quite possibly the current owner hasn't taken the proper steps (such as cost management, effective marketing, and so on) to boost its profitability. You may well be able to overcome hurdles the current owner can't. But before you make a purchase offer and then follow through on that offer, you absolutely, positively should understand many aspects of the business including, first and foremost, why the current owner wants out.

The list below describes how to discover why the current owner is selling (where appropriate, get the current owner's permission to speak with certain people):

Chat with the owner. This isn't a terribly creative, Sherlock Holmes–type method, and yes, we know that many sellers aren't going to be completely candid about why they are selling, but you never know.

Besides, you can verify the answer you get from the owner against what other sources tell you about the owner's motivations to sell.

Talk with the business owner's advisors. As we explain throughout this chapter, in the course of evaluating the worth of a business, you should be speaking with various advisors, including those you hire yourself. Don't overlook, however, the wealth of information and background that the current owner's advisors have. These advisors may include lawyers, accountants, bankers, and the business's own board of advisors or directors.

Confer with industry sources. Most industries are closely knit groups of companies, each one knowing, in general, what's going on with the other businesses in the same industry. Most importantly, the vendor salespeople or manufacturers' representatives who call on the industry can be a terrific source for information. Sure, they may not be completely candid, but your job is to read between the lines of what they have to say. (They generally won't out-and-out lie to you either. They're aware that you could be their next customer.)

Seek out customers. (Carefully!). The business's current customers usually do not know that a business is for sale, but they can provide you with the information you need to determine whether the current owner is selling from strength or from weakness.

Discuss with key employees. Some employees probably know the real answer as to why the business is for sale. Your job: Find out what they know. In your discussions with and investigations about the current owner, also reflect upon these final, critical questions: How important is the current owner to the success of the business? What will happen when he or she is no longer around? Will the business under new management lose key employees, key customers, and so on?

3.7.6 Understanding the Company's Culture

When you buy a small business, you're adopting someone else's child. Depending on the strength of its already-formed personality and how it meshes with yours, you may or may not be successful in molding that business into your image.

Eight out of 10 dentists recommend Crest. Eight out of 10 acquisitions fail to meet expectations. Why? A clash of cultures. Ninety-two percent of the survey respondents said that their deals would "have substantially benefitted from a greater cultural understanding prior to the merger." Seventy percent conceded that "too little" effort focuses on culture during integration [18].

Is your expectation compatible with their "culture"? Culture can be defined as "how we do things around here in order to succeed" [19]. To prevent future headaches, ensure that your "culture" is in line with theirs [20]. Part of the problem may be that, especially when integrating companies are in the same or similar businesses, the acquirer tends to assume they are "just like me" and dismiss the need for deep cultural analysis.

Likewise, when the acquirer and acquiree in a deal get along with each other, they tend to assume that their companies will get along equally well. No two companies are cultural twins, and companies seldom get along with each other as easily as their executives might. In fact, the survey establishes that the issue of culture comes down to two fundamental problems: understanding both cultures and providing the right amount and type of leadership.

For understandable reasons, leaders discount the impact of corporate culture when they acquire. They have other factors to consider at the time of the acquisition—market opportunities, operational and business process synergies, financial analysis, and potential profits. These factors are obviously important. In addition, "culture" is not only an amorphous concept, it is believed to be immeasurable and inherently unmanageable. Most leaders probably just assume that culture will "iron itself out" over time. However, organizational culture is too important to be left up to hope and natural evolution.

3.8 The JOBS Act and Crowdfunding

In an effort to jump-start the entrepreneurial economy, the JOBS (Jumpstart Our Business Startups) Act created a new provision in the Securities Act of 1933 Section 4(6) that allows Emerging Growth Companies (EGCs) to raise up to $1 million in any 12-month period by selling securities through authorized intermediaries, subject to certain limitations on the matter of the offering and by limiting the amount any person is permitted to invest.

Emerging Growth Companies are a new category of issuer. EGCs are those with (1) less than $1 billion total annual gross revenues in their most recent fiscal year and (2) have not had a registered public offering before December 8, 2012 [21].

The JOBS Act (signed into law April 6, 2012) facilitates financing across the spectrum from seed capital to public offerings. Below are some of the most important aspects and implications:

- Permitting "crowdfunding."
- Easing restrictions on fundraising from accredited investors.
- Easing mandatory reporting triggers under the SEC Act.
- Increasing the amount of money companies may raise in "mini-IPOs."

- Reducing many burdens on EGCs going public.
- Providing more capital to entrepreneurs and EGCs, creating jobs, and providing opportunities for nonaccredited investors to invest in both community-based businesses and entrepreneurial companies.
- For the last several years, the number of VC financings in the US has continued to drop—approximately 3500 VC led deals; VCs are raising less capital and continue to finance only larger opportunities with significant IRR potential and with exits of greater than $50 million.
- Although angel statistics are difficult to obtain, they funded nearly as much as VCs.
- Fewer than 10% of all accredited investors in the United States invest in private financings. Except as friends or family, nonaccredited investors have no exposure to private financings.
- There are 25,000,000 ECGs in the United States; many are looking for funding and banks aren't lending, and identifying investors is extremely difficult given securities laws.

3.8.1 The JOBS Act at a Glance

The JOBS Act seeks to accomplish this goal by, among other measures, relaxing certain provisions of the Sarbanes–Oxley and Dodd–Frank Acts insofar as those provisions apply to a class of newly public companies dubbed "Emerging Growth Companies." A primary goal of the legislation is to facilitate the ability of growing companies to raise capital, as shown below:

- Removes the prohibition on general solicitation in connection with transactions dealing with Rule 508 or Rule 144A, provided that sales are limited to qualifying investors.
- Allows the thresholds that trigger registration of a security under Section 12(g), including a different threshold for banks and bank holding companies.
- Provides, to a new category of ECGs, relief from requirements and other restrictions applicable to IPOs (initial public offerings) and, on a transitional basis for up to 5 years, relief from certain reporting requirements.
- Adds a crowdfunding exemption and authorizes the SC to increase the amount permitted to be raised in a Regulation A offering to $50 million in any 12-month period.
- Modifications to Rule 506 will provide substantial freedom for issuers to promote their offerings to a wider group of investors.
- Anyone who can convince the investing public that they have a good business idea can become an entrepreneur.

- Modeled in part on campaign donations, since politicians have been collecting small donations from the general public for decades.
- Another route for business funding (since VCs reject 98% of business plans).

3.8.2 Title III of the US JOBS Act

- The Act limits both the aggregate value of securities that an issuer may offer through a crowdfunding intermediary and the amount that an individual can invest.
- An issuer may sell up to an aggregate of $1,000,000 of its securities during any 12-month period.
- Investors with an annual income or net worth of up to $40,000 will only be permitted to invest $2000 and above $40,000 and less than $100,000 investors shall be entitled to invest 5% of their annual income or net worth in any 12-month period.
- Investors with an annual income or net worth greater than $100,000 will be permitted to invest 10% of their annual income or net worth.
- Investors are limited to investing $100,000 in crowdfunding issues in a 12-month period.
- Investors who purchase securities in a crowdfunding transaction are restricted from transferring those securities for a period of 1 year. This restriction is subject to certain exceptions, including transfers (i) to the issuer, (ii) to an accredited investor, (iii) pursuant to an offering registered with the SEC, (iv) or to the investor's family members.

3.8.3 Equal Access and Disclosure

Equal access to and disclosure of material information is a core principle of federal and state securities regulations. It is essential for investors to have the necessary information to appreciate the potential risks and rewards of an investment. The JOBS Act requires issuers to provide investors with a description of the following:

- *Company:* the issuer and its members, including the name, legal status, physical address, and the names of the directors and officers holding more than 20% of the shares of the issuer.
- *Offering:* the anticipated business plan of the issuer, the target offering amount, the deadline to reach the target offering amount, and the price to the public of the securities.
- *Structure:* the ownership and capital structure of the issuer, including terms of the securities of the issuer being offered.

- *Valuation:* how the securities being offered are being valued, and examples of methods for how such securities may be valued by the issuer in the future, including during subsequent corporate actions.

- *Risks:* the risks to purchasers of the securities relating to minority ownership in the issuer, the risks associated with corporate actions, including additional issuances of shares, a sale of the issuer or of assets of the issuer, or transactions with related parties.

- The intermediary crowdfunding portals are also required to make available to the SEC and to potential investors any information provided by the issuer no later than 21 days before the first day on which securities are sold to any investor.

3.8.4 Crowdfunding

Crowdfunding refers to the funding of an EGC by selling small amounts of equity to many investors. This form of crowdfunding has recently received attention from policymakers in the United States with direct mention in the JOBS Act; legislation that allows for a wider pool of small investors with fewer restrictions [22].

With the passing of the Act, the word of the day seems to be crowdfunding. While this concept has arguably been around a long time, it is still formally recognized as a new industry to many consumers, particularly those outside the United States.

Crowdfunding is, by definition, "the practice of funding a project or venture by raising many small amounts of money from a large number of people, typically via the Internet."

Crowdfunding has its origins in the concept of crowdsourcing, which is the broader concept of an individual reaching a goal by receiving and leveraging small contributions from many parties. Crowdfunding is the application of this concept to the collection of funds through small contributions from many parties in order to finance a particular project or venture [23].

Theoretically, crowdfunding allows EGCs to sell securities to anyone, without being compelled to produce the onerous amounts of information currently required by existing federal law. A number of US organizations have been founded to provide education and advocacy related to equity-based crowdfunding as enabled by the JOBS Act. They include the following:

- National Crowdfunding Association
- Crowdfunding Professional Association
- CrowdFund Intermediary Regulatory Advocates

Crowdfunding is not available to non-US companies, public companies, or investment companies, including companies exempt by Section 3(b) or 3(c) of the Investment Company Act of 1940. In addition, securities sold in a crowd-funding deal may not be transferred for 1 year from the date of purchase, except in limited circumstances.

3.8.5 Issuer Requirements

EGCs seeking to raise capital under Section 4(6) [24] are required to provide certain information to potential investors, such as

- The company
- Its business
- Officers and directors
- Major stockholders (greater than 20%)
- Terms of the offering securities being offered for sale

Importantly, the JOBS Act requires that EGCs must provide more detailed financial disclosures for larger offerings. Thus, if the aggregate amount of the offering is $100,000 or less, the issuer must only provide tax returns for the company's most recently completed fiscal year, and financial statements certified by the company's chief executive officer.

In contrast, if the aggregate amount is $100,000 to $500,000, the issuer must provide financial statements reviewed by an independent public accountant. If the aggregate amount being offered exceed $500,000, the issuer must provide audited financial statements.

3.8.6 Intermediary Requirements

The JOBS Act requires that crowdfunded offerings be conducted through authorized third-party "intermediaries" [25]. Intermediaries, crowdfunding brokers, and funding portals have significant duties under the JOBS Act to provide information to investors, reduce the risk of fraud, and, where required under the Act, ensure that investors and issuers satisfy the requirements outlined in Title III of the JOBS Act.

The JOBS Act requires these intermediaries to, among other things:

- Provide disclosures that the SEC determines appropriate by rule, including regarding the risks of the transaction and investor education materials
- Ensure that each investor (1) reviews investor education materials; (2) positively affirms that the investor understands that the investor is risking the loss of the entire investment, and that the investor could bear such a loss; and (3) answers questions that demonstrate that the investor understands the level of risk generally applicable

to investments in start-ups, emerging businesses, and small issuers and the risk of illiquidity

- Take steps to protect the privacy of information collected from investors

- Take such measures to reduce the risk of fraud with respect to such transactions, as established by the SEC, by rule, including obtaining a background and securities enforcement regulatory history check on each officer, director, and person holding more than 20% of the outstanding equity of every issuer whose securities are offered by such person

- Make available to investors and the SEC, at least 21 days before any sale, any disclosures provided by the issuer

- Ensure that all offering proceeds are only provided to the issuer when the aggregate capital raised from all investors is equal to or greater than a target offering amount, and allow all investors to cancel their commitments to invest

- Make efforts to ensure that no investor in a 12-month period has purchased crowdfunded securities that, in the aggregate, from all issuers, exceed the investment limits set forth in Title III, Section 4A of the JOBS Act; plus any other requirements that the SEC determines are appropriate.

3.8.7 Funding Portals

Title III of the JOBS Act adds a new Section 3(h) to the Exchange Act that requires the SEC to exempt, conditionally or unconditionally, an intermediary operating a funding portal from the requirement to register with the SEC as a broker.

The intermediary, though, would need to register with the SEC as a funding portal and would be subject to the SEC's examination, enforcement, and rulemaking authority. The funding portal also must become a member of a national securities association that is registered under Section 15A of the Exchange Act.

A funding portal is defined as a crowdfunding intermediary that does not (i) offer investment advice or recommendations; (ii) solicit purchases, sales, or offers to buy securities offered or displayed on its website or portal; (iii) compensate employees, agents, or others persons for such solicitation or based on the sale of securities displayed or referenced on its website or portal; (iv) hold, manage, possess, or otherwise handle investor funds or securities; or (v) engage in such other activities as the SEC, by rule, determines appropriate.

The JOBS Act directs the SEC to adopt rules to implement Title III within 270 days of enactment of the Act. The president signed the JOBS Act into law on April 5, 2012.

3.8.8 Restrictions on Funding Portals

The JOBS Act imposes several restrictions on the activities of a registered funding portal. A funding portal is *not* permitted to

- Provide investment advice or make recommendations
- Solicit purchases, sales, or offers to buy the securities offered or displayed on its website or portal
- Compensate employees, agents, or other persons for such solicitation or based on the sale of securities displayed or referenced on its website or portal
- Hold, manage, possess, or otherwise handle investor funds or securities
- Engage in any other activities the SEC determines to prohibit in its crowdfunding rulemaking

In addition, each funding portal and each crowdfunding broker is prohibited from

- Compensating promoters, finders, or lead generators for providing the intermediary with the personal identifying information of any potential investor
- Allowing its directors, officers, or partners (or any person occupying a similar status or performing a similar function) to have a financial interest in any issuer using the services of the intermediary

3.8.9 Crowdfunding Sites for Social Entrepreneurs

If money is the only thing stopping you from doing something good in the world, stop waiting and start doing some good! Nothing better symbolizes entrepreneurship than fundraising. Social entrepreneurs are no different. Today, there are a host of online resources for crowdfunding that social entrepreneurs can use to fund their projects, films, books, and social ventures. The following list presents the crowdfunding go-to sites:

- Kickstarter.com: Kickstarter is the 800-pound gorilla in crowdfunding, originally designed and built for creative arts; many technology entrepreneurs now use the site, some reporting to have raised millions of dollars. The Kickstarter funding model is an all-or-nothing model. You set a goal for your raise; if your raise exceeds the goal, you keep all the money; otherwise, your supporters don't pay and you don't get anything. This protects supporters from some of the risk of your running out of money before your project is completed.
- StartSomeGood.com: StartSomeGood is great for early-stage social good projects that are not (yet) 501(c)(3) registered nonprofits.

StartSomeGood uses a unique "tipping point" model for fundraising, allowing you to set a funding goal and a lower "tipping point" at which your project can minimally proceed and where you will collect the money you raise.

- Indiegogo.com: Indiegogo allows you to raise money for absolutely anything, using an optional "keep what you raise" model with higher fees or pay less to use an all-or-nothing funding approach.
- Rockethub.com: Rockethub is also a broad platform targeting "artists, scientists, entrepreneurs, and philanthropists" on their site, using a keep-what-you-raise model that rewards you for hitting your funding goal (or penalizes you for failing to hit it).

All of these sites are making great things happen for real people every day, advancing the arts, entrepreneurship, and philanthropy in myriad ways. Check them and others all out and then decide which one is the best for your needs.

References

1. Freear, J., Sohl, J.E., and Wetzel, W. Angels: Personal investors in the venture capital market. *Entrepreneurship and Regional Development*, 7, 85–94, 1995.
2. Carter, N.M., Brush, C., Gatewood, E., Greene, P., and Hart, M. Does enhancing women's financial sophistication promote entrepreneurial success? Paper presented at the Promoting Female Entrepreneurship: Implications for Education, Training and Policy Conference, Dundalk Institute of Technology, Ireland, 20, November 2002.
3. McCune, J.C. Bootstrapping: Cutting corners and pinching pennies to finance your business, *Bankrate.com*, Internet, 1999, http://www.bankrate.com/brm/news/biz/Cashflow_banking/19991101.asp.
4. Bhide, A. Bootstrap finance: The art of start-ups. *Harvard Business Review*, 70 (November–December), 109–117, 1992.
5. http://www.investopedia.com/terms/s/sweatequity.asp
6. Lahm, R.J. and Little, H.T., Jr. *Bootstrapping Business Start-Ups: A Review of Current Business Practices.* 2005 Conference on Emerging Issues in Business and Technology, http://paws.wcu.edu/RJLahm/teaching/entrepreneurship/Bootstrapping_Lahm.pdf.
7. http://www.angelblog.net/Startup_Funding_the_Friends_and_Family_Round.html
8. Hsu, D. and Ziedonis, R.H. Patents as Quality Signals for Entrepreneurial Ventures. Copenhagen, DRUID Summer Conference, Denmark, June 2007, http://www2.druid.dk/conferences/viewpaper.php?id=1717&cf=9.
9. Spence, M. Job market signaling. *Quarterly Journal of Economics*, 87, 355–374, 1973.

10. Tyson, E. and Schell, J. *Small Business for Dummies*, Wiley Publishing, Inc., Hoboken, NJ, 2008.
11. Sugars, B. Keeping Your Costs Down, http://www.entrepreneur.com/article /177116.
12. Fallon, N. Business News Daily, www.businessnewsdaily.com/5358-startup -budget-tips.html.
13. http://earlygrowthfinancialservices.com/where-is-your-startup-overspending/
14. http://smallbusiness.chron.com/budget-startup-business-1351.html
15. http://www.businessinsider.com/ben-horowitz-budget-process-kills-startups -2014-7
16. http://search.aol.com/aol/search?s_it=topsearchbox.search&v_t=wscreen -smallbusiness-w&q=budgeting+startups+++pdf
17. http://jeffmagnusson.com/agile-budgeting-cash-is-king/
18. Perspectives on merger integration. McKinsey, http://www.mckinsey.com/~/media /mckinsey/dotcom/client_service/Organization/PDFs/775084%20Merger%20 Management%20Article%20Compendium.ashx.
19. Schneider, W.F. Merger or acquisition failing? http://www.cdg-corp.com /documents/WES%20M%20&%20A%20article.pdf.
20. http://knowledge.senndelaney.com/docs/thought_papers/pdf/SennDelaney _cultureclash_UK.pdf
21. http://ww2.cfo.com/growth-companies/2013/10/the-jobs-act-crowdfunding -and-emerging-businesses/
22. http://www.forbes.com/sites/tanyaprive/2012/11/27/what-is-crowdfunding -and-how-does-it-benefit-the-economy/
23. http://en.wikipedia.org/wiki/Crowdfunding
24. http://en.wikipedia.org/wiki/Jumpstart_Our_Business_Startups_Act
25. http://www.sec.gov/divisions/marketreg/tmjobsact-crowdfundingintermedi ariesfaq.htm

4

Funding a Knowledge-Intensive Business

4.1 Introduction

Starting your own knowledge-intensive business is definitely not for everyone; it can be a highly stressful way to earn a living. On the positive side, you have total control over your life; there's no boss telling you what to do and when to do it. You are the master, or mistress, of your own destiny, and you will be doing what you like, when you like to do it, and how you like to do it.

However, there is a dark side; you will work longer hours and there is no guarantee that, magically, money will appear in your bank account biweekly, or monthly. That security of income suddenly disappears, as dozens of other things require paying before you can take your wage.

The majority of would-be entrepreneurs underestimate the amount of money they need to start a business. Here is a list of some of the *initial* costs you will encounter [1]:

1. All the documents, and professional help—licenses, permits, incorporation, legal fees, accountancy fees, partnership agreements, and more

2. Equipment (manufacturing, computers, printers, cash registers, alarms, chairs, desks, phones, the list goes on)

3. Inventory: goods, or raw materials, work-in-process

4. Insurance—liability, life, building, umbrella policies, and so on

5. Rent, down payments, and any leasehold improvements

6. Air conditioning, gas, oil, water, telephone, Internet, and so on

7. Staff payroll, taxes, benefits, training

8. Delivery, warehousing, courier, postage, and so on

9. Marketing costs: business cards, stationery, advertising, website, mailing lists, online, travel, accommodation, entertainment, conferences, and so on

10. Professional association memberships

In many cases, the above list will only represent the starting point of all the money you will need to fund your start-up, and all that is even before you start to pay yourself. Remember, you are unlikely to start your business one day and be able to pay all your expenses from profit the next. Cash flow is a critical component of survival, so it is vital that you have sufficient capital to bridge the gap between the day you start your business and the time your business not only can sustain itself but also make a profit. Consider the following list of undercapitalized start-ups that made it big:

- Starbucks was started by three guys in 1971 who invested $1350 each. 2015 brand value: $132 billion.
- UPS was started by a couple of teenagers who possessed one bicycle between them and $100. 2015 brand value: $40 billion.
- Apple—It's 1976, two guys make a sale, buy a bunch of parts bought on credit and deliver some computers. 2015 brand value: $200 billion.
- Gillette started in 1903 with 25 cents. 2015 brand value: $22 billion.
- Nike, in 1963, launched with $1000. 2015 brand value: $20 billion.
- Hewlett Packard started in 1938 in a garage with the princely sum of $538 dollars. 2015 brand value: $40 billion.

4.2 Starting Your Start-Up

Your start-up's demand for cash depends on the costs associated with developing and marketing your product. Entrepreneurs creating a sweat equity company in their garage and initially funded by personal savings do not need to seek, or solicit, investment capital.

In contrast, the entrepreneur who plans to start a new biopharmaceutical company must spend countless hours trying to secure large amounts of investment capital. Once the initial capital is secured, founders will immediately start planning when and how to secure the next "round" of financing.

Start-up firms are voracious in their appetite for cash, and raising money is a never-ending process, being at the mercy of the investment community. The decision to form a modest investment company or an equity investment company is largely dependent on your timeline to market launch.

While your innate desire to preserve ownership and operational control of the venture via a modest investment company is understandable, many commercial opportunities require extensive partnering, in both investment and strategy.

Most start-ups go through a predictable series of steps, before raising capital. Figure 4.1 summarizes the typical history of a start-up.

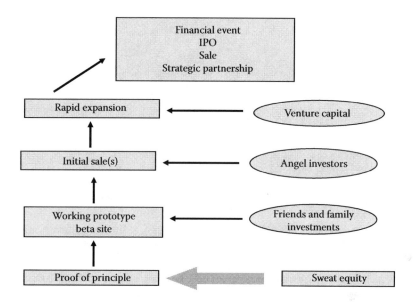

FIGURE 4.1
Typical historical development.

4.3 When Is the Best Time to Start Your Start-Up?

Entrepreneurs get so excited about forming a company that they often lose sight of the hard road ahead. It is easy to overlook the fundamentals of building a successful business. While there is no mathematical formula for determining the best time to start a new company, raising enough capital to cover the first year of operations is a good rule of thumb.

The "best" time has less to do with the stage of research than with the ability to raise capital. Innovative discoveries are generally quite far from being products and have increased chances of failure during development. The pathway from concept to product entails substantial risk. Therefore, the more embryonic the discovery, the higher the risk.

Investors prefer companies that are advanced in product development. For knowledge-intensive products, such as drugs or high technology, companies with mid-stage human clinical trials or those with successful beta tests of their software are desired.

Investors can be stratified according to their comfort levels with risks at each of the stages of the commercialization process. Those at the early (highest-risk) end are often called "seed" investors, and those at the later (lower-risk) stages are called "mezzanine" investors. It is important for entrepreneurs to clearly understand the risk profile associated with commercializing their product, since it enables them to better assess the investment climate.

4.4 Start-Up Fundraising Principles

Dig your water hole before you are thirsty.

The amount of money you plan to raise should be sufficient to accomplish key milestones that will either (1) make your start-up self-sufficient or (2) enable you to raise additional capital at *a higher valuation.* Higher valuations enable management to keep a greater percentage of the company, in anticipation of future financing rounds.

Like it or not, the entrepreneur needs to prepare for an exhaustive due diligence process. Due diligence is the analysis and evaluation conducted by firms considering an investment in your company and focuses primarily on (1) your management team, (2) the market opportunity, and (3) your technology, including intellectual property protection, usually in that order.

You should prepare a list of references and accomplishments of key management team members (including your scientific advisory board members) and your technology. Furthermore, have your patent firm prepare a status report on your patents, including a "freedom to operate" opinion, so you can verify that your products are proprietary and that you are not encumbered by the patents of others.

In summary, what do you need to attract investors?

- A great business model
- A great business plan
- A great management team
- Proprietary technology
- A growing market segment

4.5 Types of Financing for Start-Ups

So you think you are ready to commercialize your innovation? Congratulations! Now you need start-up financing—that initial infusion of money needed to turn the idea into something tangible. And that is where it becomes very tricky.

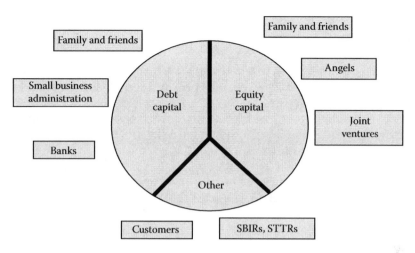

FIGURE 4.2
Types of financing for start-ups.

When you are just starting out, you are not yet at the point where a traditional lender or investor would be interested in you. So that leaves you with selling cherished assets, borrowing against your home, maxing out credit cards, dipping into a 401(k), and asking loved ones for loans. There is a lot of risk involved, including the risk of bankruptcy with your personal finances and soured relationships with friends and family [2].

The type of investors that you should seek for your start-up will depend on (1) the type of company that is being built, (2) the stage of development, and (3) the projected capital needs. The type of financing available to you will depend on

- The amount you need and how it will be used
- Your personal financial condition
- Your available collateral
- Your ability to manage a business
- Your determination, presentation skills, and ability to negotiate

Basically, start-ups can raise capital by three mechanisms: (1) equity, (2) debt, or (3) other, as shown in Figure 4.2.

4.5.1 Equity Financing Process

Equity financing is the process of raising capital through the sale of shares in an enterprise. Equity financing essentially refers to the sale of an ownership interest to raise funds for business purposes. With equity financing, a company gives investors shares in the company's ownership in exchange for capital. There is no promise to repay the investment like in a loan arrangement, nor is there an interest component.

There is, however, a cost to equity capital. In order for investors to agree to invest in the company, they expect to earn an "acceptable return" that justifies the risk of the investment.

That "acceptable return" varies over time and across industries as investors compare the potential upside, the potential risks, and the risk–reward profile of investment opportunities other than the given company. If the company fails to meet these return expectations, investors can share their ownership interest and move capital elsewhere, reducing the value of the company and hampering future efforts to raise capital [3].

Equity financing spans a wide range of activities in scale and scope, from a few thousand dollars raised by an entrepreneur from friends and family, to giant initial public offerings (IPOs) running into the billions by household names such as Google and Facebook.

While the term is generally associated with financings by public companies listed on an exchange, equity financing includes financings by private companies as well. Equity financing is clearly distinct from debt financing, which refers to funds borrowed by a business [4].

Equity financing involves not just the sale of common equity but also the sale of other equity or quasi-equity instruments such as preferred stock, convertible preferred stock, and equity units that include common shares and warrants.

A start-up that grows into a successful company will likely require several rounds of equity financing as it evolves. Since a start-up typically attracts different types of investors at various stages of its evolution, it may use different equity instruments for its financing needs.

For example, friends and family as well as angel investors—who are generally the first investors in a start-up—are inclined to favor convertible preferred shares rather than common equity in exchange for funding new companies, since the former have greater upside potential and some downside protection. Once the company has grown large enough to consider going public, it may consider selling common equity to institutional and retail investors. Later on, if it needs additional capital, the company may opt for secondary equity financings such as a rights offering or an offering of equity units that includes warrants as a "sweetener."

The characteristics of equity financing for start-ups is summarized in Table 4.1.

4.5.2 Debt Financing

In contrast, debt financing is when a company takes out a loan or issues a bond to raise capital. While there can be much complexity in the details of large corporate debt deals, the fundamentals are largely similar to common

TABLE 4.1

Equity Financing for Start-Ups

Investor Types	Characteristics
Friends and family Typical round: $10 to $100,000	Not necessarily "accredited" individuals "Passive" investment Personally interested in the technology
Angels Typical round: $50 to $500,000 Increasingly as angel groups	Accredited individuals Expertise and personal investments Bets on the jokey, not the horse
Venture Capital Typical round: $1 million to $5 million Looks for an "exit"	Professional investors LLP, General Partnerships Follow-on investments

household debts already familiar with individuals. Companies can accept long-term financing to purchase facilities, equipment, or other long-term assets, similar to a family that takes out a mortgage loan to purchase a house or a loan to buy a car.

Debt is borrowing money from an outside source with your promise to repay the principal, in addition to an agreed-upon level of interest. Although the term tends to have a negative connotation, start-up companies often turn to debt to finance their operations. In fact, even the healthiest of corporate balance sheets will include some level of debt. In finance, debt is also referred to as "leverage." The most popular source for debt financing is the bank, but debt can also be issued by a private company or even a friend or family member [5].

We can now define debt financing as: A method of financing in which a company receives a loan and gives its promise to repay the loan [6].

Debt financing includes both secured and unsecured loans. Security involves a form of collateral as an assurance the loan will be repaid. If the debtor defaults on the loan, that collateral is forfeited to satisfy payment of the debt. Most lenders will ask for some sort of security on a loan. Few, if any, will lend you money based on your name or idea alone.

In addition to secured or unsecured loans, most debt will be subject to a repayment period. There are three types of repayment terms:

1. **Short-term loans** are typically paid back within 6 to 18 months.
2. **Intermediate-term loans** are paid back within 3 years.
3. **Long-term loans** are paid back from the cash flow of the business in 5 years or less.

The most common source of debt financing for start-ups often isn't a commercial lending institution, but family and friends. When borrowing money from your relatives or friends, have your attorney draw up legal papers dictating the terms of the loan. Why? Too many entrepreneurs borrow money

TABLE 4.2

Summary Differences between Debt and Equity Financing

Debt (Bank Loan)	Equity (Angels, Venture Capital)
Emphasis on collateral and cash flow	Return on investment
Repayment starts immediately after funding	Deferred repayment
Debt return based on ability to pay	Repayment based on financial performance
Lowest risk for lender	Highest risk for investor
Lowest cost if business is successful	Higher cost if business is successful
No ownership dilution	Heavy ownership dilution
Focused on short-term expansion	Focused on long-term business prospects
Monitoring relationship	May demand board seats, plus upper management participation
Boilerplate documents	Complex documentation

from family and friends on an informal basis. The terms of the loan have been verbalized but not written down in a contract.

Lending money can be tricky for people who can't view the transaction at arm's length; if they don't feel you're running your business correctly, they might step in and interfere with your operations. In some cases, you can't prevent this, even with a written contract, because many state laws guarantee voting rights to an individual who has invested money in a business. This can create and has created a lot of hard feelings. Make sure to check with your attorney before accepting any loans from friends or family.

Table 4.2 summarizes the most common differences between debt and equity financing available to entrepreneurs.

4.6 Alternative Financing Opportunities

Most businesses don't start with bank loans or venture capital. Most actually start their organizations financed with a combination of personal resources, "bootstrapping," and help from family and friends. Only a small number of start-ups begin with a bank loan, and even less start with a venture capital infusion.

If you have little cash or personal assets and bad personal credit, bank loans are not an immediate option. Your first step may be to recruit an equity partner ("angel") or a cosigner. Creative and determined entrepreneurs routinely start businesses without bank loans.

4.6.1 Sweat Equity and Friends, Family, and Fools (3Fs)

Usually, the founders each put a great deal of time ("sweat equity"), plus some of their personal funds into the enterprise during its early years to help with initial expenses. More committed entrepreneurs, especially those without co-founders, may invest a considerable amount of their own money into the company, frequently using credit cards and home equity loans.

Also, entrepreneurs may tap their friends and families ("friends, family, and fools") as early angels to provide initial funding. Soliciting money from family and friends can be emotionally draining. It is wise to be clear upfront about your goals and intentions. A written agreement or contract will be useful.

4.6.2 Nonprofit Foundation Grants

Nonprofit foundations are often good starting places to seek funding if your mission and goals are compatible with the missions and goals of the nonprofit foundation.

Occurring more frequently in healthcare, certain nonprofit foundations may be interested in sponsoring "orphan drug" development, new cancer therapies, fighting exotic tropical diseases, and so on. For example, the Food and Drug Administration (FDA) Office of Orphan Products Development (OOPD) provides incentives for sponsors to develop products for rare diseases. The program has successfully enabled the development and marketing of more than 2800 orphan designations, and more than 400 drugs and biologic products for rare diseases have been granted FDA approval since 1983 [7].

The Humanitarian Use Device Program has been the first step in approval of more than 150 Humanitarian Device Exemption approvals [8]. Orphan status is applied to drugs and biologics that are defined as those intended for the safe and effective treatment, diagnosis, or prevention of rare diseases/disorders that affect fewer than 200,000 people in the United States, or that affect more than 200,000 persons but are not expected to recover the costs of developing and marketing a treatment drug.

The Humanitarian Use Device program designates a device that is intended to benefit patients by treating or diagnosing a disease or condition that affects fewer than 4000 individuals in the United States per year as per 21 CFR 814.3(n).

The OOPD administers two extramural grant programs. The Orphan Products Grants Program provides funding for clinical research that tests the safety and efficacy of drugs, biologics, medical devices, and medical foods in rare diseases or conditions. The Pediatric Device Consortia Grant Program provides funding to develop nonprofit consortia to facilitate pediatric medical device development.

There are a few other factors that positively influence the economics of orphan drug development: timelines are typically shorter [9], the FDA is often more flexible with approvals because of the lack of alternative treatments [10], and approved orphan drugs often require less marketing, have a faster uptake, and are generally well reimbursed.

All these considerations have made orphan drug development strategies increasingly popular with big pharma and venture capital investors—and, thus, with biotech entrepreneurs—but what financial rewards have start-up orphan drug companies actually reaped, and how likely is it that your company will draw interest from big-pocketed buyers?

Although a rare disease is defined as one that affects fewer than 200,000 people in the United States, the number of such conditions totals approximately 7000 and collectively they affect nearly 30 million Americans, or one in 10 of the population. According to the FDA, one-third of all new drug approvals over the last 5 years have been for rare diseases. In 2013, the Pharmaceutical Research and Manufacturers of America claimed that there are more than 450 new medicines for rare diseases in clinical-stage development or undergoing FDA review, including 85 for genetic disorders [11].

4.6.3 SBIR and STTR Grants

Small Business Innovation Research (SBIR) and Small Business Technology Transfer (STTR) are federal grant programs that fund research in companies with fewer than 500 employees. See Chapter 5 for more details.

These programs recognize that much of the United States' innovation occurs within the small business sector, and they aim to accelerate further innovation in specific areas of research. More than 2 billion dollars in grants are awarded each year by agencies of the federal government under published solicitations.

SBIR/STTR Awards have three phases:

- Phase I (up to $150,000), in which new concepts undergo "proof of principle"
- Phase II (up to $1 million), in which successful Phase I projects are developed into products
- Phase IIb (up to $3 million) in which the Phase II projects are moved close to commercialization

SBIR/STTR awards are made to the small business, but a portion of the funds may be subcontracted to a university, or another research entity laboratory, which can be a great source for managing proof-of-concept projects without having to pay for expensive infrastructure such as instrumentation in a private sector laboratory (up to 33% for SBIR and 60% for STTR during Phase I).

4.6.3.1 Academic Start-Ups

SBIR/STTR awards are attractive to academic start-ups for two reasons: They play to the grant-writing strengths of academic researchers and the entrepreneurial founder. These are outright grants, not equity investments (e.g., you don't have to give a piece of the company away to get the money). The major downside to the awards is that there can be a significant lag between Phase I and Phase II awards, and it may be difficult to keep research teams together (i.e., meet payroll, and keep the lights on) while the Phase II application is pending.

Many academics have been tempted to use the SBIR/STTR programs to extend their academic research instead of using the funds to build a company and develop products.

4.6.3.2 Expert Review Panels

Expert panels are utilized to review the grant applications for both technical and commercial merit. Applications that are academically focused are generally not accepted, but used in their intended manner, SBIR/STTR awards are an excellent way to fund early research in a start-up and the Phase II awards are robust. Still, a company trying to build its entire portfolio of products from SBIR/STTR grants without other investments is not likely to secure sufficient resources.

4.7 Obtaining Small Business Financing

Benjamin Franklin, Thomas Edison, Wilbur and Orville Wright—the annals of American history are filled with numerous people who created something new that changed an entire industry and even our way of life. Most people know the "famous" inventors, but many other folks invent something that becomes a business success.

Every year, *Inc.* magazine publishes its list of "The 500 Fastest Growing Companies in America." This list includes tomorrow's potential goliaths of the business world. Such companies as Apple, Microsoft, Timberland, Oracle, and Twitter have graced and then graduated from the list since its inception.

Industry	Number of *Inc.* 500 Companies Listed (2014)
Telecommunications and wireless	65
IT Services	50
Software	48
Financial Services	41
Government Services	38
Health	38
Energy	35
Pharmaceuticals and biotechnology	29

Clearly, if your start-up is any of the fastest-growing industries, you stand a better chance of getting equity financed by any of the resources that are listed in the subsequent paragraphs.

4.7.1 Angels: Investors with a Heart

Angels are individuals—usually ex-entrepreneurs who are experienced enough to understand and live with the financial risks they take—with money available to lend or invest. The angels' motives may vary: Most seek to increase their net worth, some want to help (mentor) aspiring entrepreneurs, while some simply crave a "piece of the action."

Angels typically invest capital in seed, start-up, and early-stage companies. Angels are often successful, excited entrepreneurs themselves, or retired executives who wish to "give back" their time and expertise. Angels invest their own money; that is, they are *not* money managers, and generally prefer to invest in local companies, looking to make a reasonable return on investment.

According to a 2010 report distributed by the Angel Capital Education Foundation, total start-up funding from venture capital funds, state funds, and angel investors totals approximately $20.8 billion annually. Surprisingly, friends and family contributed nearly three times that amount of capital to thousands of start-ups each year. With approximately $60 billion in start-up funding from friends and family, entrepreneurs must consider this important option as they seek to launch new businesses [12].

Angels are an *accredited investor* (an SEC definition) that includes

- **Financial position**
  - Net worth: $1 million
  - Annual personal income: $200,000
  - Family income: $300,000
- **Assumptions**
  - Knowledgeable—capable of performing own due diligence
  - Can afford to lose the entire investment
- **Implications**
  - Giving up regulated disclosure, but many are now part of Angel groups

4.7.2 Angels Classification

Angels come in many forms: Some fly in flocks (i.e., belong to angel organizations or investment groups), some work solo, some look for a piece of the company's ownership (equity), and others prefer lending (debt). Almost all angels demand personal involvement in your business, however, and in many cases, the know-how an angel can bring to the table is worth more than the capital itself.

Angels are like the highway patrol—the time that you need them the most is the time they are the most difficult to find. Movements are afoot, however, to make the identity of angels more accessible. According to the Yellow Pages Publishers Association, "angels" will soon be a Yellow Pages heading in most telephone books (along with "psychic life readings" and "body piercing").

The SBA spawned Active Capital (activecapital.org), and you'll discover a mix-and-match format designed to bring together aspiring small-business start-ups and "accredited small-business investors." The "accredited small-business investor" must have a net worth in excess of $1 million or an individual annual income in excess of $200,000 (or $300,000 joint income).

Angel investors are individuals who invest their own personal money in a fledgling enterprise. An angel investor is usually someone who has led the launch and development of successful companies, followed by a financially profitable exit. Angel investors often form groups so potential investments can be better evaluated.

Each angel typically invests between $25,000 and $100,000. If a group pools their capital, the total amount of investment can reach more than $1 million dollars. Angel investors usually come in at an earlier stage than venture capital financing.

Equity investors receive stock in the company, with the amount dependent on the value ("valuation") of the company in proportion to how much they have invested. The cash value placed on a new company ("pre-money valuation") is somewhat arbitrary and subject to negotiation, with entrepreneurs usually thinking high valuations and investors a much lower valuation.

It is inevitable that after multiple rounds of equity investment, the investors will own a majority of the shares of the company. Academics often view this outcome as "losing control" of their company (often called "Founder's syndrome" or "founderitis"), but without external investments, the company would not be able to move forward (unless you have a rich uncle).

The Founder's syndrome [13] is a difficulty faced by many organizations where one or more founders maintain disproportionate power and influence after the effective initial establishment of the project, leading to a wide range of problems for both the organization and those involved. The passion and charisma of the founder or founders, which were such an important reason for the successful establishment of the organization, become a limiting and destructive force, rather than the creative and productive force they were in the early stages [14].

Do YOU have Founder's syndrome [15]? If you answer "Yes" to most of the following questions, you may suffer from an incurable case of founderitis:

1. When you leave, will you feel skeptical that things might be managed differently?
2. Are you staying because it's "best" for the organization if you stay?

3. Do you identify with the organization as being a part of who you are?

4. Do you fear the organization will change its mission contrary to your original mission and vision?

5. Can you separate organizational issues from your personal viewpoint of the issues?

6. Do you relate to the organization as belonging to you by saying, "My organization"?

7. Do you feel as though you are indispensable and irreplaceable?

8. Do you want to stay involved long after you depart to avoid feeling a sense of great personal loss?

If you want to find an angel in your own backyard, your state or city may have an angel-matching program. Ask local bankers, accountants, financial advisors, or lawyers for their input on how to find a local angel-matching program; call your local Chamber of Commerce; or contact your state's Department of Commerce.

4.7.3 Venture Capital

Venture capital firms and organizations offer cash in exchange for equity in later-stage companies, so they are, in effect, an organized version of angel investing. According to Wikipedia, venture capital (VC) is financial capital provided to early-stage, high-potential, high-risk, high-growth start-up companies. A venture capital fund makes money by owning equity in the companies it invests in, which usually have novel technologies or business models in high-technology industries (e.g., biotechnology, IT, or software).

The typical venture capital investment occurs after the seed funding round, and the angel round(s), frequently referred to as a growth funding round (a.k.a. Series A round). The VC seeks to generate returns through an eventual realization event, such as an IPO or a trade sale of the company [16]. Venture capital is a subset of private equity.

One of the first steps toward a professionally managed venture capital industry was the passage of the Small Business Investment Act of 1958; this Act officially permitted the US Small Business Administration (SBA) to license private small business investment companies (SBICs) to help finance and manage small entrepreneurial businesses in the United States.

Before World War II, money orders (originally known as "development capital") were primarily the exclusive domain of wealthy individuals and families. Modern private equity investments began to emerge after World War II with the founding of the first two venture capital firms in 1946, American Research and Development Corporation (ARDC) and J.H. Whitney & Company.

ARDC was founded by Georges Doriot [17], the "father of venture capitalism" (and former dean of Harvard Business School and founder of INSEAD) [18], with Ralph Flanders and Karl Compton (former president of MIT), to encourage private sector investments in businesses run by soldiers returning from World War II. ARDC was the first institutional private equity investment firm that raised capital from sources other than wealthy families, although it had several notable investment successes as well. ARDC is credited with the first trick when its 1957 investment of $70,000 in Digital Equipment Corporation would be valued at more than $355 million after the company's IPO in 1968 (representing a return of more than 1200 times on its investment and an annualized rate of return of 101%) [19].

4.7.4 Venture Capital Financing

As opposed to more conservative sources of capital, which look closely at a business's past performance and its collateral before handing out cash, venture capital firms focus primarily on future prospects when looking at a business plan. Thus, venture capital is useful for a few sophisticated businesses in higher risk, higher-reward industries. Venture capital firms look for the possibility of hefty annual returns (30% or more) on their investments in order to offset the losses that are sure to occur within their high-risk portfolios.

Unfortunately, very few start-ups are in a position to take advantage of venture capital financing. The typical venture capital firm funds only 2% of the deals under consideration. Moreover, that 2% has to meet a wide range of investment criteria, such as highly attractive niches, sophisticated management, and potential for high return—criteria that the typical small business start-up cannot begin to meet. Do not be disappointed at not qualifying for venture capital funding. Venture capital is usually reserved for fast-growing "start-ups" that have a proven track record of business successes.

4.7.5 Venture Capital Firms

Venture capitalists (VCs) are professional investors and money managers who manage and invest a pool of money from high net worth individuals and institutional investors who are looking for higher returns on their investments than the average stock market returns.

There are thousands of venture firms in the United States, and each firm usually specializes in a particular industry. There are more VCs focused on high tech than life sciences, simply because an exit in a life science is usually much longer, and riskier.

VCs provide significant value to a start-up company that goes beyond monetary value. Many VCs were themselves former executives who launched and managed successful companies and they can provide valuable advice and guidance. In addition, when a VC signs up to invest in your enterprise, you are automatically getting their entire network of friends. VCs have impressive networks of associates that can help start-ups solve business-related problems.

4.7.6 Venture Capital's Management Fees

VCs make money by charging a management fee of the managed funds they raise from accredited wealthy individuals and institutional investors. It is in a VC firm's best interest to make money for their own investors, because their reputation is on the line. In turn, their reputation is based on their investment track records. If managers have below average success rates, investors are likely to choose a different money manager.

Equally important as selecting the right CEO (chief executive officer) is the proper choice of the right investors. Investors play a critical role in shaping the company, providing network, management, and so on. The quality of your seed investors will play a key role in attracting future investments.

Sometimes, the entrepreneur is in such desperate need for funding that he or she accepts investments from inexperienced investors. These investors often have unrealistic expectations, little industry-specific network and little credibility with follow-on investors. Few start-ups can survive inexperienced seed investors.

4.8 Persuasive Business Presentations

> *Leadership is the art of communication.*

As a budding entrepreneur, you might as well get used to this: As an entrepreneur, you will be giving presentations till the cows come home, and persuasive presentations will become your trademark.

A **persuasive presentation** (speech) aims to get your audience to accept your business premise by prompting them to act, think, or feel in a desired manner, without coercion or force. Figure 4.3 presents the four cornerstones of persuasive presentations.

Pathos refers to presenting your reasons to believe in something, overcoming risks, natural apprehensions, perceived problems, and so on. **Ethos** refers to your personal technical competence, goodwill, and dynamism to be trusted with investor's moneys. **Logos** are your set of rational, logical, and validated proofs. Last, **Mythos** are the combined force of ethical values, industry beliefs, and national culture that may prompt investments in you and your company.

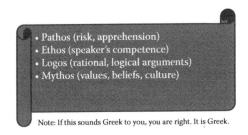

FIGURE 4.3
The four cornerstones of persuasive presentations.

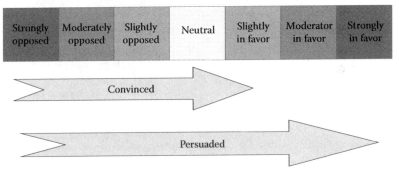

FIGURE 4.4
Degrees of convincing and persuading.

Persuasive speech is the most complicated form of verbal communication. It involves moving your audience to accept your premise from a position of deep skepticism/opposition to strongly/enthusiastically embracing your proposed solution based on its perceived benefits [20]. The entire sequence is shown in Figure 4.4.

4.8.1 Rookie Mistakes

There is an old adage that goes: "Your presentation is 20% *what* you say, and 80% *how* you say it." Most rookie entrepreneurs tend to ignore their demeanor when making presentations, believing that their data "speaks for itself."

Another hurdle is the fact that most people become tongue-tied when placed in front of an audience. Most of us "freeze" when asked to give an important presentation. Did you hear the joke about the survey that asked aspiring entrepreneurs what are their three greatest fears in life? Their answer is seen below:

1. Fear of dying
2. Fear of speaking in public
3. Fear of dying while speaking in public

Figure 4.5 presents a tongue-in-cheek list of do's and don'ts for entrepreneurs.

4.8.2 Your Elevator Pitch

> I only had one superstition. I made sure to touch all the bases when I hit a homerun.
>
> **Babe Ruth**

The **elevator pitch** derives its name from an apocryphal story: after submitting a "teaser" document to a VC, and after waiting many weeks to hear something from the VC, suddenly you get an unexpected phone call from the Managing Partner. "I am in the elevator going to a meeting. Tell me why I should fund your company now." The Partner has just asked you to three questions: Why me? Why you? Why now?

Guess what? You only have one chance of getting funded. Thus, an elevator pitch must be a concise, carefully planned, and well-practiced description about your company that anyone should be able to understand in the time it would take to ride up three floors in an elevator. Like Babe Ruth, your pitch needs to touch these bases:

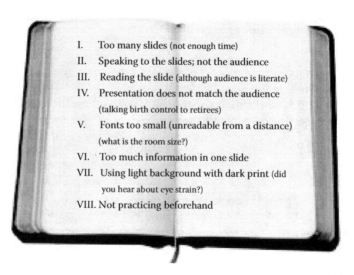

    I.   Too many slides (not enough time)
    II.   Speaking to the slides; not the audience
    III.   Reading the slide (although audience is literate)
    IV.   Presentation does not match the audience
          (talking birth control to retirees)
    V.   Fonts too small (unreadable from a distance)
          (what is the room size?)
    VI.   Too much information in one slide
    VII. Using light background with dark print (did
          you hear about eye strain?)
    VIII. Not practicing beforehand

FIGURE 4.5
How to screw up your presentation in eight easy steps.

- A burning market need and your proposed solution to the burning need
- Your team and how they are uniquely qualified to manage the company
- How you will make money for your investors
- Memorable tagline/pitch **closing**

4.8.2.1 Elevator Pitch Must-Haves

Your pitch should have a riveting **opening**; that is, it should grab the interest of your recipient. Your pitch should show **passion**—if you are not excited about your idea, no one else will be.

Brief descriptions. After your pitch be prepared to answer questions briefly. You must prepare a brief description of how the business is different from the competition, a brief description of how you will make money, a brief description of the resources you need from investors, and a brief description of the returns/payback the investor can expect.

Last three bits of advice: (1) Always use the KISS (Keep It Simple, Stupid) principle. (2) Do not use Techno-Latin, a language that only you understand. (3) Highlight marketing advantages, not merely technical benefits.

4.9 The Knowledge-Intensive Industry

The knowledge-intensive industry is vast, feverishly paced, and extremely competitive. For companies in this field, one thing is certain—today's new product is tomorrow's commodity. That is the main risk of a high-tech venture, and that is one of the challenges of a high-tech enterprise.

The term *knowledge-intensive industry* derives from the recognition of the role of knowledge and technology in economic growth. Knowledge, as embodied in human beings (as "human capital") and in technology, has been central to the economic development of many advanced countries.

The science-based system, essentially public research laboratories and institutes of higher education, carries out key functions in the knowledge-based economy, including knowledge production, transmission, and transfer.

Modern economies are more strongly dependent on the production, distribution, and use of knowledge than ever before. Output and employment are expanding fastest in high-technology industries, such as computers, electronics, biotechnology, nanotechnology, and aerospace. Knowledge-intensive service sectors, such as education, communications, and information, are growing even faster.

4.10 Employment in a Knowledge-Intensive Economy

Employment in a knowledge-intensive economy is characterized by increasing demand for more highly skilled workers. Knowledge-intensive and high-technology economies tend to be the most dynamic in terms of output and employment growth. Changes in technology, and particularly the advent of information technologies, are making educated and skilled labor more valuable, and unskilled labor much less so.

Government policies will need more stress on upgrading human capital through promoting access to a range of skills, and especially the capacity to learn; enhancing the *knowledge distribution power* of the economy through collaborative networks and the diffusion of technology; and providing the enabling conditions for organizational change at the firm level to maximize the benefits of technology for productivity.

4.11 Knowledge Codification

In order to facilitate economic analysis, distinctions can be made between different kinds of knowledge that are important in the knowledge-based economy: know-what, know-why, know-how, and know-who. Knowledge is a much broader concept than information, which is generally the "know-what" and "know-why" components of knowledge. These are also the types of knowledge that come closest to being market commodities or economic resources to be fitted into economic production functions. Other types of knowledge—particularly know-how and know-who—are more "tacit knowledge" and are more difficult to codify and measure [21].

- **Know-what** refers to knowledge about facts. How many people live in New York? What are the ingredients in pancakes? and When was the battle of Waterloo? are examples of this kind of knowledge. Here, knowledge is close to what is normally called information—it can be broken down into bits. In some complex areas, experts must have a lot of this kind of knowledge in order to fulfill their jobs. Practitioners of law and medicine belong to this category.

- **Know-why** refers to scientific knowledge of the principles and laws of nature. This kind of knowledge underlies technological development and product and process advances in most industries. The production and reproduction of know-why is often organized in specialized organizations, such as research laboratories and universities. To get access to this kind of knowledge, firms have to interact with these organizations either through recruiting scientifically trained labor or directly through contacts and joint activities.

- **Know-how** refers to skills or the capability to do something. Businessmen judging market prospects for a new product or a personnel manager selecting and training staff have to use their know-how. The same is true for the skilled worker operating complicated machine tools. Know-how is typically a kind of knowledge developed and kept within the border of an individual firm. One of the most important reasons for the formation of industrial networks is the need for firms to be able to share and combine elements of know-how.

- **Know-who** involves information about who knows what and who knows how to do what. It involves the formation of special social relationships that make it possible to get access to experts and use their knowledge efficiently. It is significant in economies where skills are widely dispersed because of a highly developed division of labor among organizations and experts. For the modern manager and organization, it is important to use this kind of knowledge in response to the acceleration in the rate of change. The know-who kind of knowledge is internal to the organization to a higher degree than any other kind of knowledge.

Learning to master the four kinds of knowledge takes place through different channels. While know-what and know-why can be obtained through reading books, attending lectures, and accessing databases, the other two kinds of knowledge are rooted primarily in practical experience. Know-how will typically be learned in situations where an apprentice follows a master and relies upon him as the authority. Know-who is learned in social practice and sometimes in specialized educational environments. It also develops in day-to-day dealings with customers, subcontractors, and independent institutes. One reason why firms engage in basic research is to acquire access to networks of academic experts crucial for their innovative capability. Know-who is socially embedded knowledge that cannot easily be transferred through formal channels of information.

4.12 Information Technology

The development of information technology may be regarded as a response to the need for handling the know-what and know-why portions of knowledge more effectively. Conversely, the existence of information technology and communications infrastructures gives a strong impetus to the process of codifying certain types of knowledge. All knowledge that can be codified and reduced to information can now be transmitted over long distances with very limited costs. It is the increasing codification of some elements of knowledge that have led the current era to be characterized as "the information society"—a society where a majority of workers will soon be producing, handling, and distributing information or codified knowledge.

The digital revolution has intensified the move toward knowledge codification and altered the share of codified versus tacit knowledge in the knowledge stock of the economy. Electronic networks now connect a vast array of public and private information sources, including digitized reference volumes, books, scientific journals, libraries of working papers, images, video clips, sound and voice recordings, graphical displays, and electronic mail. These information resources, connected through various communications networks, represent the components of an emerging, universally accessible digital library.

Because of codification, knowledge is acquiring more of the properties of a commodity. Market transactions are facilitated by codification, and diffusion of knowledge is accelerated. In addition, codification is reducing the importance of additional investments to acquire further knowledge. It is creating bridges between fields and areas of competence and reducing the "dispersion" of knowledge.

These developments promise an acceleration of the rate of growth of stocks of accessible knowledge, with positive implications for economic growth. They also imply increased change in the knowledge stock owing to higher rates of scrapping and obsolescence, which will put greater burdens on the economy's adjustment abilities.

High-tech entrepreneurs face that risk—and that challenge—with imagination, innovation, and insight, but, unfortunately, many do not—and cannot—bring the same creativity and competence to the management of their companies' business affairs.

As a result, promising high-tech companies often fail, not for lack of ideas, but for the same reasons companies in any and every industry can, and do—lack of capital when they need it most; a naive understanding of the marketplace; poor forecasts of development and production costs; mismanaged growth; inadequate tax planning; the wrong advisers, at the wrong time.

References

1. *Starting a Business 101 (Canadian Edition)*, Blue Beetle Books, http://www.small businesssuccess.ca/ebooks/meridian/pdfs/eBook-Starting-a-Business-101.pdf.
2. http://www.entrepreneur.com/article/52718

3. http://www.fool.com/knowledge-center/2015/10/24/the-key-differences-between-debt-and-equity-financ.aspx

4. http://www.investopedia.com/terms/e/equityfinancing.asp

5. http://entrepreneurs.about.com/od/financing/a/debtfinancing.htm

6. http://www.entrepreneur.com/encyclopedia/debt-financing

7. http://www.accessdata.fda.gov/scripts/opdlisting/oopd/

8. http://www.fda.gov/ForIndustry/DevelopingProductsforRareDiseases
Conditions/ucm2005525.htm

9. Meekings, K.N., Williams, C.S., and Arrowsmith, J.E. Orphan drug development: An economically viable strategy for biopharma R&D. *Drug Discov. Today,* 17, 660–664, 2012.

10. Sasinowski, F.J. Quantum of effectiveness evidence in FDA's approval of orphan drugs. *Drug Inf. J.,* 46, 238–263, 2012.

11. http://www.pharmatimes.com/article/13-10 09/US_biopharma_452_drugs_for_rare_diseases_now_in_R_D.aspx

12. http://blog.startupprofessionals.com/2010/08/friends-and-family-largest-startup.html

13. McNamara, C. Founder's Syndrome: How Corporations Suffer—And Can Recover, http://managementhelp.org/misc/founders.htm.

14. https://en.wikipedia.org/wiki/Founder's_syndrome

15. http://www.leadingtransitions.com/pdfs/Leadership%20Guide.pdf

16. http://en.wikipedia.org/wiki/Venture_capital

17. WGBH Public Broadcasting Service. Who made America?—Georges Doriot.

18. Ante, S.E. *Creative Capital: Georges Doriot and the Birth of Venture Capital.* Harvard Business School Press, Cambridge, MA, 2008. ISBN 1-4221-0122-3.

19. Venture Impact: The Economic Importance of Venture Backed Companies to the U.S. Economy. NVCA.org. Retrieved 2013.

20. Lucas, S.E. Speaking to persuade. Chapter 15, http://www.jdcc.edu/includes/download.php?action=2023&download_file_id=5274&action=2023&table_num=.

21. Smith, E.A. The role of tacit and explicit knowledge in the workplace, http://www.basicknowledge101.com/pdf/KM_roles.pdf.

5

SBIR/STTR Grants

5.1 Introduction

A **grant**, also known as a *cooperative agreement*, is a monetary award given by a *grantor* to a *grantee*. A *grant request* is an advance promise of what you or your organization (the grantee) proposes to do when the grantor fulfills your request for funding. The most distinguishing characteristic between a grant and a cooperative agreement is the degree of federal participation or involvement during the performance of the work activities. When a federal agency program officer participates in funded project activities, it is called a cooperative agreement. When the grant applicant is the sole implementer of project activities, it is called a grant.

What kind of entrepreneur applies for a grant? A person who is in need of cash flow and who is willing to roll up his sleeves, dig deep for hard-to-find information, and speak boldly and proudly about their technology, identifying current funding needs and explaining their commercialization capabilities.

What does it take to get started? First and foremost, you need to learn from knowledge and experience—part of which is presented in this chapter. Also, you should deeply desire to make a difference in the lives of others. Whether it's a grant-funded intervention or prevention or a contract bid award for delivering an excellent quality of goods or services, you should be ready to give it your full attention. It is akin to a full-blown PhD dissertation.

Some grant awards come with no strings attached, but many others require you to use the funds in a certain way. Grantors with strings attached to their funds are almost always government grantmaking agencies (local, state, and federal public sector funders). Grantors with literally no strings attached are referred to as *private sector funders*. These usually include corporate and foundation grantmakers.

What can a grant pay for? A grant award can be used for whatever the funder agency wants to fund. This means that reading the funding guidelines is critical when it comes to improving your chances for success. Remember that not following instructions to the letter is an automatic reason for rejection.

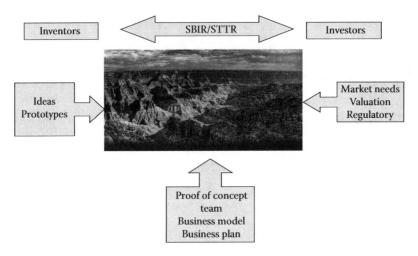

FIGURE 5.1
Bridging the "valley of death."

From an entrepreneurial perspective, Small Business Innovation Research (SBIR)/Small Business Technology Transfer (STTR) grants are frequently used to "bridge the valley of death," as depicted in Figure 5.1.

5.2 The World of SBIR/STTR Grants

The SBIR/STTR grants program's wonderfully patriotic mission is "Supporting scientific excellence and technological innovation through the investment of federal research funds in critical American priorities to build a strong national economy one small business at a time" [1].

In the words of program founder Roland Tibbetts: "to provide funding for some of the best early-stage innovation ideas—ideas that, however promising, are still too high risk for private investors, including venture capital firms" [2]. For the purposes of the SBIR/STTR programs, the term *small business* is defined as a for-profit business with fewer than 500 employees, owned by one or more *individuals* who are citizens of, or permanent resident aliens in, the United States of America [3].

Funds are obtained by allocating a certain percentage of the total extramural (research and development [R&D]) budgets of the 11 federal agencies with extramural research budgets in excess of $100 million. Approximately $2.5 billion is awarded through this program each year.

The United States Department of Defense (DoD) is the largest agency in this program, with approximately $1 billion in SBIR grants annually. More than half the awards from the DoD are to firms with fewer than 25 people and a third are to firms of fewer than 10. A fifth are minority or women-owned businesses. Historically, a quarter of the companies receiving grants are receiving them for the first time.

As of September 2015, SBIR programs are in place at the following agencies:

- Department of Agriculture
- Department of Commerce (National Institute of Standards and Technology and National Oceanic and Atmospheric Administration)
- Department of Defense
- Department of Education
- Department of Energy
- Department of Health and Human Services (National Institutes of Health [NIH])
- Department of Homeland Security
- Department of Transportation
- Environmental Protection Agency
- National Aeronautics and Space Administration
- National Science Foundation (NSF)

5.3 Before You Write Your Application

Theoretically, one would identify an unmet public health need or problem and then develop a product that significantly affects the problem. In the real world, companies develop a technology and then search for a problem where their technology can create a product. Young companies often have difficulty deciding on which problem to focus on. A grant application that does not focus on a narrow unmet public health need is unlikely to fare well in review.

You need a clear vision of the product you will make with your technology before you begin writing a grant application. It is probably not good business strategy to let NIH Funding Opportunity Announcements influence your choice of problem or product. Instead, deciding on your product and its development pathway requires both market research and strategic planning.

You need to know the size of the public health problem, current solutions and their drawbacks, and ongoing research efforts and progress. For your product or technology, you need to know its market advantages and be able to list the milestones necessary to develop the product for sale, the estimated time and costs for each milestone, and your exit strategy along the development pathway.

5.4 Purposes and Goals of SBIR/STTR Grants

The SBIR program is one of the largest examples of US government public–private partnerships. A premise of the SBIR program is that small businesses are an important front for new ideas, but that they likely will need some support in their early stages as they translate these ideas into innovative products and services for the market. Founded in 1982, the SBIR program is designed to encourage small business to develop new processes and products and to provide quality research in support of the many missions of the US government.

Today's knowledge-based economy is driven in large part by the nation's capacity to innovate. One of the defining features of the US economy is a high level of entrepreneurial activity. Entrepreneurs in the United States see opportunities and are willing and able to take on risk to bring new welfare-enhancing, wealth-generating technologies to the market. Yet, while innovation in areas such as genomics, bioinformatics, and nanotechnology presents new opportunities, converting these ideas into innovations for the market involves substantial challenges [4].

The American capacity for innovation can be strengthened by addressing the challenges faced by entrepreneurs. Public–private partnerships are one means to help entrepreneurs bring new ideas to market [5]. According to the Small Business Innovation Development Act of 1982 P.L. 106-554 signed December 21, 2000, the purposes and goals of the SBIR grant program are as follows:

- To stimulate technological innovation
- To use small business to meet federal R&D needs
- To foster and encourage participation by minorities and disadvantaged persons in technological innovation
- To increase private-sector commercialization innovations derived from federal R&D

The aims of the STTR program, Small Business Research and Development Enhancement Act of 1992 P.L. 107-50 are as follows:

- To stimulate and foster scientific/technological innovation through cooperative R&D carried out between small business concerns and research institutions (typically universities)
- Foster technology transfer between small business concerns and research institutions

The STTR program is a set-aside program designed to facilitate cooperative R&D between small business concerns and US research institutions—with immediate potential for commercialization. The STTR program provides an opportunity for small businesses to partner with academic institutions to develop products with biomedical applications (e.g., assays, research tools, medical devices, biomarkers, therapeutics, and software development).

Since the STTR program is a collaborative research effort between a small business and a research institution, this partnership can offer the following benefits:

- Enhanced credibility, which can increase the chances of winning an STTR award.
- Additional opportunity for proposal review before submission.
- Opportunity for research ideas to develop within the research institution.
- At some research institutions, the researcher can take a leave of absence to work on an SBIR/STTR project.
- SBIR applications have historically outnumbered STTR applications by more than eightfold, causing the success rate for SBIR applicants to be lower than that for STTR applicants.

5.5 Detailed Program Description

The SBIR and STTR grants are programs intended to help eligible small businesses conduct advanced R&D. Funding takes the form of contracts or grants. The recipient programs must have high potential for commercialization and must meet specific US Government R&D needs. Programs provide billions of dollars of research support to translate innovative ideas into useful commercial products.

However, these programs are highly competitive and applications to various governmental agencies (e.g., NIH, NSF, DoD, etc.) differ greatly, with success rates generally below 20% for Phase I applications. The SBIR/STTR helps government agencies to conduct innovative R/R&D that results in product, process, or service that will

- Improve human health
- Speed process of discovery
- Reduce cost of medical care/cost of research
- Improve research tools and technology

Phase I
Feasibility study
$100K–150K   12 months

Phase II
Full R&D
2-year award $500K–$1 million

Phase III
Commercialization stage
Use of non-grant funds

FIGURE 5.2
Three phases program.

5.6 Eligibility Requirements

Generally, businesses with fewer than 500 employees are eligible to receive an SBIR award. Phase I of the Agency's SBIR program determines the technical feasibility and quality of performance of the proposed innovation. Phase II awards are based on the results of Phase I and the technical merit and commercial potential of the innovation. Phase II may not complete the total R&D needed for commercialization, as shown in Figure 5.2.

Below is a summary of some of the most important eligibility requirements:

- Organized for-profit US business.
- At least 51% United States–owned and independently operated.
- Small business located in the United States.
- P.I.'s primary employment with a small business during a project or fewer employees.
- Eligibility is determined at time of award.
- No appendices allowed in Phase I.
- The PI *is* required to have expertise to oversee project scientifically and technically.
- Applications *may be* submitted to different agencies for similar work.
- Awards may *not* be accepted from different agencies for duplicative projects.

5.7 SBIR/STTR Are Sequential Programs

The SBIR/STTR program is a highly competitive three-phase program that reserves a specific percentage of federal R&D development funding for

TABLE 5.1

Three Sequential Multiphase Programs

Phases	Comments
SBIR Phase I Median Award $210K/year (FY2014)	Awards to approximately 10% of applications (FY2014)
STTR Phase I Median Award $230K/year (FY2014)	Fast-Track—Combined Phase I/II application
Competing Phase II (renewal)	For FDA-related products
	Awards up to $1M per year for 2 to 3 years
Phase III	Remaining steps of commercialization
	Not funded by government. Funded by other sources

award to small businesses in partnership with nonprofit research institutions to move ideas from the laboratory to the marketplace, to foster high-tech economic development, and to address the technological needs of the federal government.

By including qualified small businesses in the nation's R&D effort, SBIR awards are intended to stimulate innovative new technologies to help agencies meet their missions in many areas including health, the environment, and national defense. SBIR and STTR grants are sequential multiphase programs [6], as summarized in Table 5.1.

5.8 Format for Grant Application Package

The format for government grant requests varies from agency to agency, but some common threads exist in the highly detailed, structured, stylized regimen that is commonly referred to as an *application package*. These common threads include a standard cover, certification and assurances forms, narrative sections, and the budget narrative and forms. Of course, all types of government grant applications require mandatory attachments or appendices, such as financial statements and résumés of project staff.

Always follow the pagination, order of information, and review criteria guidelines. All government grants are awarded on the basis of your meeting their specific review criteria, which are written and published in each funding agency's grant application guidelines. The review criteria tell you what the peer reviewers will read and rate when they receive your grant application.

As you read through the application guidelines, highlight all narrative writing requirements and look for sections that tell you how the grant reviewers will rate or evaluate each section of the narrative. By formatting and writing to meet the review criteria, you can edge out the competition and increase your funding success rate.

5.8.1 Applicant Organization and Qualifications

Any funding source you approach will have questions about your legal name and organizational structure. Although the wording may vary slightly from one application to another, the cover documents and narratives of grant applications and cooperative agreements all ask for the same basic information. Understanding exactly what the application is asking for and knowing how to reply in the right language are critical. Keep in mind that any discrepancy in your application will be grounds for rejection.

The following list summarizes the common requirements by government funding sources [7]:

- **Legal name of the organization applying:** Be sure to list your organization's *legal* name here.
- **Type of applicant:** Check the box that best describes your organization's forming structure. For example, you can choose from state agency, county, municipal, township, interstate, intermunicipal, special district, independent school district, public college or university, Indian Tribe, individual, private, profit-making organization, and other (which you have to specify).
- **Eligibility:** Is your organization a type of applicant that isn't eligible? Search for a partner (government agency or nonprofit) that can be the lead grant applicant or RFP (request for proposal) responder. Doing so will get dollars into the front door of your organization or business because you'll be incorporated into the funding request as a subcontracting partner. So get ready to negotiate your services and products during the planning and writing period. That way, you'll have monies earmarked for you in the funding request's budget narrative and detail.

If an organization is waiting on nonprofit designation, it's common to partner with an established nonprofit to act as the fiscal agent. (An *established nonprofit* is one that has been around for more than 3 years.)

- **Year founded:** Enter the year that your organization incorporated or was created.
- **Current operating budget:** Supply the applicant organization's operating budget total for the current fiscal year.

When it comes to money, supply information that portrays the truth and nothing but the truth!

- **Employer identification number and DUNS Number:** This portion of the form asks for the seven-digit EIN (employer identification number) assigned to your organization by the Internal Revenue Service. The EIN is also called a *taxpayer reporting number.*

In addition to the EIN, federal grantmaking agencies require that all grant applicants have a nine-digit DUNS (Data Universal Numbering System) Number, an identification number that makes it easier for others to recognize and learn about your organization. You can register for a unique DUNS Number at the Dunn & Bradstreet website, www.dnb.com/US/duns_update.

The DUNS Number is a unique nine-digit identification sequence that provides unique identifiers of single business entities while linking corporate family structures together.

- **Organization's fiscal year:** Indicate the 12-month time frame that your organization considers to be its operating, or fiscal, year. The fiscal year is defined by the organization's bylaws and can correspond with the calendar year or some other period, such as July 1 to June 30.
- **Congressional districts:** On a federal grant application, you need to list all the congressional districts in which your organization is located and your grant-funded services will be implemented. You can get this information by calling the public library or surfing the Internet to locate your legislator's website—which will contain their district numbers.
- **Contact person information:** Name the primary contact in your organization for grant or cooperative agreement negotiations, questions, and written correspondence. Make your contact person an individual who helped write the grant and who's quick enough on their feet to answer tough technical questions from the funder, especially by phone.
- **Address:** Provide the current street and mailing address for the applicant organization.
- **Telephone/fax/e-mail information:** List the contact person's telephone and fax numbers (with area code) as well as an e-mail address.

5.9 The Famous (Infamous?) Grants.gov

Why do so many entrepreneurs fail to apply for government grants? The answer is that they fear the inherent complexities of federal grant applications. Federal grants are the most difficult grants for which to apply—far more difficult than foundation, corporate, or state and local government grants. Federal grants are known for their short deadlines, technically worded writing and review criteria, and quadrillions of intimidating forms. Grants.gov (which is found online at www.grants.gov) attempts to facilitate the process.

When the federal government first launched Grants.gov, it was as if every grant writer's worst fears had come true. Technology was taking over the submission process, and it wasn't readily accepted or wanted. The process would be seamless and straightforward—at least that's what the feds told everyone. But there were many glitches along the way while the online e-grant submission website was being perfected. Today, it's still a work in progress, but it is the way it must be done.

Grants.gov is a central storehouse for information on more than 1000 grant programs. It provides access to approximately $400 billion in annual awards. As you can see, there are plenty of grant programs and billions of dollars available. Even in slow economy years, grants are still awarded, and the payments keep coming, rain or shine, if you have been awarded a grant.

Throughout the Grants.gov website, you'll find tidbits of valuable information that help first-time grant writers familiarize themselves with the basic questions, such as "What is a grant?" and "Who's eligible for one?" Some of the eligible applicant categories for federal grants are the following:

- Government organizations
- Education organizations
- Public housing organizations
- Nonprofit organizations
- For-profit organizations
- Small businesses
- Individuals

5.9.1 Grants.gov Home Page

The Grants.gov home page is your gateway to everything you need to know to find federal grants, apply for federal grants, and follow-up on federal grant applications submitted.

The Grants.gov home page looks straightforward at first glance, but in reality it can be very tortuous. Many novice grant writers are intimidated by the federal grant writing process. They fear the technical instructions, lengthy writing requirements, and many forms with "I don't have a clue" types of information fields. Even the most fearless grant writer—one who can master the federal grant application research and writing process—is further aghast at the online grants. It may be best to engage a knowledgeable consultant to help with the submission.

5.9.2 Getting Registered to Apply

In order to apply for a grant from Grants.gov, you or your organization must complete the (not so easy) Grants.gov registration process. You can register as an organization or as an individual. I explain both ways in the following sections.

The registration process can take between three to five business days. It can even take as long as 2 weeks if all the steps aren't completed on a timely basis. In order to get your organization registered to submit grant applications on the Grants.gov system, you need to follow these steps:

1. **Get a Dun & Bradstreet number (DUNS Number).**

    You can do this online at www.dnb.com/US/dunsupdate. In fact, there's a link to this website on Grants.gov. This registration is free and gives you a common tracking number for doing business with the government (federal, state, and local).

2. **Register with the Central Contractor Registry (also known as the CCR).**

    What is the CCR? It's a secondary website that collects all your organization's contact information. The information requested is similar to what you submit in your annual IRS tax return, such as name of organization, address, contact person, and contact person's information including Social Security number. You'll also be asked to upload your banking information (the bank's tracking number and the organization's bank account number). This info is used to facilitate electronic banking transfers between the government and your organization.

3. **Create a username and password with the Grants.gov credential provider.**

    You'll receive a user name and password from a third-party credential provider contracted by the government. At that point, you'll be routed back to Grants.gov to complete your registration with the access point information.

4. **Grants.gov and eRA Commons: Required *early* registration for SBIR newcomers.**

    If your company is applying for an NIH SBIR grant for the first time, it must register with *both* NIH eRA Commons and Grants.gov. (eRA stands for Electronic Research Administration.) The NIH does not award grants to unregistered applicants. Unfortunately, registration cannot be done at the last minute. eRA Commons and Grants.gov require your company to register at least 4 weeks prior to the grant submission due date. To be safe, prepare to spend approximately 5 weeks [8].

A university is required to register in eRA Commons to electronically submit a grant application. Only individuals with legal signing authority at the university (e.g., dean)—known as signing officials (SOs)—can register their organizations. Once the organization is registered, the SO can register or affiliate the principal investigator (PI) in Commons.

More than 13,000 organizations are already registered in Commons. To see if your organization is already registered, check this Quick Query: Commons Registered Organizations. If your organization is not listed, SOs can register their institutions at the Register Grantee Organization link on the eRA Commons home page. The following are the three basic tasks:

1. Register the applicant organization in eRA Commons
2. Create a new PI account
3. Create new user accounts

5.9.3 Obtaining AOR Authorization

This step sounds terribly difficult, but it isn't! The E-Business Point of Contact (or E-Biz POC) at your organization must respond to the registration e-mail from Grants.gov and login at Grants.gov to authorize you as an Authorized Organization Representative (AOR). Your E-Biz POC is the executive director or person who manages finances at your organization.

Only the AOR can log on and conduct business or grant-related transactions with the federal government. At any time, you can track your AOR authorization status by logging in with your username and password that you obtained in Step 3 above.

5.10 The Bayh–Dole Act, or the Cavalry to the Rescue

The **Bayh–Dole Act** or **Patent and Trademark Law Amendments Act** (Pub. L. 96-517, December 12, 1980) is United States legislation dealing with intellectual property arising from federal government–funded research. Sponsored by two senators, Birch Bayh of Indiana and Bob Dole of Kansas, the Act was enacted by the US Congress on December 12, 1980, is codified at 94 Stat. 3015 and in 35 U.S.C. § 200–212, and is implemented by 37 C.F.R. 401.

The key change made by Bayh–Dole was in ownership of inventions made with federal funding. Before the Bayh–Dole Act, federal research funding contracts and grants obligated inventors (wherever they worked) to assign inventions they made using federal funding to the federal government [9]. Bayh–Dole permits a university, small business, or nonprofit institution to elect to pursue ownership of an invention in preference to the government [10].

If an organization (such as a grantee) elects to retain title to a subject invention for which it has obtained assignment, the organization is obligated to do the following:

- Grant to the government a nonexclusive, nontransferable, irrevocable, paid-up license to practice or have practiced for or on behalf of the United States the subject invention throughout the world.
- File its initial patent application within 1 year after its election to retain title.
- Notify the government if it will not continue prosecution of an application or will let a patent lapse.
- Convey to the federal agency, upon written request, title to any subject invention if the organization fails to file, does not continue a prosecution, or will allow a patent to lapse.
- In each patent, include a statement that identifies the contract under which the invention was made and notice of the government's rights in the invention.
- Report on the utilization of subject inventions.
- Require in exclusive licenses to use or sell in the United States that products will be manufactured substantially in the United States.
- Agree to allow the government to "march in" and require licenses to be granted, or to grant licenses, in certain circumstances, such as if the organization has not taken effective steps to achieve practical application of the invention.

Certain additional requirements apply to nonprofit organizations only. Nonprofits must also

- Assign rights to a subject invention only to an organization having as a primary function the management of inventions, unless approved by the federal agency
- Share royalties with the inventor
- Use the balance of royalties after expenses for scientific research or education
- Make efforts to attract, and give preference to, small business licensees

5.10.1 Intellectual Property Control Resulting from Federal Funding

The Bayh–Dole Act gave US universities, small businesses, and nonprofits intellectual property control of their inventions that resulted from federal government–funded research.

The Bayh–Dole Act is a significant 20th-century piece of legislation in the field of intellectual property in the United States. Perhaps the most important contribution of Bayh–Dole is that it reversed the presumption of title, permitting a university, small business, or nonprofit institution to elect to pursue ownership of an invention.

5.10.2 "March-In" Rights under the Act

Entrepreneurs need to be aware that your ownership of federally sponsored intellectual property rights has some limits. The Code of Federal Regulations (CFR) TITLE 35, PART II, CHAPTER 18, § 203 "March-in rights" states:

a. With respect to any subject invention in which a small business firm or nonprofit organization has acquired title under this chapter, the Federal agency under whose **funding agreement the subject invention** was made **shall have the right,** in accordance with such procedures as are provided in regulations promulgated hereunder to **require the contractor**, an assignee or exclusive licensee of a subject invention to grant a nonexclusive, partially exclusive, or exclusive license in any field of use to a responsible applicant or applicants, upon terms that are reasonable under the circumstances, and if the contractor, assignee, or exclusive licensee refuses such request, to grant such a license itself, if the Federal agency determines that such—

   1. action is necessary because the contractor or assignee has not taken, or is not expected to take within a reasonable time, effective steps to achieve practical application of the subject invention in such field of use;

   2. action is necessary to alleviate health or safety needs which are not reasonably satisfied by the contractor, assignee, or their licensees;

   3. action is necessary to meet requirements for public use specified by Federal regulations and such requirements are not reasonably satisfied by the contractor, assignee, or licensees; or

   4. action is necessary because the agreement required by section 204 has not been obtained or waived or because a licensee of the exclusive right to use or sell any subject invention in the United States is in breach of its agreement obtained pursuant to section 204.

b. A determination pursuant to this section or section 202 (b)(4) shall not be subject to the Contract Disputes Act (41 U.S.C. § 601 et seq.). An administrative appeals procedure shall be established by regulations promulgated in accordance with section 206. Additionally, any contractor, inventor, assignee, or exclusive licensee adversely affected by a determination under this section may, at any time within sixty days after the determination is issued, file a petition in the United States Court of Federal Claims, which shall have jurisdiction to determine the appeal on the record and to affirm, reverse, remand or modify, as appropriate, the determination of the Federal agency. In cases described in paragraphs (1) and (3) of subsection (a), the agency's determination shall be held in abeyance pending the exhaustion of appeals or petitions filed under the preceding sentence.

5.11 Recommendations for Killer Proposals

How do you ensure that your grant proposal looks more like science, and less like science fiction? Science fiction will not be funded by the government.

The following sections will discuss some of the most important principles we recommend to maximize your chances of getting your proposal funded.

5.11.1 Focus on a Market Need, Not on Your Technology

Developing a core technology that can be used to create many different products may be an outstanding business strategy, but a deadly approach for an SBIR/STTR application.

Your best grant writing strategy is to *focus* on a specific need for a specific health problem. For example, imagine that your technology enables inexpensive rapid genetic tests for susceptibility to cancer, heart disease, infectious diseases, or other health problems. Your application would probably be assigned to the National Human Genome Research Institute based on this technology but would the Genome program staff be supportive? Would scientific reviewers be supportive? How would business reviewers evaluate the product when it is not clear what specific health problem your product will test?

Conversely, consider instead an application focused on applying your genetic testing technology to a specific type of breast cancer. The application would be assigned to the National Cancer Institute. Cancer reviewers are likely to be enthusiastic about an innovative product that affects their area. Business reviewers are likely to be enthusiastic about the potential sales of an innovative product addressing a major health problem.

Because you focused on a single use, you could submit additional SBIR/ STTR applications for other uses based on the same core technology. I strongly suggest you direct your applications to different review groups and different institutes. For example, an application on cardiac screening could be directed to the National Heart, Lung, and Blood Institute and one on asthma could be directed to the National Institute of Allergy and Infectious Diseases. In each application, it is critical to focus on the public health significance of the product in that specific area, plus the financial impact of the product in the market and to your company.

Examples of focusing on a single area include the following:

- Neuropharmacology
- Respiratory sciences
- Cardiovascular sciences

5.11.2 Specific Aims (Significance, Innovation, and Approach)

Begin your Specific Aims section with a paragraph briefly describing the problem and why it is significant. Then, briefly describe the current status of solutions and unmet public health needs. Check the IC's web pages for background information that may help you. Describe your product in the next paragraph. Hypothesize why your product is an innovative solution to the problem.

Present your Specific Aims in bullet format. Describe two to four measurable Specific Aims for Phase I research and, for each, the criteria by which success will be judged. Make your Specific Aims "end points" as opposed to a "best effort." Your Specific Aims may be milestones, or, if appropriate, each of your Specific Aims may be subdivided into milestones.

A review committee should easily be able to determine if your Specific Aims have been achieved and agree that successfully accomplishing them justifies Phase II funding. Propose a timeline for achieving your Specific Aims in table or graphic format. Do not propose more work than reviewers would think reasonable to achieve in Phase I. Estimate the additional time and funding necessary to bring your product to market after the completion of Phase I.

5.11.3 Significance (A Major, Unsolved Public Health Problem)

Describe the significance of the public health problem. My advice is to appeal to reviewers by focusing on a single disease even if your technology has multiple applications. Describe the number and composition of the population affected. Give references to supporting statistical data. Provide background on the current solutions to the problem, their limitations, and the discoveries needed. Show reviewers you know the field by the breadth of your knowledge of both published and unpublished work by others, some of whom could be your reviewers.

5.11.4 Innovation (Your Specific Product)

Describe why your product is innovative. Does it work better, faster, or at lower cost than what is currently available? What are its public health implications? Estimate your product's potential financial projections. How are you protecting your intellectual property? Explain why the Phase I milestones outlined in Specific Aims will justify a Phase II award. Describe milestones projected for Phase II and the progress necessary for your company to either sell the product or license the further development to another organization. Spend considerable effort on this section because it greatly affects your score.

5.11.5 Preliminary Studies (Why Your Approach Is Likely to Succeed)

Although the SBIR/STTR solicitation states that "Preliminary data are not required," do not be misled. Most applications include good preliminary data. Review committees are likely to have greater enthusiasm for proposals with highly encouraging preliminary data. Poorly presented or poorly interpreted preliminary data will likely result in your proposal not being "competitive." You can kiss a "noncompetitive" proposal goodbye.

Include preliminary studies that support the feasibility of your project. They may consist of your own publications and those of others, as well as unpublished data from your laboratory. To improve your "Investigator" score, emphasize work you have accomplished that indicates you can direct the proposed research and achieve your Specific Aims. Interpret results critically and evaluate alternative meanings but do not overinterpret. You can be assured that critical members of the review committee will look for explanations other than the ones you propose.

The Preliminary Studies section of your Research Plan should convince reviewers that your approach could work. Reviewers may also use your work described in this section to assess the investigator criterion. Be aware that the Phase I progress report in your Phase II application will list the milestones proposed and achieved in Phase I.

5.11.6 Research Design (What You Will Call Success)

The Research Design section of your Research Plan should spell out in detail what you are going to do, how you are going to do it, and your criteria for success. Reviewers will use this section to evaluate your approach and innovation. Make it easy for reviewers by organizing this section by Specific Aims and include a timeline in table or diagram format to quickly convey your entire project to reviewers.

Give a rationale for each set of experiments. Convince reviewers that your methods are appropriate to your Specific Aims. If your methods are innovative, show how you have changed existing or proven methods while avoiding technical problems. Also, do not forget to provide supporting data and references.

Describe the kinds of results you expect and how they will support continuation of your project. Present other possible outcomes and contingency plans. Define the criteria for evaluating the success or failure of each set of experiments. If possible, include statistical analysis as reviewers are impressed by statistics.

Describe hazards anticipated and precautions you propose. Spell out your sources of important reagents and equipment, as well as details of any use of animals or human subjects. Be sure to follow NIH guidelines. Explain how credible collaborators will participate in your proposed research. Your research proposal should include letters that describe collaborators' agreements with you, including their expert role on the project and hours to be committed.

5.11.7 Project Summary/Abstract (Your Chance to Blow Your Own Horn)

Your title and project summary/abstract are very important components of your application because all reviewers read them and they contain information relating to all five review criteria. Compose your abstract last because your plans may change as you write other components. Hone your abstract to summarize everything in your application in the 30 lines allowed. Include no proprietary information because your abstract will become public if you receive an award.

Write a few sentences each on the public health problem, issues with current solutions, how your product would address unmet needs, a summary of your approach, collaborators and unique resources, Phase I Specific Aims, and how anticipated results will justify Phase II and further product development. Conclude with the additional time and funding necessary to bring your product to market after the completion of Phase I.

The required Project Narrative is a description in three sentences or less of the relevance of your project to public health.

5.11.8 Final Words of Wisdom

Rudolph [11], in his "How to write a winning SBIR grant application in 3 easy lessons," recommends the use of the following procedure:

- Follow the guidelines for each section.
- Provide enough detail so that reviewers fully understand what you plan to do, how you will do it, how you will *know* that you have done it, and the importance of doing it.

- Make the proposal easy to read—white space between paragraphs, descriptive subject headers every paragraph or two, figures and charts to illustrate your points.
- Read the review criteria (in the *Application Guide*) and clearly address each major point. Reviewers use a checklist—make it easy for them to find the information they need to evaluate your proposal.
- Make sure the budget, budget justification, and all other sections match and support the proposed work.
- Get strong letters of support from collaborators, business partners, and prospective customers.
- Ask somebody else to proofread the proposal and criticize it before you can consider it as final. Two heads are better than one.

5.11.9 Practical Answers to Frequently Asked Questions

The following are practical answers to frequently asked questions about the SBIR and STTR grant programs [12]:

- PI's role

    The PI plans and directs the project and plays a central role in leading the technical aspects of the project. The PI will usually serve as the primary contact for the federal agency's SBIR/STTR program and works to ensure that the project is concurrent with the guidelines of that federal agency's SBIR or STTR program.

    Under SBIR program requirements, all PIs must be primarily employed (more than 50%) by the small business at the start and during the performance period of the grant.

    Under STTR program guidelines, the PIs do not need to be primarily employed by the small business that is submitting the proposal. However, the PI is still required to have a formal appointment with or commitment to the small business that is submitting the proposal. As in SBIR projects, PIs involved in STTR projects are responsible for the overall scientific and technical direction of the project. Each agency has specific requirements on the percentage of work effort that the PI should contribute to the STTR project. It is important to carefully examine STTR agency solicitations for information about the required PI work effort.

- Fast-track applications

    The Fast-Track mechanism for SBIR and STTR applications allows for an expedited decision-making and award process specifically aimed at scientifically meritorious applications with high potential for commercialization. In the Fast-Track review process, both Phase

I and Phase II proposals are submitted and reviewed together. The Fast-Track application must contain a product development plan (commercialization plan) that addresses specific topics.

- Multiple participating agencies

Your proposal can be tailored to match the interests, priorities, and unique requirements of specific agencies. (Since each agency has different needs and areas of emphasis, it is important to custom tailor each proposal to fit the agency.)

Caution: The agencies do require that you disclose in each proposal whether you are submitting a "similar or related idea" to other agencies. It is important to disclose not only how multiple proposal submissions may be similar but also how they are different. If there are substantial and important differences between the proposals that are submitted to multiple agencies, and more than one agency wants to give you an award, it is possible to accept multiple awards, as long as the agencies agree.

However, if the proposals are duplicative, and multiple agencies are interested in giving your company an SBIR/STTR award, then you can legally only accept one offer.

- Submitting the same proposal multiple times

The agencies differ considerably on how they view multiple proposals on one topic in their solicitation. They may have different rules about submitting the same idea in multiple proposals, and whether an idea can be submitted for consideration under both SBIR and STTR programs. It is important to read the specific agency's solicitation guidelines carefully before submitting your proposal multiple times to the same agency.

- Solicitation process for grant proposals

Each of the participating federal agencies lists solicitations that address specific research topics one to four times per year. These federal agencies won't accept unsolicited proposals that do not correlate with their proposed research topics of interest.

Research topics for some agencies are more focused than others. For example, the DoD can be very specific in their solicited research topics. Research topics for the NIH and the NSF tend to be more general in scope, which often allows SBIR applicants to submit proposals that serve their particular research areas of interest while still meeting the overall science and technology areas outlined by such agencies.

Each agency releases its solicitation lists at different times during the year. A schedule of each federal agency's annual SBIR program solicitation dates can be found at the SBIR.gov website. Through the SBIR.gov website, prospective applicants can filter their searches by agency and keywords. An alternative resource that can be used to track seasonal solicitation dates by agency is SBIR Gateway's Phase I Solicitation Finder located at www.zyn.com/sbir/scomp.htm.

- Differences between a solicitation and a presolicitation announcement

  SBIR solicitations are specific requests for proposals released by the federal agencies participating in the program, which may result in the award of Phase I SBIR funding agreements.

  SBIR presolicitation announcements, released by SBA, contain pertinent data on SBIR solicitations such as research topic areas that are about to be released by the participating federal agencies.

- Goals of the federal agencies that participate in the SBIR program

  The DoD uses SBIR as a procurement solution to mission requirements; they are interested in obtaining solutions that result from the SBIR applicant's R&D efforts. The NIH and NSF use SBIR grants for general societal benefit; they normally are not viewed as the end customer for the technology that is created with SBIR awards. The Department of Energy uses SBIR as both a procurement tool to meet mission requirements and for general societal benefit.

- Reviewers of grant proposals

  Depending on agency, SBIR/STTR proposals may undergo an internal review, an external review, or a review that incorporates both internal and external reviewers. With internal reviews, agency members review the SBIR proposal. External reviews involve a review by people outside of the agency, such as university personnel or other experts in the field.

  The DoD, the Department of Advanced Research Projects Agency, and the Department of Transportation all use an internal review process. NASA uses both internal reviewers and at least two independent reviewers. The NIH uses dual review systems composed of an external peer review panel, an advisory panel, and an internal review group. The NSF uses ad hoc external review panels. US Department of Agriculture proposals are reviewed by a separate review panel for each topic area; proposals are subsequently reviewed by an ad hoc review panel.

- Ensuring that your proposal meets a reviewer's expectations

  SBIR/STTR applications are evaluated on the basis of the following core review criteria:

  - Exceptional Technical Merit
  - Team Qualifications
  - Value to Agency

- High Potential for Commercialization
- Cost/Cost Realism

   Each SBIR agency has different priorities in terms of these evaluation criteria. For specific agency SBIR and STTR review criteria, consult SBIR program information on agency websites and contact agency SBIR/STTR program leaders.

- Dwell time from proposal to award notification

   After the close of SBIR/STTR solicitations, the amount of time that lapses before award winners are notified can vary between 3 and 6 months, depending on the agency. Information about the SBIR/STTR award selection and notification time frame can typically be found in the agency solicitation or on the SBIR/STTR program section of the agency website. Links to the SBIR home pages of SBIR agencies can be found at SBIR.gov or on the SBIR Gateway website at www.zyn.com/sbir.

- What are your chances of getting funded?

   The good news: Your Uncle Sam has deep pockets. The bad news: Your Uncle has very short arms. The success rate for Phase I applications is between 10% and 15% [13].

   The award rate describes the chance of an individual application being funded and is the number that more closely reflects institute and center paylines (which can vary rather significantly from one institute or center to another).

$$\text{AWARD RATE} = \frac{\text{Number of awards in a fiscal year}}{\text{Applications reviewed}(\textbf{including resubmissions} \text{ in that fiscal year})}$$

   The funding rate reflects the number of investigators who seek and obtain funding. Each principal investigator (PI)* is counted once, whether they submit one or more applications or receive one or more awards in a fiscal year.

$$\text{FUNDING RATE} = \frac{\text{Number of unique PIs* receiving funding in a fiscal year}}{\text{Number of unique PIs* with applications reviewed in that fiscal year}}$$

*includes those on multiple PI applications

   The **success rate** describes the likelihood of a project or an idea getting funded, rather than of the success of the individual application submission.

$$\text{SUCCESS RATE} = \frac{\text{Number of awards in a fiscal year}}{\text{Applications reviewed}(\textbf{excluding resubmissions} \text{ in that fiscal year})}$$

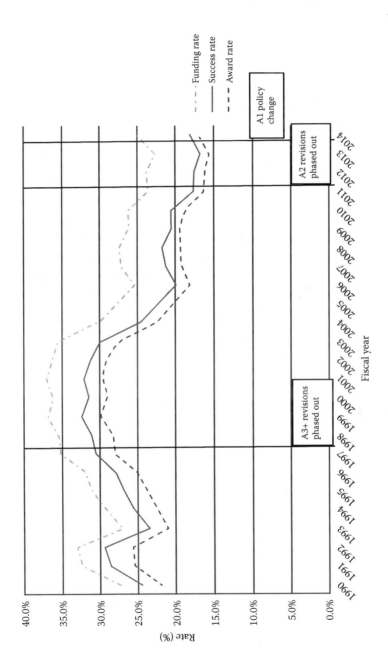

FIGURE 5.3

Award, success, and funding rates for research project grants (fiscal years 1990–2014). Excludes awards made with American Recovery and Reinvestiment Act (ARRA) funds, and ARRA-solicited applications.

Being awarded a grant is becoming increasingly harder. The government's own statistics show the history of awards as well as success and funding rates from 1990 to 2014. This is graphically shown in Figure 5.3 (not in constant dollars).

- The intriguing "Omnibus" Solicitation

  The Omnibus, or Omnibus Solicitation, is a long (more than 100 pages) report in which each NIH institute and center describes its high priorities for SBIR funding. It is published annually, usually in January, and it's free.

  Why do they call it the Omnibus? Because nobody wants to call it by its full title, a definite a double mouthful: "Omnibus Solicitation of the National Institutes of Health, Centers for Disease Control and Prevention, Food and Drug Administration, and Administration for Children and Families for Small Business Innovation Research (SBIR) and Small Business Technology Transfer (STTR) Grant Applications: NIH, CDC, FDA, and ACF Program Descriptions and Research Topics."

  The reason to read the Omnibus is that NIH institutes and centers are *not* peas in the same SBIR pod. In practice, for example, SBIR funding limits are different among NIH institutes. Some seem willing to make much higher SBIR Phase I and Phase II grant awards than others. Others offer million-dollar post-Phase II SBIR grants for certain projects (generally drug and medical device research). The Omnibus tells which do and which don't.

- Annual SBIR/STTR informational conferences

  Every year, funding agencies host daylong SBIR conference to help newcomers learn more about SBIR funding possibilities. Attending a conference isn't essential by any means to winning SBIRs, but they usually have several good presentations by grantees who have won multiple SBIRs, and they're good occasions to buttonhole grant officials to ask questions. Every year, the conferences are held in a different city.

References

1. Small Business Innovation Research (SBIR) and Small Business Technology Transfer (STTR) Programs at the NIDCR. Nidcr.nih.gov. 2011-03-25. Retrieved 2011-06-02.
2. http://www.gpo.gov/fdsys/pkg/CHRG-111hhrg48735/pdf/CHRG-111hhrg 48735.pdf
3. http://en.m.wikipedia.org/wiki/Small_Business_Innovation_Research

4. Venture Funding and the NIH SBIR Program. Committee for Capitalizing on Science, Technology, and Innovation, *An Assessment of the Small Business Innovation Research Program*; Charles W. Wessner, ed., National Research Council, http://www.nap.edu/download.php?record_id=12543#.

5. National Research Council, *Government-Industry Partnerships for the Development of New Technologies: Summary Report*, Charles W. Wessner, ed. The National Academies Press, Washington, DC, 2002.

6. http://qb3.org/sites/qb3.org/files/pictures/docs/Milman%20Presentation%202012011-09-20.pdf

7. Browing, B.A. http://www.dummies.com/store/product/Grant-Writing-For-Dummies-5th-Edition.productCd-1118834666,navId-322436.html.

8. http://sciencesherpa.com/guide-to-nih-sbir-grant-tips-and-resources/

9. Stevens, A. The enactment of Bayh–Dole. *Journal of Technology Transfer*, 29, 93–99, 2004.

10. Emerging energy and intellectual property—The often unappreciated risks and hurdles of government regulations and standard setting organizations. *The National Law Review*. Husch Blackwell. 2012-05-22. Retrieved 2012-07-02.

11. http://rudolphbiomed.com/2011/07/how-to-write-a-winning-sbir-grant-application-in-3-%E2%80%9Ceasy%E2%80%9D-steps/

12. http://asbtdc.org/sbir-faq/

13. Rockey, S. http://nexus.od.nih.gov/all/2015/06/29/what-are-the-chances-of-getting-funded/?utm_source=nexus&utm_medium=email&utm_content=nihupdate&utm_campaign=jun.

6

Marketing and Marketing Research on a Shoestring

Advertising is what you pay for, publicity is what you pray for.

6.1 Introduction

What is marketing? The concept of marketing is confusing to many people. Is marketing sales, public relations, branding, or advertising? The simple answer is that marketing is a mix of all of these things. Marketing encompasses everything you do to put your product or service in front of your *potential* customers [1].

We do not emphasize the word *potential* without reason. One thing that many companies and business owners do wrong in their marketing efforts is to think of the entire world (universe) as their potential client base. This is an inappropriate way to go about marketing your company or yourself [2].

Last, it is important to recognize that, in marketing, there are two major forms of advertising and promotion; there is one that is directed to individuals (Business to Consumer) and one that is directed to businesses (Business to Business [B2B]).

Business to Consumer is when a company wants to sell a product or a service directly to a consumer (an individual person). B2B, on the other hand, is when a company wants to sell a product or service to another company [3].

Marketing research is any organized effort to gather information about target markets or customers. It is a very important component of business strategy [4]. Marketing research is a key factor in maintaining competitiveness over competitors. Marketing research provides critical information to identify and analyze the market need, market size, and your competition.

Information is power. Marketing research, which includes social and opinion research, is the systematic gathering and interpretation of information about individuals or organizations using statistical and analytical methods and techniques of the applied social sciences to gain insight or support decision-making.

Start-ups and small, underfunded companies are often stuck in a chicken-or-egg type dilemma when it comes to marketing research: They need good marketing research information in order to make key decisions to grow the company; however, they need money to do the research to get good market information to make the fundamental decisions to commercialize products and make them profitable.

It is a common dilemma that confounds many start-up founders. They have great ideas, great products, and great people. They need actionable marketing information in order to move their companies forward, but they lack the resources to obtain that information. Fortunately, start-ups and small, resource-poor companies can obtain good, usable marketing information inexpensively through a number of unconventional methods and sources discussed in this chapter.

6.2 A Small Business Is Not a Little Big Business

In their article in the *Harvard Business Review*, Welsh and White remind us that a small business is not a little big business [5]. An entrepreneur is not a multinational conglomerate but a struggling, underfinanced, and under-staffed individual. To survive, an entrepreneur must apply principles differ-ent from those of a president of a large and established corporation.

The authors argue that the traditional assumption among mangers has been that small businesses can use essentially the same managerial princi-ples "as the big boys," only on a suitably reduced scale. The basic assumption is that small businesses are like big businesses except that small companies have lower sales, smaller assets, and fewer employees.

Nothing could be further from the truth. Smallness creates what the authors call a special condition referred to as **resource poverty**. Resource poverty distinguishes small firms from their larger counterparts and thus requires critically different management styles and strategies. This can be summarized as shown in Table 6.1.

TABLE 6.1

"Resource Poverty" Applicable to Small Companies

Strategies	Disadvantage(s) Compared to Established Businesses
Executive salaries	Represents a much larger percentage of overall costs
Human resources	Difficulty in attracting expensive but necessary talent
	Salaries versus stock options "skin in the game"
Business activities	Cannot afford large personnel expenditures in accounting, finance, marketing, sales, promotions, etc.
	Product launch expenses
External environment	Government regulations, industry standards
	Seasonal sales variations
	Insurance and banking needs
	Stakeholder demands
Internal environment	Cash flow management
	Reaching break-even point

As we can see from Table 6.1, small businesses do not have the resources compared to big businesses, so how can they operate and survive? The owners of small businesses need to wear many hats and have multiple skill sets. From finance to accounting, from marketing to human resources, from operations to negotiations, the small business person needs to understand all the elements of doing business.

Thus, where and how does the small business owner have the time to fulfill all these fundamental needs and functions, while at the same time creating the necessary innovations? Churchill and Lewis [6] identified eight factors, four related to the enterprise and four related to the owner, as follows:

A. Company-related factors:
1. Financial resources, including cash and borrowing power
2. Personnel resources, relating to numbers, depth, and quality
3. Systems resources, relating to information, planning, and control
4. Business resources, relating to customer relations, market share, supplier relations, manufacturing, technology, and company position in its industry

B. Owner-related factors:
1. Personal goals and business goals
2. Operational abilities relating to marketing, inventing, producing, and distribution
3. Managerial ability and willingness to delegate responsibility
4. Strategic abilities in matching strengths and weaknesses of the company

Also, the entrepreneur's salary in a small business represents a much larger fraction of revenues than in a big company, often such a large fraction that little is left over to pay additional managers or to reward investors. Similarly, small businesses cannot usually afford to pay for the kind of accounting and bookkeeping services they need, nor can new employees be adequately tested and trained in advance.

6.2.1 Difference between Marketing, Advertising, and Public Relations

Marketing, advertising, public relations—what do all those terms even mean? Although we could break these terms down into stodgy textbook definitions, we think noted humorist and marketing professional S.H. Simmons [7,8] put it in a more relatable context by analyzing these related fields through the prism of wooing a foxy lady:

> *If a young man tells his date she is intelligent, looks lovely, and is a great conversationalist, he's saying the right things to the right person and that is*

*marketing. If the young man tells his date how handsome, smart, and success-ful he is, that is **advertising**. If someone else tells the young woman how hand-some, smart, and successful her date is, that's **public relations**.*

According to Chron [9], marketing is the overall process of communicating and delivering products to a target audience through the marketing mix of product, price, place, and promotion. Promotion is a combination of commu-nication activities that include advertising and public relations. Deciding on what resources to apply to each of these promotion areas is a result of other factors identified in an overall marketing plan.

Advertising is a means of communication to a target audience using mostly paid media such as television, radio, the Internet, and print publications. Successful advertising programs include themes that communicate company mission, branding, and services, as well as specific product information. The media for advertising are chosen based on what market research has identified as the most successful way of reaching a target audience and the financial resources that can be applied to advertising based on the marketing budget.

Public relations is a communication method used by businesses to convey a positive image to a target audience and the general pub-lic. Public relations methods can include press releases, community involvement, and speaking at public forums on issues important to a target audience. Small companies with small advertising budgets can use public relations as an inexpensive medium to establish the company name and communicate a brand image. Successful public relations programs highlight company accomplishments and posi-tive contributions to community.

To summarize: Advertising is paid media, public relations is earned media. This means you convince reporters or editors to write a positive story about you or your client, your candidate, brand, or issue. It appears in the editorial section of the magazine, newspaper, TV station, or website, rather than the "paid media" section where advertising messages appear. Hence, your story has more credibility because it was independently verified by a trusted third party, rather than purchased [10].

6.3 Marketing Research Fundamentals

Marketing research is the best way of getting an overview of consumers' wants, needs, and beliefs. The research can be used to determine how a product should be marketed. Peter Drucker [11] eloquently argued that marketing research is the "quintessence of the marketing effort."

There are two major types of marketing research. Primary research is subdivided into quantitative/qualitative research and secondary research.

- **Primary research.** This is research you compile yourself or hire someone to gather for you.
- **Secondary research.** This type of research is already compiled and organized for you. Examples of secondary information include reports and studies by government agencies, trade associations, or other businesses within your industry. Most of the research you gather will most likely be secondary.

Regardless of whether you perform primary or secondary marketing research, the following are the critical factors that should be investigated:

- **Market information.** Through marketing information you can uncover the prices of different products in the market, as well as the supply-and-demand situation. Market researchers have a wider role than previously recognized by helping their clients to understand social, technical, and even legal aspects of markets.
- **Market segmentation.** Market segmentation is the division of the market or population into subgroups with similar motivations. It is widely used for segmenting on geographic differences, personality differences, demographic differences, technographic differences, use of product differences, psychographic differences, and gender differences. For B2B segmentation, firmographics is commonly used.
- **Market trends.** Market trends are the upward or downward movement of a specific market, during a period. Determining the market size may be more difficult if one is starting with a new innovation. In this case, you will have to derive the figures from the number of potential customers, or customer segments.
- **SWOT analysis.** SWOT is a written analysis of the Strengths, Weaknesses, Opportunities, and Threats to a business entity. Not only should a SWOT be used in the creation stage of the company, it could also be used throughout the life of the company. A SWOT may also be written up for the competition to understand how to develop the marketing and product mixes.
- **Marketing effectiveness.** Marketing effectiveness is the quality of how marketers go to market with the goal of optimizing their spending to achieve good results for both the short term and the long term. It is also related to Marketing ROI (return on investment)

and Return on Marketing Investment [12]. Marketing effectiveness includes the following:

- Customer analysis
- Choice modeling
- Competitor analysis
- Risk analysis
- Product research
- Advertising the research findings
- Marketing mix modeling
- Simulated test marketing
- Clearly identifying your target market
- Determining your target market potential
- Preparing, communicating, and delivering satisfaction to your customers

6.4 Marketing Research for Business/Planning

Needs, wants, and demands

Companies can't give job security. Only customers can.

Jack Welch
CEO General Electric

Marketing theory divides human necessities into three basic parts: needs, wants, and demands. **Needs** comprise some of the most basic and fundamental necessities of life such as food, shelter, protection, good health, and so on. These needs are not created by marketing, since they already exist in society.

Wants are desires for things that satisfy deeper requests, such as gourmet foods, sports cars, vacations to exotic locales, and so on. Advanced societies are continually reshaping wants by societal forces such as schools, families, business corporations, healthcare alternatives, and so on. Entrepreneurial companies are very active in satisfying consumer wants with innovative solutions and approaches. Needs are few; wants are many. Remember the old adage that "People don't know what they want, only what they know."

Demands are wants for specific high-quality, high-priced products/services that deliver superior performance. Entrepreneurial firms shine in this marketing sphere. Most of the innovations carry a hefty price tag, thus satisfying the demands of affluent customers, who are willing and able to

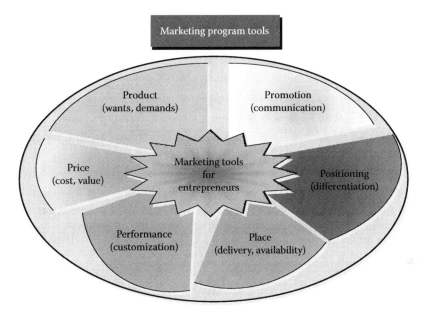

FIGURE 6.1
Marketing program tools.

buy these offerings. If we use the 80/20 rule, 20% of customers purchase 80% of the demand offerings.

Start-ups can market and promote their products by utilizing the marketing program tools shown in Figure 6.1.

6.5 Acquiring Marketing Research Information

You can use various methods of market research to find out information about markets, target markets and their needs, competitors, market trends, and customer satisfaction with products and services. Your businesses can learn a great deal about your customers, their needs, how to meet those needs, and how your business is doing to meet those needs.

6.5.1 Primary Research Information

Acquire your marketing research information from all of the following sources:

- Set your marketing budget.
- Determine what information you needed.
- Set a timeline for your research.

- Analyze the secondary research material you located.
- Locate, read, and learn existing information about the target market, industry, competition, and product/service.
- Find all relevant facts.
- Organize a lot of critical information that was missing.
- Conduct primary research.
- Design research tools, who you would talk to and what you would ask them.
- Analyze the results of the primary research and secondary research data.
- Integrate this information into the business plan by adjusting the marketing strategy (pricing, advertising, product/service alterations) to give credibility to your sales projections.

Did you use any of the following tools to conduct your primary research?

- Telephone surveys
- Interviews
- Focus groups
- Mailed questionnaires

Did you find out the answers to any of these questions from your primary market research?

- Is there a need for your product?
- What price will your customers pay?
- How often do they buy a product or service like yours?
- How do they buy it now?
- What makes them want to buy it?
- What company do they usually buy it from?
- What do they like about the product or service?
- What don't they like about it?

Did you include the following information on your competitors thru competitive analysis?

- A list of all key competitors
- Location
- Years in business

- Product/service sold
- Pricing schedule
- Hours of operation
- Customer profile
- A description of their marketing strategies
- Size of company
- Marketing/promotional strategy
- Your observations
- An analysis of their strengths and weaknesses
- A strategy on how you will deal with these competitors

Where did you get the information on your competitors?

- I hit the pavement and visited my competition personally, and I observed their setup, customers, staff, and professionalism.
- I collected any material I could find from them.
- I asked their customers (primary research).
- I used secondary sources such as the Yellow Pages, trade associations, and newspapers to gather information.
- I looked at their website.

What steps did you take to conduct a strategic competitive analysis? Did you

- Develop a thorough list of all the competition you will face in the industry.
- Search for direct competitors who offer products or services that are essentially the same as yours.
- Search for indirect competitors who are businesses that offer products or services that can be substituted for yours.
- Identify each competitor's strengths.
- Identify each competitor's weaknesses.
- Identify your top three competitive advantages.
- Identify your top three weaknesses.
- Develop a strategy for dealing with competitors.
- Work out some best-case/worst-case scenarios on paper.
- Make sure your pricing, positioning, and marketing strategies are flexible enough to deal with these situations.

6.5.2 Secondary Research Information

The vast majority of research you can find will be secondary research. While large companies spend huge amounts of money on market research, the good news is that plenty of information is available for free to entrepreneurs on a tight budget. The best places to start? Your local library and the Internet [13].

Secondary data are outside information assembled by government agencies, industry and trade associations, labor unions, media sources, chambers of commerce, and so on, and found in the form of pamphlets, newsletters, trade and other magazines, newspapers, and so on. It is termed secondary data because the information has been gathered by another, or secondary, source. The benefits of this are obvious—time and money are saved because you don't have to develop survey methods or do the interviewing.

Secondary sources are divided into three main categories:

1. **Public.** Public sources are the most economical, as they're usually free, and can offer a lot of good information. These sources are most typically governmental departments, business departments of public libraries, and so on.

2. **Commercial.** Commercial sources are equally valuable, but usually involve costs such as subscription and association fees. However, you spend far less than you would if you hired a research team to collect the data firsthand. Commercial sources typically consist of research and trade associations, organizations like SCORE (Service Corps of Retired Executives) and Dun & Bradstreet, banks and other financial institutions, publicly traded corporations, and so on.

3. **Educational.** Educational institutions are frequently overlooked as viable information sources, yet there is more research conducted in colleges, universities, and polytechnic institutes than virtually any sector of the business community.

Government statistics are among the most plentiful and wide-ranging public sources of information. Start with the Census Bureau's helpful *Hidden Treasures—Census Bureau Data and Where to Find It!* In seconds, you'll find out where to find federal and state information. Other government publications that are helpful include the following:

- *Statistical and Metropolitan Area Data Book.* Offers statistics for metropolitan areas, central cities and counties
- *Statistical Abstract of the United States.* Data books with statistics from numerous sources, government to private
- *U.S. Global Outlook.* Traces the growth of 200 industries and gives 5-year forecasts for each

Don't neglect to contact specific government agencies such as the Small Business Administration. They sponsor several helpful programs such as SCORE and Small Business Development Centers, which can provide you with free counseling and a wealth of business information. The Department of Commerce not only publishes helpful books like the *U.S. Global Outlook* but also produces an array of products with information regarding both domestic industries and foreign markets through its International Trade Administration branch. The above items are available from the US Government Printing Office.

One of the best public sources is the business section of public libraries. The services provided vary from city to city, but usually include a wide range of government and market statistics, a large collection of directories including information on domestic and foreign businesses, as well as a wide selection of magazines, newspapers, and newsletters.

Almost every county government publishes population density and distribution figures in accessible census tracts. These tracts will show you the number of people living in specific areas, such as precincts, water districts, or even 10-block neighborhoods. Other public sources include city chambers of commerce or business development departments, which encourage new businesses in their communities. They will supply you (usually for free) with information on population trends, community income characteristics, payrolls, industrial development, and so on.

Among the best commercial sources of information are research and trade associations. Information gathered by trade associations is usually confined to a certain industry and available only to association members, with a membership fee frequently required. However, the research gathered by the larger associations is usually thorough, accurate, and worth the cost of membership. Two excellent resources to help you locate a trade association that reports on the business you're researching are *Encyclopedia of Associations* (Gale Research) and *Business Information Sources* (University of California Press) and can usually be found at your local library.

Research associations are often independent but are sometimes affiliated with trade associations. They often limit their activities to conducting and applying research in industrial development, but some have become full-service information sources with a wide range of supplementary publications such as directories.

Educational institutions are very good sources of research. Research there ranges from faculty-based projects often published under professors' bylines to student projects, theses, and assignments. Copies of student research projects may be available for free with faculty permission. Consulting services are available either for free or at a cost negotiated with the appropriate faculty members. This can be an excellent way to generate research at little or no cost, using students who welcome the professional experience either as interns or for special credit.

Look in the *Encyclopedia of Associations* (Gale Cengage Learning), found in most libraries, to find associations relevant to your industry. You may also want to investigate your customers' trade associations for information that can help you market to them. Most trade associations provide information free of charge.

Did you use any of the following tools in your secondary research?

- Census information
- Trade associations
- Chamber of Commerce
- Market profiles
- Libraries
- Lifestyles profiles
- Local magazines/newspapers
- Going on line

6.5.2.1 Marketing Research Online

You may already be conducting online market research for your business—but you may not know it. Some of the easiest to use and most common tools are located right at your fingertips. Web searches, online questionnaires, customer feedback forms—they all help you gather information about your market, your customers, and your future business prospects.

The advent of the Internet has presented small businesses with a wealth of additional resources to use in conducting free or low-cost market research. The following pages will describe the different types of tools to conduct online market research, go over the general categories of market research, and advise you on how to create the best online searches and questionnaires [14].

These days, entrepreneurs can conduct much of their market research without ever leaving their computers, thanks to the universe of online services and information. Start with the major consumer online services, which offer access to business databases. Here are a few to get you started [15]:

- *KnowThis.com* is a marketing virtual library that includes a tab on the site called "Weblinks." The tab contains links to a wide variety of market research web resources.

- *BizMiners.com* lets you choose national market research reports for 16,000 industries in 300 US markets, local research reports for 16,000 industries in 250 metro markets, or financial profiles for 10,000 US industries. The reports are available online for a nominal cost.

- *MarketResearch.com* has more than 250,000 research reports from hundreds of sources consolidated into one accessible collection that's updated daily. No subscription fee is required, and you pay only for the parts of the report you need with its "Buy by the Section" feature. After paying, the information is delivered online to your personal library on the site.

6.6 Your Start-Up Marketing Plan

Without marketing, no one will ever know that your business exists—and if customers do not know you are in business, you will not record any sales. When your marketing efforts are working, however, and customers are streaming through the door, an effective customer service policy will keep them coming back for more. So now it is time to create the plans that will draw customers to your business again and again.

A marketing plan consists of the strategies and devices you are going to use to effectively communicate to your target audience. A customer service plan focuses on your customer's requirements and the ways of filling those requirements. The two must work in concert.

Descriptions of your market and its segments, the competition, and prospective customers should be in your business plan. This is the start of your marketing plan. On the basis of this information, you can begin choosing the communication channels to use to get the word out about your business: social media, blogs, e-mail newsletters, Web banners, pay-per-click ads, radio, TV, billboards, direct mail, fliers, print ads, seminars, technical conferences, live presentations to audiences, webinars, and other venues. Then, prioritize your tactics and begin with the ones that your research has shown to be the most effective for your audience.

For your customer service plan, think about what it'll take to develop relationships with your customers that can be mutually beneficial for years to come. Since repeat customers are the backbone of every successful business, in your customer service plan, you'll want to outline just how you're going to provide complete customer satisfaction. Consider money-back guarantees, buying incentives, and the resolution of customer complaints. Determine what your customer service policy will say, how you'll train your employees to attend to the needs of your customers and how to reward repeat customers. Remember, this is just the beginning: Your program should evolve as the business grows.

To begin attracting your first customers, it's helpful to create a profile of the end user of your product or service. Now's the time to get in the habit of "talking up" your business—telling everyone you know about it. Ask for referrals from colleagues, suppliers, former employers, and other associates. You can improve the quality of your referrals by being specific in your request. For example, an insurance broker developed a successful referral network by asking existing clients if they knew anyone who was "in a two-income professional family with young children," rather than just asking if they knew anyone who needed insurance.

Consider offering free consultations or an introductory price to first-time buyers. Consider joining forces with a complementary business to get them to help you spread the word about your new venture. For example, a carpet cleaner might offer incentives to a housecleaning service if they'd recommend them to their regular customers. Once you've done work for a few satisfied customers, ask them for a testimonial letter to use in your promotions.

6.7 Guerrilla Marketing

The term *guerilla marketing* is often used to describe the most inexpensive, small-scale, and short-term marketing techniques. It can be defined as marketing that uses creativity and effort to maximize sales impact at the lowest cost. It is a low-budget approach to marketing that relies on ingenuity, cleverness, and surprise rather than traditional techniques [7].

The concept of guerrilla marketing was invented as an unconventional system of promotions that relies on time, energy, and imagination rather than a traditional big marketing budget. Typically, (1) guerrilla marketing campaigns are unexpected and unconventional, (2) they are potentially interactive, and (3) specific customers are targeted in unexpected places. The objective of guerrilla marketing is to create a unique, engaging, and thought-provoking concept to generate buzz, and consequently turn viral.

One way of differentiating your "resource poor" start-up company inexpensively is to use a marketing concept known as guerrilla marketing. This concept was introduced by Jay Conrad Levinson [16] with the intention of helping small companies make big marketing splashes but only using a very limited budget.

Levinson teaches that marketing encompasses everything you do to promote your business, from the moment of conception to the point at which customers buy your product or service and begin to patronize your business on a regular basis. The key words to remember are *everything* and *regular* basis.

The meaning is clear: Marketing includes the name of your company, the determination of whether you will be selling directly or through distributors, your method of manufacturing, the location of your business headquarters, your advertising method, your sales training, your sales presentation, your telephone inquiries, web address effectiveness, your customer-based problem solving ability, your expected growth plan, and your follow-up. If you gather from this that marketing is a complex process, you are right. If you do not see guerrilla marketing as an iterative, circular process, it will be a straight line that leads directly to the nearest bankruptcy court.

According to Hutter and Hoffmann [17], three aspects distinguish guerrilla marketing from traditional marketing, namely, (1) surprise, (2) diffusion, and (3) low cost effect. A guerrilla marketing campaign should be surprising to your competition, meaning it should not follow the traditional marketing norms. Guerrilla marketers create and execute seven "strategies" as follows:

1. Purpose of your strategy
2. How you will achieve this purpose, focusing on the benefits to the consumer
3. Define your target market (or markets)
4. Define the guerrilla marketing weapons you will employ
5. Clearly focus on your niche market
6. Explain your identity (see below)
7. Calculate your budget, expressed as a percentage of your expected gross revenues

Take a moment to understand the crucial difference between your *image* and your *identity*. Image implies something artificial, contrived, and not genuine. Conversely, identity describes what your business is really all about.

6.7.1 Guerilla Marketing Tactics

Never *assume* that a large market exists for your wonderful new product. Create it! Guerrilla marketing is as different from conventional marketing as guerrilla warfare is from conventional warfare. Below are some tactics that are easy to understand, easy to implement, and outrageously inexpensive:

- Organize technical demonstrations
- Develop a sales script (your elevator speech)
- Sell at every opportunity
- Sponsor memorable events
- Speak at many technical occasions
- Ask for referrals from colleagues
- Create samples (touchy-feelies)
- Create specification sheets
- Create an unforgettable award
- Collect testimonials
- Get a journalist to write about your company/technology
- Show great interest in customer needs
- Create and distribute timely white papers

- Create a widely circulated newsletter
- Cooperate with other businesses
- Exhibit at important trade shows
- Get yourself published. Write an e-book.
- Join and participate
- Organize community hospital-oriented projects.
- Fake publicity stunts
- Attention-getting press releases

6.7.2 Apple's Guerrilla Marketing

By any measure, Apple is unquestionably one of the world's most successful retailers. Even though Apple never sold directly to consumers before it opened the first store in a mall in Tyson's Corner, Virginia, Apple has achieved some incredible bragging rights for its retail channel [18].

Apple operates more than 380 retail stores that employ more than 40,000 people and plays host to more than a million visitors every day. Apple's retail operations are on track to generate more than $20 billion in 2012. Amazingly, Apple's stores average more than $7000 per square foot, which is more than twice the former gold standard, Tiffany & Company. It is estimated that Apple's Fifth Avenue store generates more than $35,000 per square foot, making it the highest grossing retailer in New York City—ever! Apple stores are now the highest-performing stores in retail history.

6.7.2.1 Humble Beginnings

It wasn't always that way. Apple experienced massive failures in the 1990s when selling its products through retailers such as Sears and CompUSA. Its computers were muscled out of view and its brand so weakened that many retailers refused to properly market or stock Apple's computers. Even though Apple entered the retail business largely as a defensive move to gain more control of the customer experience, the climate then was anything but welcoming. Gateway was operating direct-to-consumer retail stores and failing fast. Apple had to learn how to do retail its products differently.

Less than 2 years after Apple opened its retail stores, Gateway declared bankruptcy, shut down all of its shops and laid off more than 2500 workers. Three years later, CompUSA shuttered its 23-year-old chain of stores. Thus, while there was little expectation and no guarantee that Apple might succeed selling its own computers in this challenging retail climate, amazingly, somehow it managed to survive.

6.7.2.2 Unconventional Thinking

But how did Apple survive the disappearance of its two retail distributors? Consider the following questions:

- How did a company with no experience in retail become the fastest in US history to reach annual sales of $1 billion during the worst financial crisis in modern times?
- How did a company with only four products become the most profitable retailer in history while creating an experience that is now the standard by which all others are measured?
- Why did a company that was losing money decide to enter the retail market against the recommendations of every expert and where all retail businesses were going out of business?
- How did Apple entice millions of people to visit their stores and pay full price when all their products are readily available at other retailers and even tax-free online at Amazon.com?

Clearly the answer to these questions is that Apple had to think differently about retail and make their stores more than just a place people go to buy things. They had to devise a way to enrich the lives of the people who shop at the Apple stores and do more than simply deliver a transactional experience. In short, they had to reinvent retail.

Did you know that Apple rarely invents anything new? Entire books are written about how Steve Jobs borrowed ideas for Apple from other places like Xerox and Sony, famously embracing the motto "Good artists borrow. Great artists steal." Apple clearly didn't invent the PC, the MP3 player, downloadable music, or the mobile phone. The Mac, iPod, iTunes, and iPhone were all successful because Apple had ample time to improve upon existing designs and functionality. As a consequence of being late to these markets, Apple was forced to adopt a stunningly different (guerrilla) marketing strategy than anyone else. And that is guerrilla marketing at its best!

6.8 Your Marketing Plan

Firms that are successful in marketing invariably start with a marketing plan. Large companies have plans with hundreds of pages; small companies can get by with a half-dozen sheets. Put your marketing plan in a three-ring binder. Refer to it at least quarterly, but better yet monthly. Leave a tab for putting in monthly reports on sales/manufacturing; this will allow you to track your performance as you follow the plan [19].

The guerrilla plan should cover 1 year. For small companies, this is often the best way to think about marketing. Things change, people leave, markets evolve, customers come and go. Later on, we suggest creating a section of your plan that addresses the medium-term future—2 to 4 years down the road. But the bulk of your plan should focus on the coming year.

You should allow yourself a couple of months to write the plan, even if it's only a few pages long. Developing the plan is the "heavy lifting" of marketing. While executing the plan has its challenges, deciding what to do and how to do it is marketing's greatest challenge. Most marketing plans kick off with the first of the year or with the opening of your fiscal year if it's different.

Who should see your plan? The answer: All the players in your company. Firms typically keep their marketing plans very, very private for one of two very different reasons: Either they're too skimpy and management would be embarrassed to have them see the light of day, or they're solid and packed with information... which would make them extremely valuable to the competition.

You cannot do a marketing plan without getting many people involved. No matter what your size, get feedback from all parts of your company: finance, manufacturing, personnel, supply, and so on—in addition to marketing itself. This is especially important because it will take all aspects of your company to make your marketing plan work. Your key people can provide realistic input on what's achievable and how your goals can be reached, and they can share any insights they have on any potential, as-yet-unrealized marketing opportunities, adding another dimension to your plan. If you're essentially a one-person management operation, you'll have to wear all your hats at one time—but at least the meetings will be short!

What's the relationship between your marketing plan and your business plan or vision statement? Your business plan spells out what your business is about—what you do and don't do, and what your ultimate goals are. It encompasses more than marketing; it can include discussions of locations, staffing, financing, strategic alliances, and so on. It includes "the vision thing," the resounding words that spell out the glorious purpose of your company in stirring language. Your business plan is the US Constitution of your business: If you want to do something that's outside the business plan, you need to either change your mind or change the plan. Your company's business plan provides the environment in which your marketing plan must flourish. The two documents must be consistent.

6.8.1 The Benefits of a Marketing Plan

Based on marketing research, a marketing plan, on the other hand, is replete with meaning. It provides you with several major benefits. Let's review them.

- **Rallying point:** Your marketing plan gives your troops something to rally behind. You want them to feel confident that the captain of the vessel has the charts in order, knows how to run the ship, and has a port of destination in mind. Companies often undervalue the impact of a "marketing plan" on their own people, who want to feel part of a team engaged in an exciting and complicated joint endeavor. If you want your employees to feel committed to your company, it's important to share with them your vision of where the company is headed in the years to come. People don't always understand financial projections, but they can get excited about a well-written and well-thought-out marketing plan. You should consider releasing your marketing plan—perhaps in an abridged version—companywide. Do it with some fanfare and generate some excitement for the adventures to come. Your workers will appreciate being involved.

- **Chart to success:** We all know that plans are imperfect things. How can you possibly know what's going to happen 12 months or 5 years from now? Isn't putting together a marketing plan an exercise in futility... a waste of time better spent meeting with customers or fine-tuning production? Yes, possibly, but only in the narrowest sense. If you don't plan, you're doomed, and an inaccurate plan is far better than no plan at all. To stay with our sea captain analogy, it's better to be 5° or even 10° off your destination port than to have no destination in mind at all. The point of sailing, after all, is to get somewhere, and without a marketing plan, you'll wander the seas aimlessly, sometimes finding dry land but more often than not floundering in a vast ocean. Sea captains without a chart are rarely remembered for discovering anything but the ocean floor.

- **Company operational instructions:** Your child's first bike and your new VCR came with a set of instructions, and your company is far more complicated to put together and run than either of them. Your marketing plan is a step-by-step guide for your company's success. It's more important than a vision statement. To put together a genuine marketing plan, you have to assess your company from top to bottom and make sure all the pieces are working together in the best way. What do you want to do with this enterprise you call the company in the coming year? Consider it a to-do list on a grand scale. It assigns specific tasks for the year.

- **Captured thinking:** You don't allow your financial people to keep their numbers in their heads. Financial reports are the lifeblood of the numbers side of any business, no matter what size. It should be no different with marketing. Your written document lays out your game plan. If people leave, if new people arrive, if memories falter, if events bring pressure to alter the givens, the information in the written marketing plan stays intact to remind you of what you'd agreed on.

- **Top-level reflection:** In the daily hurly-burly of competitive business, it's hard to turn your attention to the big picture, especially those parts that aren't directly related to the daily operations. You need to take time periodically to really think about your business—whether it's providing you and your employees with what you want, whether there aren't some innovative wrinkles you can add, whether you're getting all you can out of your products, your sales staff, and your markets. Writing your marketing plan is the best time to do this high-level thinking. Some companies send their top marketing people away to a retreat. Others go to the home of a principal. Some do marketing plan development at a local motel, away from phones and fax machines, so they can devote themselves solely to thinking hard and drawing the most accurate sketches they can of the immediate future of the business.

Ideally, after writing marketing plans for a few years, you can sit back and review a series of them, year after year, and check the progress of your company. Of course, sometimes it is hard to make time to review the marketing history (there is that annoying real world to deal with), but looking back can provide an unparalleled objective view of what you've been doing with your business life over a number of years.

6.8.2 Researching Your Market

Whether you're just starting out or if you've been in business for years, you should always stay up-to-date with your market information. Below, we discuss the best methods for finding your relevant data [20].

The purpose of market research is to provide relevant data that will help solve the marketing problems a business will encounter. This is absolutely necessary in the start-up phase. Conducting thorough market surveys is the foundation of any successful business. In fact, strategies such as market segmentation (identifying specific segments within a market) and product differentiation (creating an identity for your product or service that separates it from your competitors') would be impossible to develop without market research.

Your market research should be designed to answer two major questions: (1) what are your target market needs, and (2) your proposed solutions to answer those needs, as depicted in Figure 6.2.

Whether you're conducting market research using the historical, experimental, observational, or survey method, you'll be gathering two types of data. The first will be "primary" information that you will compile yourself or hire someone to gather. Most information, however, will be "secondary," or already compiled and organized for you. Reports and studies done by government agencies, trade associations, or other businesses within your

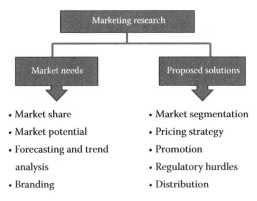

FIGURE 6.2
Marketing research. (Modified after Naresh K. Malhotra. *Marketing Research: An Applied Orientation*, Pearson Education, Upper Saddle River, NJ, 2000.)

industry are examples of the latter. Search for them, and take advantage of them.

When conducting market research on a shoestring, there are basically two types of information that can be gathered: exploratory and specific. Exploratory research is open-ended in nature, helps you define a specific problem, and usually involves detailed, unstructured interviews in which lengthy answers are solicited from a small group of respondents. Specific research is broader in scope and is used to solve a problem that exploratory research has identified. Interviews are structured and formal in approach. Of the two, specific research is more expensive.

There are basically three avenues you can take: (1) direct mail, (2) phone surveys, and (3) personal interviews. These are discussed below.

Direct Mail

If you choose a direct-mail questionnaire, be sure to do the following in order to increase your response rate:

- Make sure your questions are short and to the point.
- Make sure questionnaires are addressed to specific individuals and they're of interest to the respondent.
- Limit the questionnaire's length to two pages.
- Enclose a professionally prepared cover letter that adequately explains what you need.
- Send a reminder approximately 2 weeks after the initial mailing. Include a postage-paid self-addressed envelope.

Unfortunately, even if you employ the above tactics, response to direct mail is always low, and is sometimes less than 5%.

Phone Surveys

Phone surveys are generally the most cost-effective, considering overall response rates; they cost approximately one-third as much as personal interviews, which have, on average, a response rate that is only 10%. The following are some phone survey guidelines:

- At the beginning of the conversation, your interviewer should confirm the name of the respondent if calling a home, or give the appropriate name to the switchboard operator if calling a business.

- Pauses should be avoided, as respondent interest can quickly drop.

- Make sure that a follow-up call is possible if additional information is required.

- Make sure that interviewers don't divulge details about the poll until the respondent is reached.

As mentioned, phone interviews are cost-effective but speed is another big advantage. Some of the more experienced interviewers can get through up to 10 interviews an hour (however, speed for speed's sake is not the goal of any of these surveys), but five to six interviews per hour is more typical. Phone interviews also allow you to cover a wide geographical range relatively inexpensively. Phone costs can be reduced by taking advantage of cheaper rates during certain hours.

Personal Interviews

There are two main types of personal interviews:

1. **The group survey.** Used mostly by big business, group interviews can be useful as brainstorming tools resulting in product modifications and new product ideas. They also give you insight into buying preferences and purchasing decisions among certain populations.

2. **The depth interview.** One-on-one interviews where the interviewer is guided by a small checklist and basic common sense. Depth interviews are either focused or nondirective. Nondirective interviews encourage respondents to address certain topics with minimal questioning. The respondent, in essence, leads the interview. The focused interview, on the other hand, is based on a preset checklist. The choice and timing of questions, however, are left to the interviewer, depending on how the interview goes.

When considering which type of survey to use, keep the following cost factors in mind:

- **Mail.** Most of the costs here concern the printing of questionnaires, envelopes, postage, the cover letter, time taken in the analysis and presentation, the cost of researcher time, and any incentives used.
- **Telephone.** The main costs here are the interviewer's fee, phone charges, preparation of the questionnaire, cost of researcher time, and the analysis and presentation of the results of the questioning.
- **Personal interviews.** Costs include the printing of questionnaires and prompt cards if needed, the incentives used, the interviewer's fee and expenses, cost of researcher time, and analysis and presentation.
- **Group discussions.** Your main costs here are the interviewer's fees and expenses in recruiting and assembling the groups, renting the conference room or other facility, researcher time, any incentives used, analysis and presentation, and the cost of recording media such as tapes, if any are used.

6.9 Competitive Intelligence

The Society of Competitive Intelligence Professionals defines Competitive Intelligence as "the process of ethically collecting, analyzing, and disseminating accurate, relevant, specific, timely, foresighted, and actionable intelligence regarding the implications of the business environment, competitors and the organization itself."

Competitive intelligence (CI) is the selection, collection, interpretation, and distribution of publicly held information that is strategically important to a firm. A substantial amount of this information is publicly accessible via the World Wide Web, periodic company SEC filings, the patent literature, company promotional campaigns, and so on.

The knowledge-intensive world is ruled by hypercompetition. Hypercompetition is a rapid and dynamic competition characterized by unsustainable advantage. It is the condition of rapid escalation of competition based on price-quality positioning, competition to protect or invade established product or geographic markets, and competition based on vast scientific knowledge, deep pockets, and the creation of even deeper pocketed alliances [21].

The knowledge base for managing in this hypercompetitive environment is called Competitive Intelligence. CI is a process that provides you insights into what might happen in the near future. This process requires that we go from data to information to intelligence. Here is a basic example:

Data → Prices for our products have dropped by 5%

Information → New offshore facilities enjoy significantly lower labor costs

Intelligence → Our key competitor is about to acquire a facility in China that will…

The differences between data, information, and intelligence can be subtle, but very real:

Data → Unconnected pieces of information: Nice to know, but so what!

Information → Increased knowledge derived by understanding the relationships of data: Interesting, but how does it relate to what I do! The knowledge-intensive business world is driven by hypercompetition.

Intelligence → Organizing the information to fully appreciate the implications and impact on the organization: Oh really, then we better do something!

A formalized CI program should

- Anticipate changes in the marketplace
- Anticipate actions of competitors
- Discover new or potential competitors
- Learn from the successes and failures of others
- Increase the range and quality of acquisition targets
- Learn about new technologies, products, and processes that affect your business
- Learn about political, legislative, or regulatory changes that can affect your business
- Enter new businesses
- Look at your own business practices with an open mind
- Help implement the latest management tools

6.9.1 CI Is a Top Management Function

CI is not for everyone. In fact, most companies do not use CI. Despite the fact that most executives rely on the flow of information for decision-making, only a handful of companies have a fully functional, integrated CI process in place. Why is that? Perhaps the most important reason is attitudinal: the way executives think about CI [22]. Have you ever heard some of the comments listed below? Or perhaps you have said them yourself!

- CI is spying; it is unethical. I don't want any part of it.
- It was not part of my school curriculum. It must not be important.
- CI is a cost center. We do not have a budget for it.
- How do I quantify CI's cost/benefit ratio?
- Nothing happens in this industry that I don't know already.
- If I don't know it, is it not worth knowing.
- We tried it before, and it didn't work.
- I am too busy to review all this garbage.

CI requires authorization by the highest echelons of management. CI is a top management function. It can provide vital analysis of competitor capabilities, plans, intentions, and limitations. It spotlights industry structure and trends. It may also reveal political, economic, and social forces affecting your company.

The CI life cycle is iterative, consisting of four major functions: (1) planning and direction, (2) information collection, (3) analysis and forecast, and finally (4) information and dissemination, as shown in Figure 6.3.

CI is particularly useful in industries with long development and approval cycles, such as the pharmaceutical and biotechnology industries. These industries are faced with long research and development times—sometimes 10 to 15 years for innovative drugs—coupled with uncertain and hugely

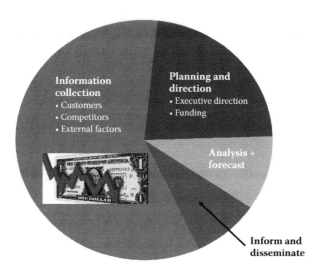

FIGURE 6.3
The CI life cycle.

expensive clinical trials. This allows continual tracking of a drug's progress by competitors through the public FDA approval process.

Thus, pharmaceutical/biotechnology companies utilize CI during the years of drug development to help determine if a new drug development should be continued, or dropped. Likewise, it allows companies to monitor a competitor's activities and decide whether to initiate their own drug development for a specific indication.

6.9.2 CI Should Be Actionable

CI differs from data and information since it requires some form of analysis. The purpose of this analysis is to derive some meaning from the piles of data and information that bury everyone. By going through analysis and filtering, we can refine it enough so that someone can act on it and understand their options, giving them an opportunity to make forward-looking decisions.

Note that **Information** is factual. It is numbers, statistics, bits of data, and interesting stories that seem important. **Intelligence**, on the other hand, is an *actionable* list of data that have been analyzed, filtered, and distilled. This is what we call intelligence know-how.

Thus, when you present CI to your staff, they should draw a conclusion and make an important decision quickly. Therefore, CI should put conclusions and recommendations up front with supporting research behind the analysis. CI should not simply present the facts, declaring what we found, but instead make a statement, saying this is what we believe is about to happen.

CI involves the use of public sources to develop data on your competition, competitors, and the market environment. It can then transform those data into actionable policies (intelligence). In this context, "public" means all the information you can legally and ethically identify, obtain, locate, deduce, and access [23].

CI is also known by several other names: competitor intelligence, business intelligence, strategic intelligence, marketing intelligence, competitive technical intelligence, technology intelligence, and technical intelligence, depending on what specific information is being targeted [24].

The development of CI usually proceeds in a five-phase predetermined cycle, as seen below:

1. **Establish your needs.** Clearly identify the information needed on the competition, or the competitive environment.
2. **Collect data.** Assemble raw data, using legal and ethical means, from public sources.
3. **Analyze the data.** Convert data into useful information.
4. **Communicate intelligence.** Convey the finished intelligence to the decision-maker(s) for their use.
5. **Actionable intelligence.** Provide strategic direction to decision-maker(s) in a timely manner.

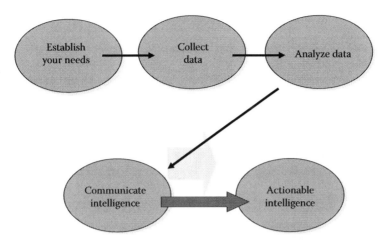

FIGURE 6.4
Five-phase intelligence cycle.

These phases are visually summarized in Figure 6.4.

6.9.3 Market Intelligence

Market intelligence is focused on the very current activities in the marketplace. You can look at it as the qualitative side of the quantitative data research you have conducted in many retail markets. The primary beneficiaries of market intelligence are usually the marketing department, market research, and the sales force. To a lesser degree, market intelligence serves those in market planning by providing retrospective data on the success and failure of their own sales efforts.

Market intelligence's focus is on sales, pricing, payment, and financing terms, as well as on promotions being offered and their effectiveness. Market intelligence's time horizon typically runs from 3 to 6 months back to no more than 6 months in the future. Sometimes, however, the horizon is actually measured in terms of weeks, or even days, rather than months.

References

1. http://www.moderndaymarketing.co.uk/SpecialReportWebOpt.pdf
2. Heasman, L. Modern Day Marketing, http://www.moderndaymarketing.co.uk/SpecialReportWebOpt.pdf.
3. Gummesson, E. and Polese, F. B2B is not an island! *Journal of Business & Industrial Marketing*, 24(5), 337–350, 2009.

4. https://en.wikipedia.org/wiki/Market_research
5. Welsh, J.A. and White, J.F. A small business is not a little big business. *Harvard Business Review*, 50(4), 9172, https://hbr.org/1981/07/a-small-business-is-not-a -little-big-business/ar/4.
6. Churchill, N.C. and Lewis, V.L. The Five Stages of Small Business Growth Harvard Business Review, Reprint 83301, Boston. May–June 1983.
7. Margolis, J. and Garrigan, P. Guerrilla Marketing for Dummies, p. 12, Wiley Publishing Inc., Hoboken, NJ, 2008.
8. Heuring, E. and Heuring, J. Brief History of the Simmons Hardware Company, 2010. http://www.thckk.org/history/simmons-hdwe.pdf.
9. http://smallbusiness.chron.com/difference-between-marketing-advertising -public-relations-sales-promotion-22873.html
10. Forbes/entrepreneurs, July 8, 2014. http://www.forbes.com/sites/robertwynne /2014/07/08/the-real-difference-between-pr-and-advertising-credibility/.
11. Drucker, P.F. *Management: Tasks, Responsibilities, Practices*. Harper & Row, Australia, p. 864, 1974. ISBN 0-06-011092-9.
12. https://en.wikipedia.org/wiki/Marketing_effectiveness
13. http://www.entrepreneur.com/article/217388
14. http://www.inc.com/guides/biz_online/online-market-research.html
15. https://bookstore.entrepreneur.com/product/start-your-own-business-6th -edition/
16. Levinson, J.C. *Guerrilla Marketing*. Houghton Mifflin Company, New York, 1933.
17. Hutter, K. and Hoffmann, S. Guerrilla marketing: The nature of the concept and propositions for further research. *Asian Journal of Marketing*, 1–16, 2011.
18. Chazin, S. The secrets of Apple's retail success, http://www.marketingapple .com/Apple_Retail_Success.pdf.
19. How to create a marketing plan. Entrepreneur, www.entrepreneur.com /article/43018.
20. http://www.entrepreneur.com/article/43024
21. http://en.wikipedia.org/wiki/Hypercompetition
22. Kahaner, L. *Competitive Intelligence*. Touchstone Books, Rockefeller Center, New York, 1996.
23. McGonagle, J.J. and Vella, C.M. *Bottom Line Competitive Intelligence*. Quorum Books, Westport, CT, 2002.
24. What is competitive intelligence and why should you care about it? Chapter 2, http://search.aol.com/aol/search?enabled_terms=&s_it=wscreen-smallbusiness -w&q=competitive+intelligence+++pdf.

7

Establishing Your Dream Team

7.1 Introduction

It is well established that teams outperform individuals, especially when performance requires multiple skills, judgments, and experiences. One of your first tasks is to establish a "dream team" of specialists as a cohesive organization.

Organizations generally consist of groups of people who work together for the achievement of common goals. A **team** comprises any group of people linked in a common purpose. However, a group in itself does not necessarily constitute a team. Teams are especially appropriate for conducting tasks that are high in complexity and have many interdependent subtasks, such as the development and commercialization of knowledge-intensive products. Last, **teamwork and team building** are an organized effort to improve your overall team effectiveness.

There are five reasons why your dream team is particularly important during the start-up phase:

1. Complex tasks—the necessary allocation of tasks is only possible with a team that displays complementary skills.
2. New sorts of problems continually arise—a well-functioning team, well deployed, will find the optimal solution.
3. External investors—are betting their money in you and your team.
4. Shared vision—it is ultimately the people behind the idea who will make it successful.
5. Shared burden—the team has the advantage that the whole burden is shared across the team; if one member drops out, the whole enterprise does not collapse.

Building your start-up is a process that requires a wide variety of talents that are rarely all found in a single person. Because your idea is innovative, there are no standard solutions for the problems that will arise. A group of people with complementary skills will always solve problems better than any individual ever could.

7.2 Hiring Your Dream Team

More than anything else, the hiring of your dream team will decide the ultimate fate of your company. In the author's experience, at the board level (during our formative years), we spent more time dealing with "people issues" than any other subject.

For their technical team, entrepreneurs should select people whose talents are recognizably complementary to their own weaknesses. To select the optimal executive team, you start by objectively understanding yourself, what you know, and what your weakest areas of expertise are. This is easier said than done, since self-criticism is as rare as rain in the desert, particularly after you have climbed to the top of the ladder by talent, perseverance, and guts, as shown in Figure 7.1.

In hiring your technical team, you will need to initially decide between a heterogeneous or a homogenous group [1].

- The members of a *heterogeneous executive team* are diverse in terms of their abilities and experiences.
- In contrast, the members of a homogeneous executive team are similar to one another in terms of their abilities and experiences.

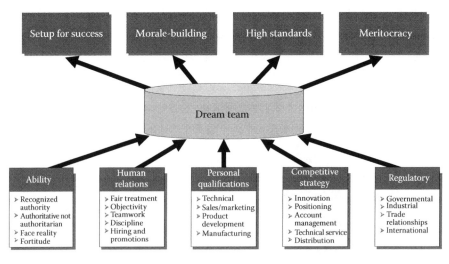

FIGURE 7.1
Your dream team. Select executives with complementary skills to yours.

Heterogeneous teams are traditionally favored by investors because (1) the shared intense effort is required by a start-up; (2) the loss of one member is less likely to result in start-up abandonment; (3) the team concept allows expertise across major functional areas: marketing, finance, operations, sales, and so on; and (4) a skilled team lends credibility to the start-up and lowers risks to investors [2].

7.2.1 Teamwork Not Titles

A real team is a small number of people with complementary skills, committed to a common vision. The vision includes (1) a common purpose, (2) an agreed approach, (3) performance standards, and (4) realistic goals for which they hold themselves mutually accountable [3]. Goals at the executive team level are assigned based on individual skills (specialization), regardless of formal titles.

7.2.2 Team Discipline

The technical team must be goal oriented. Goals specify in advance what each member must accomplish and periodically evaluate the degree to which members have met those goals. This is illustrated in Figure 7.2.

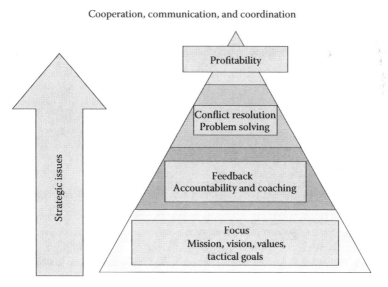

FIGURE 7.2
Dream team goals. Be crystal clear about your goals to reach profitability.

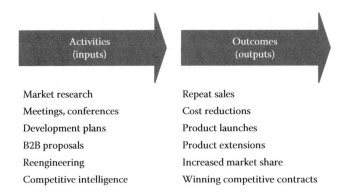

Activities (inputs)	Outcomes (outputs)
Market research	Repeat sales
Meetings, conferences	Cost reductions
Development plans	Product launches
B2B proposals	Product extensions
Reengineering	Increased market share
Competitive intelligence	Winning competitive contracts

FIGURE 7.3
Activities versus outcomes. Concentrate on outcomes (and be specific).

7.2.3 Focus on Outcomes, Not Activities

What gets measured gets done.

In most large companies, the vast majority of objectives is really nothing more than activity-based goals. In his 1999 book, Douglas K. Smith laid out a guide for evaluating and realigning goals to achieve specific outcomes. *Activities are not objectives. Activities are how we achieve the objectives, the outcome-based goals* [4].

It is not enough to say: "This week I will visit a minimum of four customers." That is **activity**. It should be: "This week, out of the four customers, I will get a large purchase order from at least one." That is **outcome**. Figure 7.3 illustrates some important differences between activities and outcomes.

7.3 Teamwork and Team Building

Tuckman and Jensen [5] (Four-Phase Model) identified a life cycle of stages through which most teams experience, namely, forming, storming, norming, performing, and adjourning. According to this view, the team begins with the forming stage, where members are just beginning to associate themselves with the team. At this stage, the team lacks a clear vision, purpose, and structure, whereas in the storming stage, members realize the complexity of the problem and might get polarized into subgroups. In the norming stage, team members form lasting relationships with other colleagues and the team clearly defines the specific expectations from individual members in terms of both actions and behaviors. The fourth stage of team development is the

TABLE 7.1

Tuckman and Jensen Teambuilding Model

Stage	Characteristics
1. Forming	• Excessive caution • Uncertainty of goals and procedures • Avoidance of conflict • Search for direction
2. Storming	• Interpersonal conflict • Power struggles • Criticisms of fellow members • Challenges to goals • Questioning previous decisions
3. Norming	• Cohesion • Mutual support • Willingness to consider conflicting alternatives • Sharing knowledge
4. Performing	• Full involvement • Acceptance of other views • Voluntary efforts • Warm relationships and fusion • Group creativity at maximum
5. Adjourning	• Acceptance of team breakup • Sadness in the face of team success • Team asked to "stand down" and disperse

performance stage, where the team is set to perform the task after which the team lapses into an adjourning stage where it does not possess the kind of energy demonstrated in the performance stage [6]. This is illustrated in Table 7.1.

7.4 Intellectual Capital Management

Savvy founders realize that start-up market value multiples associated with its intangible assets (staff, patents, trademarks, trade secrets, brandings, etc.) are often many times higher than the multiples associated with the cash flows generated from its tangible assets in isolation [7].

The challenge facing start-ups is to implement business practices and systems to manage, leverage, and exploit these intellectual assets, compared to traditional accounting approaches.

Intellectual capital management is composed of several related "assets" as defined below:

- Human Capital—the people element of an organization. It includes owners, employees, contractors, suppliers, and those who collectively bring to the organization their individual abilities (i.e., know-how,

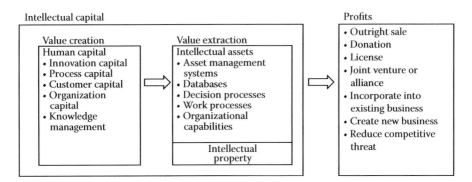

FIGURE 7.4
Intellectual capital overview.

experience, skills, creativity). Human capital is one of the two major elements comprising intellectual capital.

- Intellectual Assets—the tangible or physical description of specific knowledge to which an organization may assert ownership rights (i.e., documents, databases, processes, inventions, programs). Intellectual assets are the other major element comprising intellectual capital.

- Intellectual Property—the subset of intellectual assets for which legal protection has been obtained (i.e., patents, trademarks, copyrights, trade secrets).

- Intellectual Capital—the collective elements of human capital and intellectual assets... the "knowledge" of an organization that can be converted into profit.

Intellectual capital management, then, is the processes and structures used to undertake the two activities of "value creation" and "value extraction" from any organization and, with the concepts above, could be generally conceived of as shown in Figure 7.4.

7.4.1 Human Capital

Human capital is the composite of knowledge, habits, and social and personality attributes, including creativity, embodied in the ability to perform labor so as to produce economic value for an organization [8].

It is a measure of the economic value of your staff's skill set. This measure builds on the basic production input of labor measure where all labor is thought to be equal. The concept of human capital recognizes that not all labor is equal and that the quality of employees can be improved by investing in them. The education, experience, and abilities of your staff have an economic value for employers [9].

Economist Theodore Schultz [10] invented the term in the 1960s to reflect the value of our human capacities. He believed that human capital was like any other type of capital; it could be invested in through education, training, and enhanced benefits that will lead to an improvement in the quality and level of production, thus increasing enterprise value.

Human capital is an intangible asset—it is not owned by the firm that employs it and is generally not fungible. Specifically, individuals arrive at 9 a.m. and leave at 5 p.m. (in the conventional office model), taking most of their knowledge and relationships with them in their heads.

Human capital, when viewed from a time perspective, consumes time in one of key activities:

1. Technical knowledge (activities involving one employee)
2. Collaboration (activities involving more than one employee)
3. Processes (activities specifically focused on the knowledge and collaborative activities generated by organizational structure—such as silo impacts, internal politics, etc.)
4. Absence (annual leave, sick leave, holidays, etc.)

Despite the lack of formal ownership, start-ups can gain from high levels of training, in part because it creates a corporate culture or vocabulary teams use to create cohesion.

Studies of human capital proliferated in the 1980s after US manufacturers realized that Japanese firms often bested them on price and quality in large part because of their human relations policies, such as teamwork production methods, employee involvement in decision-making, job rotation, and pay for performance [11].

One of the first studies to consider investment outcomes found positive correlations to return on assets and return on investment among 495 business units drawn from a sample of private-sector US employers and a suite of alternative pay systems, including profit-sharing, gain sharing, employee stock options, employee stock ownership plans, and production incentive or bonus plans [12].

7.4.2 Knowledge Management

Knowledge management (KM) [13] is the process of capturing, developing, sharing, and effectively using organizational knowledge to enhance enterprise value. It refers to a multidisciplinary approach to achieving organizational objectives by making the best use of knowledge [14].

In our context, knowledge refers to the theoretical or practical understanding of a subject. It can be implicit (as with practical skill or expertise) or explicit (as with the theoretical understanding of a subject).

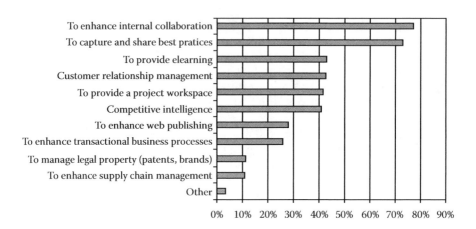

FIGURE 7.5
Objective for knowledge management efforts. (Source: IDC, 2002.)

KM efforts typically focus on organizational objectives such as improved performance, competitive advantage, innovation, the sharing of lessons learned, integration, and continuous improvement of the organization [15].

Knowledge teams are multidisciplinary, cross-functional, and hubs of knowledge to the entire organization. Knowledge teams provide start-ups with two keys: (1) share existing knowledge ("knowing what you know") and (2) provide knowledge for innovation ("creating and converting").

A 2002 IDC report [16] cited various objectives for KM efforts as seen in Figure 7.5.

KM efforts overlap with organizational learning and may be distinguished from that by a greater focus on the management of knowledge as a strategic asset and a focus on encouraging the sharing of knowledge. It is an enabler of organizational learning [17]. In summary, the KM cycle [18] can be illustrated in Figure 7.6.

7.4.3 Your Seven Knowledge Levers

Companies are increasingly recognizing the contribution of knowledge to their bottom line if effectively managed. But what are the key levers of a knowledge-based strategy that realize these benefits [19]? This section outlines seven such levers that can be used to create value for your knowledge-based business:

- Customer knowledge—*the most vital knowledge*
- Knowledge in products—*"smarts" add value*

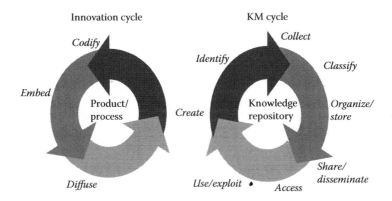

FIGURE 7.6
Knowledge cycle.

- Knowledge in processes
- Know-how when needed most—*sharing best practices*
- Organizational memory—*do we know what we know?*
- Knowledge in relationships—*who you know*
- Knowledge assets—*intellectual capital*

Customer Knowledge. Meeting or, even better, exceeding customer's expectations is a key strategic benefit. Customers provide useful feedback on products and services and how their needs are evolving. They are the major source of ideas for improved products and services. Most companies know a lot less about their customers and their markets than they claim. Too much reliance is placed on traditional market research and customer satisfactions surveys that tell them little of the real customers' concerns, desires, wishes, and desires. You need a deep intuitive understanding of customers' latent and unidentified needs.

Knowledge in Products and Services. "Intelligent" or "smart" products can command premium prices and be more beneficial to users. One example is the "intelligent" oil drill that bends and weaves its way to extract more oil than ever from the pockets of oil in underground formations. Customization also adds value and creates a more personalized offering. Hotel chains or car rental companies, for example, can make suitable rooms or cars available by knowing the customer's preferences. In creating new products, companies use a lot of knowledge, gleaned from market research and prototype testing. Yet only a fraction of the knowledge generated makes it into the final product. Smart organizations will create opportunities out of this knowledge.

Knowledge in Processes. In many companies, there are often differences in performance levels of 3:1 or more between different groups performing the same process. The detail and knowledge used is different. If this knowledge of best practice can be diffused and learned, then overall performance will improve. Every business process contains embedded knowledge. It is the result of thinking and codifying what was formerly a series of ad hoc tasks into something that is systematic and routine. The processes are also surrounded by the skills and knowledge of the person applying them and the experts who developed them. Making this knowledge more widely accessible is part of exploiting this lever.

Know-How When Needed Most. "Our most valuable asset is people," according to many academic reports, although the actual way people are treated and managed often belies this claim. The challenge is to turn individual know-how into organizational knowledge. Many organizations apply this lever through a "learning organization" program that stimulates personal development and organizational learning. Another aspect of this lever is to understand what motivates knowledge workers and reward them accordingly.

Organizational Memory. Much knowledge flow in organizations is transitory. It occurs in conversations, meetings, and e-mails. This strategic lever is a way of addressing the issue of knowing "what we know" or once knew. It helps avoid repeating the mistakes of the past, and in drawing lessons from similar situations elsewhere. Organization memory exists in many forms—processes, databases, artifacts, documents, but above all the minds of people. Sometimes overlooked are archives owned by outsiders, such as researchers, customers, or former employees. They may have retained detail that your own company lost as people left.

Knowledge in Relationships. Such depth of knowledge is not easily replaced overnight. Companies have many relationship webs involving customers, suppliers, employees, business partners, shareholders, and so on. These relationships involve sharing knowledge and understanding—not just of needs and factual information but also of deeper knowledge such as behaviors, motivations, personal characteristics, ambitions, and feelings. Such knowledge is often highly personal, but is easily lost during restructuring.

Knowledge Assets. Knowledge is one of the intangible assets of a company that do not appear in its balance sheet. The core of this lever is the adage "what you can measure you can manage." Many economists have argued that knowledge is now a critical resource that needs such an approach. However, most business managers have not turned this concept into practice. While accountants and auditors pore over detailed figures about every piece of physical plant and machinery, the major contributor to the value of their business, intellectual capital, gets scant attention. It so happens that changes in intellectual capital are usually lead indicators of future financial performance—an important reason for taking their measurement and management seriously.

7.4.4 Intellectual Property Management

Historically, intellectual property (IP) has been approached from three different perspectives—research and development (R&D), legal, and business. Because of the legal complexities, IP has largely been the purview of legal counsel, where focus is typically on legal registrations of patents and trademarks and providing support to R&D or business units. R&D departments generally measure IP performance by the number of inventions and by product support and enhancement.

7.5 Accountants and Lawyers

Remember that accountants and lawyers are cost centers. Necessary, indispensable, and crucial, but cost centers nevertheless. The founder must carefully select the proper accounting/legal team. By proper, I mean professionals who are familiar with the special circumstances surrounding start-ups. Engage only those individuals that are "specialized" in the intricacies of start-ups.

7.5.1 Accountants

Neither accountants nor lawyers academically "specialize" in start-ups, but in practice, the representation of start-ups becomes a *de facto* specialization for both professions. For example, a small business accountant will (1) help you with your business plan, (2) set up an inexpensive accounting system such as QuickBooks, and (3) patiently guide you through the intricacies of accounting jargon and Generally Accepted Accounting Practices. You will need all of this for your initial funding, plus all the necessary periodic reports to your investors.

7.5.2 Lawyers

The small business lawyer will help you navigate the process of incorporation and represent your small business during legal negotiations. Perhaps the lawyer will agree to be paid in installments tied to specific milestones. Bob Loblow, a small business lawyer, blogs that lawyers should be selected based on three criteria: local, right sized, and start-up focused [20].

The Walker Corporate Law Group listed the "Top 10 reasons why entrepreneurs hate lawyers" [21]:

- #10—"Because they don't communicate clearly or concisely"
- #9—"Because they don't keep me informed"

- #8—"Because they are constantly over-lawyering"
- #7—"Because they have poor listening skills"
- #6—"Because inexperienced lawyers are doing most of the work"
- #5—"Because they spend too much time on insignificant issues"
- #4—"Because they don't genuinely care about me or my matter"
- #3—"Because their fees are through the roof"
- #2—"Because they are unresponsive"
- #1—"Because they are deal-killers"

7.6 Managing Managers

Be a coach, not a referee.

As founder, one of your most pressing goals should be to make sure that your managers have all the tools necessary to perform their jobs well. Managers need to understand not only the "what" but also the "why" behind your business plan. Give them a sincere sense of ownership in the organization and its future. Figure 7.7 summarizes the complex issue of managing managers.

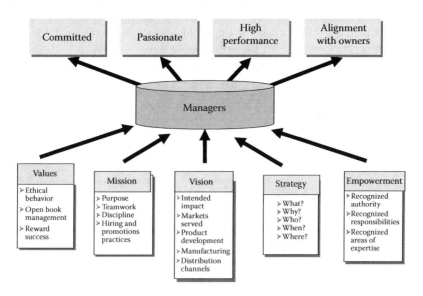

FIGURE 7.7
Managing managers.

7.6.1 How Is Managing Managers Different from Managing Projects?

We must all row in the same direction.

You will find that effective mangers need to know less about "how" and more about "why." Managers should be evaluated primarily on team-based financial success, rather than products, schedules, or activities. Their opinions should carry extra weight along with responsibility and corresponding authority.

7.6.2 A Roadmap for Managing Managers Effectively

Don't bring me problems; bring me solutions.

Bruce McGraw listed the following important leadership skills for senior managers [22]:

- Set the vision. It is essential that you communicate the long-term goals of your department or organization to your managers clearly and often. A shared vision provides the touchstone to help your managers make decisions and solve problems.
- Network with other managers and technical resources to get things done across your organization.
- Set straightforward, measureable objectives for each manager and project under your authority. Have short-term and long-term goals for each person who reports to you and reinforce those goals in monthly or quarterly meetings.
- Talent management—hiring, giving effective feedback, and developing talent for the project work.
- Demonstrating accountability and holding team members and project managers accountable.
- Influencing others—up (your leaders), across (your peers), and down (your project managers and team).
- Facilitate problem solving. It may be tempting to jump in and solve a problem yourself. You have been there and solved that problem successfully before. However, your managers need to learn and they need to put their own stamp on projects.
- Do not micromanage. Let me say that again—do not micromanage. Rather, offer advice and ask leading questions to help clarify a situation and your subordinate manager's options. You are also in a better position than before to break down barriers to solving problems by using your position and influence.

- Be a role model. Social learning theory, also called social cognitive theory, supports the idea that people learn new behaviors and change existing ones based not just on their experience but also on their observations of significant others, such as senior managers. Your values, priorities, and even your mode of dress may be copied.

7.7 The Firing Line

Regardless of how careful you are in hiring your dream team, it may be necessary to dismiss an important team member. No matter the reason, whether poor work performance, inability to act as a team member, or an economic downturn, firing someone is very unpleasant for you and the executive.

As founder, even if the firing is well deserved, in actuality, terminating an executive is never easy considering the disruptions suffered by both the employee and your own team. It is frequently highly emotional, confrontational, and may even carry legal consequences if the employee has not been given enough chances to correct their weaknesses before being dismissed [23].

7.7.1 At-Will Employment versus Employment Contracts

At-will employment is generally described as follows: "Any hiring is presumed to be 'at will'; that is, the employer is free to discharge individuals 'for good cause, or bad cause, or no cause at all,' and the employee is equally free to quit, strike, or otherwise cease work" [24].

At-will employment [25] is a term of art used in US labor law for contractual relationships in which an employee can be dismissed by an employer for any reason (i.e., without having to establish "just cause" for termination) and without warning [26]. When an employee is acknowledged as being hired "at will," courts generally deny the employee any claim for loss resulting from the dismissal. The rule is justified by its proponents on the basis that an employee may be similarly entitled to leave his or her job without reason or warning [27].

7.7.2 Employment Contracts for Key Employees

The doctrine of at-will employment can be overridden by a written contract or civil service statutes (in the case of government employees). As many as 34% of all US employees apparently enjoy the protection of some kind of "just cause" or objectively reasonable requirement for termination that takes them out of the pure "at-will" category, including the 7.5% of unionized private-sector workers, the 0.8% of nonunion private-sector workers protected by union contracts, the 15% of nonunion private-sector workers with individual express contracts that override the at-will doctrine, and the 16% of the total workforce who enjoy civil service protections as public-sector employees [28].

A written employment contract is a document that you and your employee sign, specifying the terms of your relationship. You don't enter into a written contract with every employee you hire. In fact, written employment contracts are generally the exception, rather than the rule. In some situations, however, it makes good sense to ask a key employee to sign a contract. According to the NOLO legal encyclopedia [29], the employment contract can address many aspects of the employment relationship, such as

- Duration of the job (1 year, 2 years, or indefinitely)
- Information about the employee's responsibilities
- The benefits (such as health insurance, vacation leave, disability leave, etc.) the employee will receive
- Grounds for termination
- Limitations on the employee's ability to compete with your business once the employee leaves
- Protection of your trade secrets, client lists, and other sensitive information
- Your ownership of the employee's work product (e.g., if the employee writes books or develops patentable inventions)
- A method for resolving any disputes that arise about the agreement

7.7.3 How to Fire an Employee Correctly

If you have a problem with an employee, you have two choices: (1) try to coach them and work with them to improve their performance, or (2) fire them. Firing an employee can be costly and cause your employee a great deal of emotional and financial difficulties. Done the wrong way, firing someone can also open you or your organization to liability and lawsuits. Unfortunately, however, there are situations where terminating an employee is your best and only option [30].

The following 10 steps are considered appropriate when dealing with troublesome employees:

1. **Set your expectations clearly and concisely.** Discuss with your employees any behavior that could be grounds for termination.
2. **Conduct regular performance appraisals.** Communicate regularly how you view their performance, and how to improve any deficiencies.
3. **Act quickly and decisively when problems are noticed.** Quickly communicate performance problems as soon as you are aware of them, and coach your employee on how to improve their behavior, and what needs to be rectified [31].

4. **Humanely consider personal factors.** Health problems, death in the family, divorce or other relationship trauma, moving stress, and financial troubles are all part of life and can understandably cause otherwise valuable employees to temporarily lose focus.

5. **Focus on the problem and keep copious records.** Have the problem employee sign a document outlining the conversation to cover yourself and the company. It should specifically state that the employee is not admitting fault, but has been told that job performance is not satisfactory and may result in termination.

6. **Termination meeting.** State your case and the reason(s) for termination. You've given the employee ample time to correct any failings, and that hasn't happened.

7. **Aftermath of termination.** You don't need to delineate your reasons— if they need reiteration, they can be stated in a letter. In this case, the less you say the better.

8. **Separation legal details.** Explain the severance package you are offering, if any. If necessary, remind them of any legally binding agreements the employee has signed, such as an agreement not to disclose company secrets. If you are asking the terminated employee to sign legal documents, allow him or her a few days to take the documents home and review them.

9. **Offer assistance.** If the employee worked in good faith, but simply lacked the skills necessary for the job or the right temperament for your company, you may offer to provide a recommendation regarding his or her reliability, attitude, teamwork, and whatever parts of the job were successfully performed.

10. **Separate the person from the problem.** Keep it professional, and not personal. It will help the employee's self-esteem and ability to secure other employment.

References

1. Building a New Venture Team. Chapter 6, http://foba.lakeheadu.ca/hartviksen /3215/Management%20Team.ppt.
2. Allen, K.R. *Launching New Ventures: An Entrepreneurial Approach.* ISBN-10: 053848179X.
3. Katzenbach, J.R. *Teams at the Top.* Harvard Business School Press, McKinsey & Company, Inc., 1998.
4. Smith, D.K. *Make Success Measurable!* John Wiley & Sons, Inc., 1999.
5. Tuckman, B.W., Developmental Sequence in Small Groups, http://openvce.net /sites/default/files/Tuckman1965DevelopmentalSequence.pdf.

6. Smith, M.K. and Bruce W. Tuckman—Forming, storming, norming and performing in groups, the encyclopedia of informal education, www.infed.org/thinkers/tuckman.htm.

7. http://www.nortonrosefulbright.com/files/the-management-of-intellectual-capital-pdf-329kb-99687.pdf

8. https://en.wikipedia.org/wiki/Human_capital

9. http://www.investopedia.com/terms/h/humancapital.asp#ixzz3hTs35Ct3

10. Schultz, T.W. Investment in Human Capital, *The American Economic Review*, 51:1, 1–17, 1961.

11. Task Force on Human Capital Management. 2003. Accounting for People Report. UK Department for Trade and Industry, http://webarchive.national archives.gov.uk/20090609003228/http://www.berr.gov.uk/files/file38839.pdf.

12. Mitchell, D. and Lawler, E. *Alternative Pay Systems, Firm Performance and Productivity*. Center for Effective Organization Publication G 89-6 (149). School of Business Administration, University of Southern California, 1989.

13. https://en.wikipedia.org/wiki/Knowledge_management

14. http://web.archive.org/web/20070319233812/http://www.unc.edu/~sunnyliu/inls258/Introduction_to_Knowledge_Management.html

15. Gupta, J. and Sharma, S. *Creating Knowledge Based Organizations*. Idea Group Publishing, Boston, 2004. ISBN 1-59140-163-1.

16. http://www.providersedge.com/docs/km_articles/IDC_KM_Study_April_2002.pdf

17. Nonaka, I. The knowledge creating company. *Harvard Business Review*, 69(6), 96–104, 1991.

18. http://www.umsl.edu/~lacitym/evekmbif7.ppt

19. Seven Ways to Create Value through Knowledge, May 2002, http://www.skyrme.com/kshop/kmseven_p4.pdf.

20. Loblow, B. http://www.bothsidesofthetable.com/2010/01/21/how-to-work-with-lawyers-at-a-startup/.

21. Walker, S.E., Top 10 reasons why entrepreneurs hate lawyers, http://venture hacks.com/articles/hate-lawyers.

22. McGraw, B. Managing Managers Requires Good Leadership Skills, May 12, 2011, http://fearnoproject.com/2011/05/12/managing-managers-requires-good-leadership-skills/.

23. Muenz, R. The Firing Line. *Lab Manager*, December 2014, http://www.labmanager.com/leadership-and-staffing/2014/11/the-firing-line#.VOJDYz-DiqQ.

24. Rothstein, M.A., Knapp, A.S., and Liebman, L. *Cases and Materials on Employment Law*. Foundation Press, New York, p. 738, 1987.

25. http://en.wikipedia.org/wiki/At-will_employment

26. Shepherd, J. *Firing at Will: A Manager's Guide*. Apress Media, 3–4, 2011.

27. Epstein, R. *In Defense of the Contract at Will*, 57 U. Chi. L. Rev. 947, 1984.

28. Verkerke, J.H. Discharge, in Dau-Schmidt, K.G., Harris, S.D. and Lobel, O., eds., *Labor and Employment Law and Economics*, vol. 2 of *Encyclopedia of Law and Economics*, 2nd ed., pp. 447–479. Northampton: Edward Elgar Publishing, 448, 2009.

29. http://www.nolo.com/legal-encyclopedia/written-employment-contracts-pros-cons-30193.html

30. How to fire an employee. Wikipedia, http://www.wikihow.com/Fire-an-Employee.

31. Cliff, E. The right way to fire someone. *Entrepreneur*, September 2006, http://www.entrepreneur.com/article/166644.

8

Strategic Planning for Start-Ups

Plans are nothing. Planning is everything.

Dwight D. Eisenhower

8.1 Introduction

Strategic planning is a tool for organizing the present on the basis of the projections of the desired future. That is, a strategic plan is a roadmap to lead an organization from where it is now to where it would like to be in 5 or 10 years.

It is necessary to have a strategic plan for your chapter or division. In order to develop a comprehensive plan for your chapter or division that would include both long-range and strategic elements, we suggest the methods and mechanisms outlined in this manual.

Your plan must

Be simple to follow.

Be written logically and purposefully.

Be clear to everyone.

Be based on the real current situation.

Have enough time allowed to give it a time to settle. It should not be rushed.

Over the past decades, you may have witnessed an explosion in the use of management tools and techniques—everything from Six Sigma to benchmarking. Keeping up with the latest and greatest, as well as deciding which tools to put to work, is a key part of every leader's job. But it's tough to pick the winners from the losers.

As new management tools appear every year, others seem to drop off the radar screen. Unfortunately, there is no official scorekeeper for management tools. Thus, choosing and using "fad management" tools can become a risky and potentially expensive gamble, leaving many business leaders stymied and confused [1].

Since 1993, Bain & Company, a leading management consulting company, launched a multiyear research project to get the facts about management tools and trends. The objective of the study was to provide managers with information to identify and integrate tools that improve bottom-line results as well as understand their strategic challenges and priorities.

Bain systematically assembled a database that now includes nearly 8000 businesses from more than 70 countries in North America, Europe, Asia, Africa, the Middle East, and Latin America. The *Bain & Company's 2005 Management Tools* survey received responses from a broad range of international executives. To qualify for inclusion in the study, a tool had to be relevant to senior management, topical as evidenced by coverage in the business press, and measurable. Bain focused on the most discussed management tools as shown in Table 8.1.

Would you like to know the surprising results? Out of all the management tools surveyed, 79% of respondents preferred strategic planning, followed closely by customer relationship management at 75%. In fact, strategic planning is a long-time favorite tool, having been used by more than half of companies in every survey since Bain started this project. Not surprisingly, the most popular tools are the ones that create the highest returns and results-oriented ratings [2]. See Table 8.2 for more details.

TABLE 8.1

Most Frequently Discussed Management Tools

1. Activity-based management	14. Mission and vision statements
2. Balanced scorecard	15. Offshoring
3. Benchmarking	16. Open market innovation
4. Business process reengineering	17. Outsourcing
5. Change management programs	18. Price optimization models
6. Core competencies	19. Radio frequency identification (RFID)
7. Customer relationship management (CRM)	20. Scenario and contingency planning
8. Customer segmentation	21. Six sigma
9. Economic value added analysis	22. Strategic alliances
10. Growth strategies	23. Strategic planning
11. Knowledge management	24. Supply chain management
12. Loyalty management	25. Total quality management
13. Mass customization	

Source: Modified after Bain & Company (2005). http://www.bain.com/management_tools /Management_Tools_and_Trends_2005.pdf.

TABLE 8.2

Top Five Management Tools Ranked by Usage Rate

Management Tool Name	Usage (%)
Strategic management	79
Customer relationship management	75
Benchmarking	73
Outsourcing	73
Customer segmentation	72

Source: Modified after Bain & Company (2005). http://www.bain.com/management_tools /Management_Tools_and_Trends_2005.pdf.

8.2 Strategic Planning for Start-Ups

Strategic planning is the process used by an organization to visualize its desired future and develop the necessary steps and operations to achieve those aims. It directs managers to determine how they will be expected to behave. In order to determine the direction of the organization, it is necessary to understand its current position and the possible avenues through which it can pursue a particular course of action. Generally, strategic planning deals with at least one of three key questions [3]:

1. "What do we do?"
2. "For whom do we do it?"
3. "How do we excel?"

The key components of "strategic planning" include an understanding of the firm's vision, mission, values, and strategies [4]. (Often a "Vision Statement" and a "Mission Statement" may encapsulate the vision and mission.)

- **Vision:** Outlines what the organization wants to be, or how it wants the world in which it operates to be (an "idealized" view of the world). It is a long-term view and concentrates on the future. It can be emotive and is a source of inspiration. For example, a charity working with the poor might have a vision statement which reads "A World Without Disease."

- **Mission:** Defines the fundamental purpose of an organization or an enterprise, succinctly describing why it exists and what it does to achieve its vision. For example, the charity above might have a mission statement as "providing jobs for the homeless and unemployed."

- **Values:** Beliefs that are shared among the stakeholders of an organization. Values drive an organization's culture and priorities and provide a framework in which decisions are made. For example, "Knowledge and skills are the keys to success" or "Give a man bread and feed him for a day, but teach him to farm and feed him for life." These example maxims may set the priorities of self-sufficiency over shelter.

- **Strategy:** Strategy, narrowly defined, means "the art of the general"— a combination of the ends (goals) for which the firm is striving and the means (policies) by which it is seeking to get there. A strategy is sometimes called a roadmap—which is the path chosen to plow toward your end vision. The most important part of implementing the strategy is ensuring that the company goes in the right direction, which is toward the end vision.

Unlike operational planning—which stresses how to get things done—and long-range planning—which primarily focuses on translating goals and objectives into current budgets and work programs—strategic planning is concerned with identifying barriers and issues to overcome. Managers are more likely to act on the assumption that current trends will continue into the future (steady-state management), while entrepreneurs need to anticipate new trends and possible surprises that represent both opportunities and threats.

8.3 Your Value Chain Analysis

The term **value chain** was first used by Michael Porter in *Competitive Advantage: Creating and Sustaining Superior Performance* [5]. The value chain analysis describes the activities that an organization must undertake and links them to its competitive strength and position.

The value chain concept revolves around the notion that an organization is more than just an agglomeration of machinery, equipment, facilities, technology, and human resources. Only when these support activities are aligned with primary activities will customers be persuaded to buy its products or services. The combination of all these factors becomes the source of competitive advantage. This is illustrated in Figure 8.1.

Notice the important distinction between primary and support activities. **Primary activities** are those directly involved with the creation or delivery of your product or service. **Support activities** help improve effectiveness or efficiency of the operation. **Profit margin** is the ability of the organization to

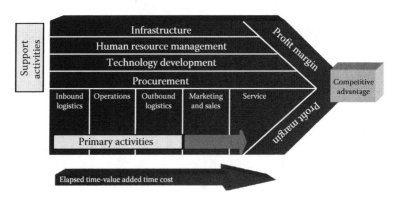

FIGURE 8.1
Porter's value chain. (Source: Modified after Porter 1985.)

successfully deliver a product/service at a price that is higher than the combined costs of all the activities in the value chain. The numerical difference between price and cost is your profit margin.

You should perform your competitive advantage analysis within your value chain by

- Analyzing which costs are related to every single activity
- Determining the optimal price of your product/service to your customer
- Identifying potential cost advantages you may have over your competitors
- Analyzing how your product/service potentially adds value (lower cost, higher performance, user-friendly, just-in-time delivery, etc.) to your customer's value chain

---

8.4 Your Value Proposition

> Killing two stones with one bird.

A **value proposition** is a promise of worth to be delivered and a belief from the customer that profit will be experienced. A value proposition can apply to an entire organization, or parts thereof, or customer accounts, or products or services. Creating a value proposition is a part of business strategy [6]. Developing a value proposition is based on a review and analysis of the benefits, costs, and value that an organization can deliver to its customers, prospective customers, and other constituent groups within and outside the organization. It is also a positioning of value, where Value = Benefits − Uncertainty (includes economic risk) [7].

Why should anyone buy anything from you? What do you have to offer? New products are "new" and therefore untested; generally, they cannot attract customers. The value proposition is best quantified by the value equation as shown in Figure 8.2 [8].

In order to attract their customers, entrepreneurs need to develop a compelling value proposition. As seen in Figure 8.2, a customer would be persuaded to buy your new product/service if (a) the benefits outweigh his costs/risks and (b) it solves a major serious problem. Figure 8.3 presents a stepwise process for establishing your value proposition.

$$\text{Value} = (\text{seriousness of problem} + \text{benefits}) - (\text{cost of solution} + \text{risks})$$
$$\text{Value} = (\text{benefits}) - (\text{implementation uncertainties})$$

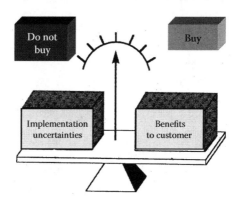

FIGURE 8.2
Value equation. (Modified after Rackham, *Spin Selling*, McGraw-Hill Book Co © 1998.)

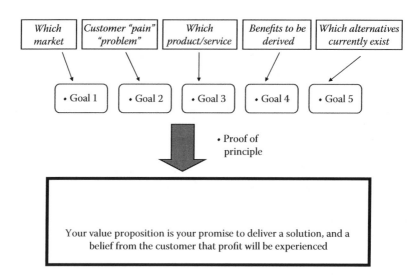

FIGURE 8.3
Value proposition.

Examples of value propositions (also called company slogans):

Coke	The pause that refreshes
FedEx	The world on time
E. F. Hutton	When E. F. Hutton speaks, people listen
American Express	Don't leave home without it
Lexus	The passionate pursuit of perfection
IBM	Global solutions for a small planet
Apple	The power to be your best
DeBeers	A diamond is forever
Visa	It is everywhere you want it to be
Intel	Intel inside
AT&T	Reach out and touch someone
BMW	The ultimate driving machine
FOX	Fair and balanced
CNN	The most trusted name in news
Clairol	Only her hairdresser knows for sure

8.5 SWOT Analysis

A **SWOT** analysis is a strategic planning tool used to evaluate the **S**trengths, **W**eaknesses, **O**pportunities, and **T**hreats involved in a project or in a business venture. It involves specifying the objective of the business venture or project and identifying the internal and external factors that are favorable and unfavorable to achieving that objective. The technique is credited to Albert Humphrey [9], who led a research project at Stanford University in the 1960s and 1970s using data from Fortune 500 companies.

- **Strengths:** attributes of the organization helpful to achieving the objective
- **Weaknesses:** attributes of the organization harmful to achieving the objective
- **Opportunities:** *external* conditions helpful to achieving the objective
- **Threats:** *external* conditions harmful to achieving the objective

A generic SWOT analysis is presented in Figure 8.4.
Your SWOT analysis should be conducted as follows:

- **Step 1.** The present. List all your current strengths and weaknesses.
- **Step 2.** The future. List all future opportunities and strengths.

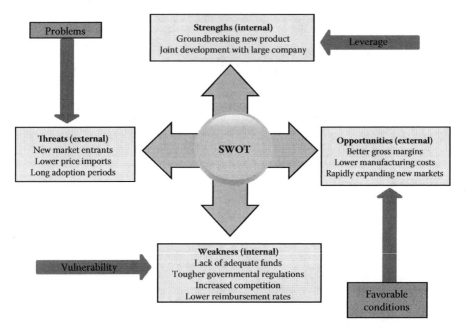

FIGURE 8.4
Generic SWOT analysis.

- **Step 3.** Your action plan. Address all four areas individually.
- **Step 4.** Develop an operational plan, complete with specific tasks and dates of completion.

8.6 Recognizing Growth Stages

Small business success doesn't just happen. Some fairly predictable but not very orderly (chaotic) stages characterize its evolution. Most entrepreneurs caught up in the day-to-day goings on in a business don't recognize these stages until they've passed, though. Time to open your eyes. The following sections describe the three stages of business evolution.

8.6.1 The Start-Up Years

The start-up years are the years when survival motivates your thoughts and actions. Everything that happens within the business is dominated by you; words such as *delegation, team,* and *consensus* generally are not yet part of the business's vocabulary. These are the hands-on years. For some owners, they're the most enjoyable years of the business; for all owners, they're an integral part of the learning process.

The work during this time is exceptionally hard—often the physically and emotionally draining kind of hard. The hours are long and sometimes tedious, but by the end of the day, you can see, touch, and feel the progress you've made. The gratification is instantaneous. The duration of this first stage can vary greatly. Some businesses may fly through the start-up stage in less than a year, but most spend anywhere from 1 to 3 years growing out of the stage. Others—oftentimes those in the more competitive niches—spend as many as five or more years in the start-up stage.

You'll know you've graduated from the start-up stage when profitability and orderliness become a dependable part of your business. The hectic days of worrying about survival are replaced by the logical, orderly days of planning for success.

8.6.2 The Growth Years

The growth years are the years when your business achieves some sense of order, stability, and profitability. Your evolving business has survived the mistakes, confusion, and chaos of the start-up years, and now optimism, camaraderie, and cooperation should play an important role in the organization.

Key employees surface, efficient administrative systems and controls become part of the business's daily operating procedures, and the need to depend on you for everything disappears.

The business of doing business remains fun for most small business owners in this stage, because increasing sales translate into increasing profits every small business owner's dream. The balance sheet puts some flesh on its scraggly bones as you generate cash as a result of profitability. You learn to delegate many of those unpleasant tasks that you performed in the past.

Survival is no longer your primary motivator. At last, the daily choices that you make can be dictated by lifestyle goals instead of survival. We have further good news: This stage can last a long time if the growth is gradual and remains under control, and if you manage the business and its expanding population of employees properly.

8.6.3 The Transition Years

The third stage, the transition years, can also be called the restructuring stage or the diversification stage. This is the stage when something basic to the success of the growth years has changed or gone wrong. As a result, in order for the business to survive, a strategic change in direction, or transition, is required.

Many factors can bring about the transition period, but the following are the most common:

- Relentless growth: This is because relentless sales growth requires relentless improvement in the business's employees, systems, procedures, and infrastructure—and many businesses simply can't keep up with such pressures.

- Shrinkage of sales and the disappearance of profits, or even prolonged periods of stagnation: This is the opposite of growth. The causes for this shrinkage or stagnation can come from anywhere and everywhere, and they often include such uncontrollable factors as new competitors, a changing economy, new technology, and changes in consumer demand.

8.7 How to Think Like an Executive

You decided to start your own company because you are a specialist in some technical field. Your technical expertise allowed you to innovate a new product that you want to commercialize as soon as possible.

You were the acknowledged specialist as a researcher/inventor. Surprisingly, as an owner, you must now become the great generalist. Being a generalist means knowing your specialty, but also knowing (and appreciating) about all the other specialties needed to build a successful company. Now, you must think like an executive, not like a specialist, a researcher, or an inventor.

8.7.1 The Great Irony

There is only one generalist job in a start-up and that is the job of the owner/inventor. However, there is no generalist path that gets you there. Ironically, it takes a specialist path to prepare you for the generalist's top job (i.e., the executive).

First, you must be a specialist in some advanced technical field, such as medical science, pharmacology, engineering, life sciences, computer science, telecommunications, and the like. As an owner/inventor, you must be able to become an orchestra conductor, not just a great instrument player, and still perform a brilliant job in your specialty. This is graphically depicted in Figure 8.5.

8.7.2 Your Team Depends on You

Your team members want to know the mission, vision, direction, and status of the company on a periodic basis, and that can only come from the communications ability of the owner/inventor. As top dog, you must be the ultimate communicator, coach, counselor, pacifier, and arbiter, particularly during conflicts, as shown in Figure 8.6.

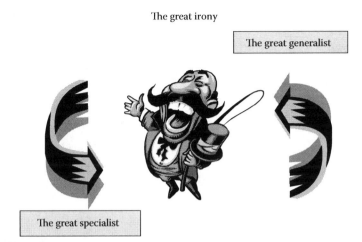

FIGURE 8.5
You, as the greatest generalist.

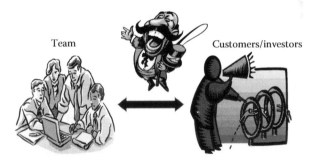

FIGURE 8.6
You, the great communicator.

Each team member wants to know how they fit into the overall organizational structure, and what is their future as the organization grows. You must provide the tools, resources, and empowerment to your team to allow them to do their specialized jobs.

8.7.3 Sole Proprietorship or Partnership?

Sole ownership is always the least conflictive and most popular of the options for starting a company, assuming that you have access to the necessary funds to launch your business, industry knowledge, and energy to make a go of the business by yourself. Sure, the leverage and financial benefits that partners and shareholders bring to the table can be worth their weight in potential opportunities, but decision-making in shared ownership situations requires consensus, and consensus can take a lot of time. Besides, consensus doesn't always represent your own personal best interests, and when your name is on the dotted line, your personal best interests should be at or near the top of the reasons for making decisions.

8.7.3.1 Being the Sole Owner

Being the sole owner has the following advantages:

- It's generally easier, quicker, and less expensive. No lawyers are required to write partnership agreements and assist in determining answers to all the questions that partnership agreements require.
- The profits (or losses) are totally yours.
- You have no need to seek consensus. Your way is the only way.
- You don't waste time catering to the often-aggravating demands of shareholders, minority or otherwise. There's no possibility of shareholder lawsuits.

Being the sole owner also has the following disadvantages:

- You have no one to share the risk with you.
- Your limited skills will have to make do until you can hire someone with complementary skills.
- Single ownership can be lonely. Many times, you'll wish you had someone with whom to share the problems and stress. You may be able to do this with trusted, senior employees. Of course, if you have good friends or a strong marriage partner, these people can be a source of much needed support.

Still confused as to whether you want to do it alone or share ownership? Answer the following questions to help with the decision.

8.7.3.2 Partnership?

Do you absolutely, positively need a partner? To provide cash? Knowledge? If you do, that settles the issue; if you don't, continue with the following questions:

- Are you capable of working with partners or shareholders? Will you have a problem sharing the decisions and the profits as well as the risks?
- Does your business fit the multiple ownership profile? In other words, does this business have room for two partners, and is it a business that has the growth potential to support two partners? Will a partner have an important role in the organization? Would his or her complementary skills enhance the business's chance for success?

- What are the legal requirements of multiple ownership? Can you live within these legal parameters?

- What do you have in common with other business owners who have opted for multiple ownership? Where do you see conflicts? Ask your banker, accountant, or attorney for the names of other business owners who have opted for multiple ownership. Interview those owners. Get their feedback on the list of pluses and minuses.

- What's the likelihood of finding a partner with complementary skills and a personality compatible with yours? This ability depends on how wired into the business community you are and the line of work you're going into. If you have a lot of business contacts and know exactly what you want, finding a partner may be easy. More typically, it isn't.

If you opt for multiple ownership, you'll live with the decision for a long, long time. If you elect sole ownership at the start, however, you can always seek partners later if you feel that you need them for the business success that you desire.

Partners make sense when they can bring needed capital to the business along with complementary management skills. Unfortunately, partners also present the opportunity for turmoil, and, especially in the early stages of a business's growth, turmoil takes time, burns energy, and costs money—all of which most small-business founders lack.

A partnership in the right hands will outperform a sole proprietorship in the right hands, any day. Having *minority shareholders* (any and all shareholders who collectively own less than 50%) can also make sense, especially after the business is out of the blocks and has accumulated value.

However, minority shareholders can be a pain; they have legal rights that often run counter to the wishes of the majority. Because majority shareholders are ceded the right to make the final decisions, courts have determined that minority shareholders must have an avenue of appeal. Thus, minority shareholders, particularly in our litigious society, sometimes look to the courts whenever they feel their rights of ownership are being violated. Unfortunately, shareholder suits are a sign of the times.

Occasionally, especially where venture capital financing is involved, the founder of the business may find himself or herself working for majority shareholders. Fortunately, this situation rarely occurs because the typical small business founder has already proven that taking orders from others is not exactly one of his or her inherent strengths. We've found that, on the infrequent occasions when this situation does occur, more often than not the founder of the company is the first one to get the boot when the going gets tough, as the chief financiers step in to protect their investment. That's why we strongly recommend that you find a way to retain majority control.

8.7.3.3 Getting a Business Partner

Here's a fact that not everyone knows: According to studies, partnerships outperform sole proprietorships by a wide margin. We're not talking rocket science here; this statement is nothing more than a simple fact of life: two heads are better than one!

Sometimes, one plus one equals significantly more than two if the partners can blend their skills and talents. In other words, synergy. (Google, Apple Computer, and Hewlett Packard are examples of companies that began as partnerships.)

So, why may a partnership make sense to you? Here are some reasons:

Although you're probably aware of your own strengths, your human nature lets you more easily overlook your weaknesses. Ask those who know you well—family, friends, and current or previous coworkers—what complementary skills you should seek in a business partner. Consider the following advantages:

- Additional capital: Two savings accounts are better than one.
- Greater problem-solving capacity.
- More flexibility: One partner goes on vacation or gets sick, the other one minds the store.
- Ease of formation: Legally speaking, partnerships are easier and less expensive to form than corporations.
- Less risk: Profits aren't the only thing partnerships share.

How do you find a partner (or partners)? The same way you locate a key employee, a consultant, or a mentor. Clearly identify your need (in this case, the skills you're looking for) and then network your available resources.

When forming a partnership, you're beginning what you hope will be a long-term relationship—a long-term relationship that oftentimes rivals marriage in terms of complexity. If you're smart, you can determine a way to test the chemistry of the partnership before you get too far involved, and cannot get out.

Want to read a business partner joke? Here is one for you [10]:

> A very successful businessman had a meeting with his new son-in-law. "I love my daughter, and now I welcome you into the family," said the man. "To show you how much we care for you, I'm making you a 50–50 partner in my business. All you have to do is go to the factory every day and learn the operations."
>
> The son-in-law interrupted, "I hate factories. I can't stand the noise."

"I see," replied the father-in-law. "Well then you'll work in the office and take charge of some of the operations."

"I hate office work," said the son-on-law. "I can't stand being stuck behind a desk all day."

"Wait a minute," said the father-in-law. "I just made you a half-owner of a highly profitable corporation, but you don't like factories and won't work in a office. What am I going to do with you?"

"Easy," said the young man. "Buy me out!!!"

8.8 Competitive Intelligence

According to Jane Hodges in *MoneyWatch* [11], there is nothing unethical about CI. Most of the time, it simply involves gathering together pieces of a puzzle that are available to anyone—if they have the time and the determination to find them.

But because the search can be tedious, it is tempting to look for shortcuts to get the needed information, especially when time is tight. When that happens, legal and ethical lines may be crossed. Table 8.3 lists some of the most common tactics that may get you into trouble.

Modern CI is often divided into four different, but overlapping, types: (1) strategic, (2) competitor, (3) tactical, and (4) technical.

TABLE 8.3

Competitive Intelligence Tactics to Avoid

Tactics	Description
Pretext	Approaching a source under false identity or deceptive pretense
Dumpster mining (diving)	Surreptitiously gathering discarded key documents through garbage or empty raw material pails on dumpsters
CDA, NDA bypassing	Encouraging a source to violate terms of a noncompete or nondisclosure agreement (NDA) they signed with their employer
Acquiring trade secrets	Finding the proprietary advantage to a competitor's success, specifically when it's a closely guarded secret, such as stealing formulas or software proprietary codes
Paying sources for proprietary information	Giving cash to someone who can tell you what you want to know about a competitor
Enticement recruitment	Deliberately targeting competitor's key employees with the purpose of obtaining trade secrets
Computer hacking	Penetrating competitor's computer systems to gain access to proprietary information on pricing, business plans, customer lists, etc.

8.8.1 Strategic Intelligence

Strategic intelligence is CI supporting strategic, as distinguished from tactical decision-making. This means providing higher levels intelligence on the competitive, economic regulatory, and political environment in which you firm operates now and in which it will operate in the future.

Who and What Does Strategic Intelligence Help?
Strategic intelligence is typically used by senior managers and executives who make and then execute overall corporate strategy. Its most common applications are in the development of the following:

- Long-term (3- to 5-year) strategic plans
- Capital investment plans
- Political risk assessments
- Merger and acquisition, joint venture, and corporate alliance policies and plans
- Research and development planning

What Does Strategic Intelligence Focus on?
Strategic intelligence usually focuses on the overall strategic environment. A firm's direct competitive environment and its direct competitors are, of course, included in that focus. It should also include its indirect competitors. In addition, strategic intelligence should develop CI on the long-run changes caused by, as well as affecting, all of the forces driving industry competition, including the following:

- Suppliers
- Customers
- Substitute products or service
- Potential competitors

You conduct strategic CI analysis when you must focus on many critical factors, such as technology trends, regulatory developments, and even political risks that, in turn, affect these forces. Strategic intelligence's focus is less on the present than it is on the past, and is primarily on the future. The time horizon of interest typically runs from 2 years in the past to 5 or even 10 years in the future.

- In terms of an interest in the past, you will be collecting and analyzing data so that your firm can evaluate the actual success (or failure) of its own strategies and of those of your competitors. This, in turn permits you to better weigh options for the future. You are looking to the past to learn what may happen in the future.

- With respect to the future, you are seeking a view of your firm's total environment: competitive, regulatory and political. As with radar, you are looking for warnings of impending problems, and alerts to upcoming opportunities—always in time to take needed action.

Who and What Does Competitor Intelligence Help?

Competitor intelligence is most often used by strategic planning operations or by operating managers within strategic business units. It may also be useful to product managers, as well as to those involved with product development, new business development, and mergers and acquisitions.

What Does Competitor Intelligence Focus on?

Competitor intelligence usually helps you answer a wide variety of key business questions, including ones such as these:

- Who are our competitors right now?
- Who are our potential competitors?
- How do our competitors see themselves? How do they see us?
- What are the track records of the key people at our competitors? What are their personalities? What is the environment in their own company? What difference do these people make in terms of our ability to predict how these competitors will react to our competitive strategy?
- How and where are our competitors marketing their products/ services? What new directions will they probably take?
- What markets or geographic areas will (or won't) be tapped by our competitors in the future?
- How have our competitors responded to the short- and long-term trends in our industry in the past? How are they likely to respond to them in the future?
- What patents or innovative technology have our competitors or potential competitors recently obtained or developed? What do those changes and innovations mean to us?
- What are our competitors' overall plans and goals for the next 1–2 years in the markets where they currently compete with us? What are their plans and goals for their other firms and how will those affect the way they run their business competing with us?
- Competitor intelligence's time horizon typically runs from 6 to 12 months in the past to 1–2 years in the future.

Who and What Does Technical Intelligence Help?
Technical intelligence is particularly useful if you are involved with your firm's research and development activities. Using basic CI techniques, those practicing technical intelligence now often can determine the following:

- Competitors' current manufacturing methods and processes
- A competitor's access to, use of, and dependence on, outside technology, as well as its need for new technology
- Key patents and proprietary technology being used by, being developed by, or being acquired by competitors
- Types and levels of research and development conducted by competitors, as well as estimates of their current and future expenditures for research and development
- The size and capabilities of competitors' research staff

8.8.2 Business Intelligence

"Business intelligence" is a particularly difficult term to deal with. At one time, this term was actually used by some CI professionals to describe CI in a very broad way, and to describe only intelligence provided in support of corporate strategy by others. Now, its use seems to have been fully co-opted by those involved with data management and data warehousing. There, it can refer to

- The software used to manage vast amounts of data
- The process of managing that data, also called data mining
- The output of either of the first two

In summary, virtually all of the reported applications and successes of business intelligence deal with processes that are internally oriented, from process control to logistics, and from sales forecasting to quality control. The most that can be said of its relationship to intelligence is that data mining and related techniques are useful tools for some early analysis and sorting tasks that would be impossible for human analysts.

8.8.3 Ten Commandments of CI

In 1988, Fuld and Company [12] published its "Ten Commandments of Legal and Ethical Intelligence Gathering":

1. Thou shall not lie when representing thyself.
2. Thou shall observe thy company's legal guidelines.

3. Thou shall not tape record a conversation.

4. Thos shall not bribe.

5. Thou shall not plant eavesdropping devices.

6. Thou shall not mislead anyone in an interview.

7. Thou shall neither obtain nor give price information to thy competitor.

8. Thou shall not swap misinformation.

9. Thou shall not steal a trade secret.

10. Thou shall not knowingly press someone if it may jeopardize that person's job or reputation.

References

1. Olsen, E. *Strategic Planning for Dummies*. Wiley Publishing Inc., Hoboken, NJ, 2007.
2. http://www.bain.com/management_tools/Management_Tools_and_Trends _2005.pdf
3. Renger, R. and Titcomb, A. A three step approach to teaching logic models. *American Journal of Evaluation*, 23(4), 493–503, 2002.
4. Wikipedia, https://en.wikipedia.org/wiki/Strategic_planning
5. Porter, M.E. *Competitive Advantage: Creating and Sustaining Superior Performance*. The Free Press, 1985.
6. Value proposition, http://en.wikipedia.org/wiki/Value_proposition
7. Kaplan, R.S. and Norton, D.P. Strategy maps: Converting intangible assets into tangible outcomes. *Harvard Business Press*, 2004. ISBN 978-1-59139-134-0. Retrieved September 21, 2011.
8. Rackham, N., McGraw-Hill Book Co., Toronto, ON, 1988.
9. Humphrey, A. SWOT Analysis for Management Consulting. *SRI Alumni Newsletter* (SRI International), 2005.
10. http://www.notboring.com/jokes/work/5.htm
11. Hodges, J. Thou shall not steal your competitors secrets. *Moneywatch*, March 28, 2007, http://www.cbsnews.com/news/thou-shalt-not-steal-thy-competitors -secrets.
12. http://cdn2.hubspot.net/hub/17073/file-13332891-pdf/resource-center/fuld -and-company-new-competitor-intelligence-excerpt.pdf

9

Virtual Organizations

9.1 Introduction

The adoption of the Internet for business use has led toward the emergence of "virtual" organizations. The five primary motives of enterprises to "go virtual" are summarized as follows:

- Reduced costs and enhanced productivity
- Increased satisfaction, closer teamwork, greater flexibility, and the retention of valued employees
- Decentralization of control, with increased flexible working patterns
- Empowerment of the workforce, improved decision making, and increased outsourcing
- Paradigm shift from hierarchical organizational structures to flatter organizations

If you founded a traditional company, then everyone on your team would work out of the same office, you would install a water cooler, a fruit smoothie stand, and a snack station where your employees could catch up on the latest gossip. You would recognize each person by first name, and you would ask about each other's kids, pets, hobbies, and other goings-on. You'd host annual picnics and holiday parties.

When your business is virtual, that whole "bonding" thing gets a little more complicated.

There are no water coolers to gather around. You rarely if ever see your employees in person, and you probably don't know their spouses' names, let alone the names of their kids and pets, or what they do in their free time. There are no annual picnics or holiday parties, because you all live in different cities and/or countries. Figure 9.1 presents an example of a virtual organization.

As a business owner managing a virtual team, your challenge is to look past physical distance and still create a cohesive and conscious virtual

Example of a "virtual" organization

- The technology completed by a virtual team
- The authors are in California and New York
- The prototype is made in Massachusetts
- The pilot production is made in China
- The proof of concept is performed in Ohio
- Deadlines are coordinated by the team leader in Massachusetts

FIGURE 9.1
Virtual organizations have no boundaries.

Traditional	Virtual
• Employee recruitment and utilization at one location only	• Employee recruitment in any geographical location
• Communications and brainstorming are face to face and frequent	• Communication via telephone, e-mail, videoconferencing, social networking, etc.
• Fixed work hours	• Flexible work hours
• Work limited to work place	• Work performed from any suitable location

FIGURE 9.2
Traditional versus virtual companies.

culture—a company culture tailored to the needs of your virtual business and remote employees.

Figure 9.2 summarizes some of the most glaring differences between traditional and virtual companies.

9.2 Is a Virtual (Boundaryless) Company in Your Future?

Virtual or boundaryless companies are those in which the boundaries, including vertical, horizontal, external, and geographic boundaries, are dynamic. Table 9.1 shows the most important characteristics of virtual companies.

Virtual organizations are not for everyone. Going virtual sounds easy and straightforward, but before deciding to "go virtual," you must consider the advantages and disadvantages shown in Table 9.2.

9.2.1 Functional (Bricks and Mortar) or Virtual?

Functional or traditional organizational structures employ a familiar power dynamic: Somebody leads, others follow, with extra managers selected to

TABLE 9.1

Characteristics of Virtual Companies

Management	Divisional Structure
Simplest, highly informal	Organized around products, projects, or markets
Coordination of tasks by direct supervision	Executives help determine product–market and financial objectives
Few rules and regulations, informal evaluation and reward system	Largely autonomous and self-directed Requires "self-starters"
Collaborative work is usually conducted virtually rather than face to face	80% of work time spent communicating, and 20% of work is accomplished independently
Project manager could be located in the United States, while the developers are in Asia	Changes the traditional concept of the "office" and "bricks-and-mortar"

TABLE 9.2

Going Virtual Pros and Cons

Advantages	Disadvantages
Shifts employees focus from activities to results	Reduces personal contact with decision makers, isolating crucial communications
Reduces real estate expenses	Disperses employees, making personal communication difficult
Provides access to global markets and presents a local face to global clients	Potential intercultural or policy clashes between teams
Allows employees a more flexible schedule	Blurs the separation between work and personal life
Opportunity to hold meetings and establish presence despite distance or location	Specialized equipment is not accessible to multiple users
Work environment without geographical boundaries	Requires technology such as telephones, Internet tools, computers
Maximum personal autonomy	No daily face-to-face contact with co-workers or supervisors

help run things smoothly, efficiently, and predictably. Many companies still use this structure of top boss, middle management, and employees because it provides control and stability. Functional structures divide technical activities into semiautonomous groups composed of highly specialized individuals, as shown in Figure 9.3.

In contrast to functional structures, virtual companies perform most of their business transactions through the Internet and e-commerce, typically do not have headquarters or an office space, and operate with a very small staff. Most aspects of their business, including research and development, marketing, and sales, are typically outsourced. Staff interactions are conducted by telecommunications, and the primary managerial role of the virtual company is to monitor and manage the outsourced activities.

- Structure provides a means of balancing two conflicting forces
  - Need for the division of tasks into meaningful groupings
  - Need to integrate the groupings for efficiency and effectiveness

FIGURE 9.3
Traditional forms of organizational structure.

By minimizing their infrastructure ("bricks and mortar"), the virtual company keeps its operating costs to a minimum. A simple definition of globalization is the interweaving of markets, technology, information systems, and telecommunications networks in a way that is shrinking the world from a size medium to a size small, according to Thomas L. Friedman, author of *The World Is Flat: A Brief History of the Twenty-First Century*, which is an international bestselling book that analyzes globalization, primarily in the early 21st century.

A **"virtual"** business employs electronic means to transact business as opposed to a traditional brick-and-mortar business that relies on face-to-face transactions with physical documents and physical buildings. By minimizing their infrastructure (bricks and mortar), the virtual company keeps its operating costs to a minimum.

9.2.2 Networking Technologies

Web 2.0 networking technologies—wikis, blogs, YouTube, Skype, Facebook, MySpace, Twitter, Dig, and the like—were fringe technologies or did not exist a decade ago. Now, they are mainstream, and businesses worldwide are rapidly adopting them. Video communications are beginning to replace time-consuming, time-intensive business travel, and instantaneous communications regardless of distance are on the horizon.

Common communication tools utilized when working virtually:

- Conference calls
- OnSync
- WebEx
- Highrise
- eBuddy
- Google Docs
- MPK20
- Facetime
- GoToMeeting

9.3 Virtual Management

The term *virtual management* is quite recent and was brought about by the rise of the Internet, globalization, outsourcing, telecommuting, and virtual teams. Its management is frequently composed of widely dispersed groups and individuals who rarely, if ever, meet face to face [1]. Traditional forms of organizational structures historically provided management with a ready-made means to balancing two conflicting forces, as shown in Figure 9.4.

Due to developments in information technology within the workplace, along with a need to compete globally and address competitive demands, organizations have embraced virtual management structures. Virtual teams are typically composed of team members who are not located face to face, and their communication is mediated through information and communication technologies (e.g., video conferencing, e-mail, and intranets). Virtual teams represent an important emerging organizational structure that facilitates collaboration between team members located almost anywhere in the world. It is estimated that 41 million corporate employees globally will spend at least 1 day a week as a virtual worker and 100 million will work from home at least 1 day a month.

The implementation of a virtual team structure has been shown to produce many benefits including reduced real estate expenses, increased productivity, access to global markets, and environmental benefits owing to a reduction in airline flights. Virtual teams are also becoming increasingly popular with workers who want to work at home, which can increase employee engagement. Furthermore, as a result of using appropriate communication media, a virtual team is not limited to members from the same physical location or organization. As such, team members can be assembled according to the skills and backgrounds required, from anywhere in the world, enabling the organization to become more flexible and to compete globally.

The virtual management could be introduced as a part of the virtual human resource development (VHRD) [2]. The VHRD model is an approach

* Functional structure
  - An organizational form in which the major functions of the firm, such as production, marketing, R&D, and accounting, are grouped internally.

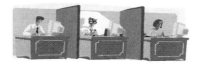

FIGURE 9.4
Traditional companies follow a "functional structure."

of utilizing the captured knowledge and information inside the enterprise environment (top management, external expertise, knowledge worker, workforce), and leveraging this knowledge to a dynamic e-content for developing and enhancing the human capital competitive advantage. This model focuses on rendering the human capital with the skills needed and driving their performance to face any future situation and solve it, by capturing the knowledge object during the interaction activities between the users and reuse it in producing a dynamic e-content for the training and development purpose and in the same adding value for the enterprise competitive advantage.

As with face-to-face teams, management of virtual teams is a crucial component in the effectiveness of the team. However, compared to leaders of face-to-face teams, virtual team leaders face the following difficulties: (a) logistical problems, including coordinating work across different time zones and physical distances; (b) interpersonal issues, including an ability to establish effective working relationships in the absence of frequent face-to-face communication; and (c) technological difficulties, including appropriate technology and ease of use. In global virtual teams, there is the added dimension of cultural differences that affect a virtual team's functioning.

9.4 Virtual Management Factors

An extensive study conducted by Jury [3] examined what factors increase leader effectiveness in virtual teams. This study identified five factors that are essential for effective leadership of virtual teams:

1. Time savings and increased productivity
2. Extended market opportunity on global scale
3. Accessing wider talent pool
4. Increased job satisfaction
5. Organizational flexibility and cost savings

There are numerous features of a virtual team environment that may affect the development of follower trust and the team members have to trust that the leader is allocating work fairly and evaluating team members equally.

Virtual team leaders need to spend more time than conventional team counterparts being explicit about expectations, because the patterns of behavior and dynamics of interaction are unfamiliar. Moreover, even in information-rich virtual teams using video conferencing, it is hard to replicate the rapid exchange of information and cues available in face-to-face discussions. In order to develop role clarity within virtual teams, leaders should focus on developing (a) clear objectives and goals for tasks, (b) comprehensive milestones for deliverables, and (c) communication channels for seeking feedback on unclear role guidance.

While technology choice is important for the development of role clarity, virtual team leaders should be aware that information overload may result in situations when a leader has provided too much information to a team member [4]. Virtual team leaders need to become virtually present in order to closely monitor team members and notice any changes that might affect their ability to undertake their tasks.

Because of the distributed nature of virtual teams, team members have less awareness of the wider situation of the team or dynamics of the overall team environment. Consequently, as situations change in a virtual team environment, such as adjustments to task requirements, modification of milestones, or changes to the goals of the team, it is important that leaders monitor followers to ensure that they are aware of these changes and make amendments as required.

Finally, when examining virtual teams, it is crucial to consider that they differ in terms of their virtuality. Virtuality refers to a continuum of how "virtual" a team is [5]. There are three predominant factors that contribute to virtuality, namely, (a) the richness of communication media; (b) distance between team members, in both time zones and geographical dispersion; and (c) organizational and cultural diversity.

9.5 Virtual Team

A virtual team (also known as a geographically dispersed team, distributed team, or remote team) [6] is a group of individuals who work across time, space, and organizational boundaries with links strengthened by webs of communication technology, or teleworking [7]. Powell, Piccoli, and Ives define virtual teams in their literature review article as "groups of geographically, organizationally and/or time dispersed workers brought together by information and telecommunication technologies to accomplish one or more organizational tasks" [8].

Members of virtual teams communicate electronically and may never meet face to face. Virtual teams are made possible by a proliferation of fiber-optic technology that has significantly increased the scope of off-site communication. Virtual teams allow companies to procure the best talent without geographical restrictions. According to Hambley et al., "virtual teams require new ways of working across boundaries through systems, processes, technology, and people, which requires effective leadership... despite the widespread increase in virtual teamwork, there has been relatively little focus on the role of virtual team leaders" [9].

In addition, you must add the "hidden costs" associated with hiring in-house personnel, that is, health and insurance benefits, taxes, payroll, office furnishings, equipment, training, and so on. Adding these expenses to a traditional staffer's salary actually increases the final monetary outlay by 2 to 2 1/2 times. This does not include the portion of the day the in-house staff is usually nonproductive owing to breaks, lunch, inefficiency, lack of work assignments, and so on.

Are *global teams, virtual transnational teams,* or *multicultural teams* different names for the same work unit? To be considered virtual, a team must have the following three attributes:

- It is a functioning team—individuals who are interdependent in their tasks, share responsibility for outcomes, see themselves as an intact social unit embedded in one or more social systems, and collectively manage their relationships across organizational boundaries [10].
- The members of the team are geographically dispersed.
- The team relies on technology-mediated communications rather than face-to-face interaction to accomplish their tasks.

The advent of virtual workers—employees whose primary work location is in a nontraditional location—has increased 50% over the last 10 years. Access to high-speed Internet connections, software solutions that enable remote collaboration, and improved telephone conferencing systems all allow employees to work seamlessly with colleagues around the world [11].

9.6 Strategies for Virtual Organization Success

According to Thompson and Caputo [12], reducing real estate costs and maintenance fees will lower operating expenses and increase profit margins. However, no organizational transition is without risk. Having a human capital management strategy for recently staffed or newly transitioned virtual workers is critical to ensuring a successful immediate and long-term return on investment.

Effective implementation is based on key elements, including the selection, management, and engagement of virtual workers, sound HR policies, and communication and change management support. Effective elements in implementing a virtual workforce include the following:

- Determining readiness for a virtual workforce
- Identifying jobs that lend themselves to work virtually

- Selecting employees who can work remotely
- Managing the virtual workforce
- Ensuring that virtual workers are engaged
- Establishing policies for the virtual work environment
- Developing a change management and communication strategy

9.7 Determining Your Readiness for a Virtual Workforce

Founders must consider a number of factors before instituting or expanding virtual work programs. Failing to adequately plan for the transition can introduce a significant amount of risk and hidden cost that can eat away at the program's anticipated return on investment. The following questions can help determine if an organization is ready for a virtual work program:

- Does the senior management team vocally support virtual work?
- Can we measure and manage virtual workers' engagement?
- Have virtual work–specific HR policies been established?
- Is there a space reduction or hoteling plan in place?
- Is there a plan for measuring virtual worker performance?
- Have we detailed the changing structure and tasks of virtual jobs?
- Is there a communication plan in place?
- Can managers be trained on how to manage virtual workers?

9.8 Overcoming the Inherent Difficulties

Teams by their very nature are interdependent [13]. Although they specify responsibilities and hire members with complementary skills, the ultimate purpose of teams is to coordinate work toward a common goal. Teams must have a shared understanding of the goals and the processes that will help them achieve that goal. In virtual teams, separated by geographical distance (and time zone differences), the process of developing a shared understanding is more challenging.

Figure 9.5 summarizes the pros and cons of virtual organizations, from a managerial perspective.

Pros	Cons
• Enables cost sharing and skills	• Potential loss of operational control
• Creates a "best of everything"	• Loss of control over emerging technology
• Encourages knowledge sharing	• Requires difficult-to-acquire managerial skills
• Accelerates organizational learning	• Potential loss of control over a critical supplier
• Smaller capital commitment	

FIGURE 9.5
Pros and cons of virtual organizations.

While the traditional teams, also known as conventional or colocated teams, consist of individuals working in close physical proximity, the term "virtual teams" refers to a group of individuals who are separated by physical distance while united by a shared goal. Generally, the virtual teams consist of talent across geographies, cultures, languages, and different time zones [14].

The "group dynamics" experienced by the members of virtual teams are complex, since members of virtual teams rely solely on electronic communication and collaboration technology to facilitate interactions among them. For a virtual team, the challenges experienced by a traditional team increase manifoldly. Below are the major differences between traditional and virtual teams:

- **Selection of team members.** Virtual team members are frequently selected based on their functional skills, but performing in a virtual team environment is not easy for everyone. However, lack of direct human interactions and social focus in a virtual setting might lead to isolation and seclusion.

- **Organization structure.** Compared to the traditional teams, virtual teams support flatter organization structure with blurred lines of authorities and hierarchies. This is required to survive in hypercompetitive market, deliver results faster, and encourage creativity—which are the primary objectives for forming a virtual team.

- **Leadership style.** In virtual team setting, managers cannot physically control the day-to-day activities and monitor each team member's activities; therefore, they need to delegate a little more as compared to traditional teams. The command-and-control military leadership style is giving way to the more democratic and coaching style of today.

- **Knowledge exchange and decision taking.** Often in traditional teams, information is exchanged and discussed during informal discussions. But in case of virtual teams, members have very limited or no informal access to information. Hence, there is a need for more frequent updates on project status and to build a shared database to provide all the important information to the team. Considering the time zone differences in global virtual teams, it becomes difficult to schedule meetings.

- **Relationship building.** When traditional team members meet face-to-face in the workplace every day, they develop close social ties with each other. They develop rapport with each other when they interact, discuss, and reach a consensus. In a virtual team, the interactions tend to be more task-focused. Further, lack of verbal cues and gestures (body language) in virtual settings complicates communication.

- **Psychological "social contract."** A psychological social contract refers to an unwritten relationship between an employer and its staff concerning mutual expectations and work outcomes. Misunderstanding or gaps in communication result in violation of the unspoken psychological "social contract" with negative effects on the team's effectiveness. Virtual teams experience difficulties in building trust, cohesion, and commitment among their members.

In summary, members of virtual teams (1) must rely heavily on mediating technologies for their day-to-day communications, (2) do not share the same work context, and (3) are not geographically proximate. These three factors conspire to inhibit knowledge sharing and shared understanding on virtual teams.

References

1. http://en.wikipedia.org/wiki/Virtual_management
2. Hanandi, M. and Grimaldi, M. Internal organizational and collaborative knowledge management: A virtual HRD model based on Web 2.0. *The International Journal of Advanced Computer Science & Applications*, 1(4), 11–19, 2010.
3. Jury, A.W. Leadership Effectiveness within Virtual Teams: Investigating Mediating and Moderating Mechanisms. PhD Thesis, School of Psychology, The University of Queensland, 2008.
4. Jury, A.W. Key themes for effective virtual team leaders. Illuminations. Australian Psychological Society, 5–7, 2008.
5. Kirkman, B.L., Rosen, B., Gibson, C.B., Tesluk, P.E., and McPherson, S.O. Five challenges to virtual team success: Lessons from Sabre Inc. *Academy of Management Executive*, 16(3), 67–79, 2002.
6. http://blog.hubstaff.com/5-steps-to-becoming-a-better-virtual-employee-an -employers-perspective/

7. Jones, C. *Teleworking: The Quiet Revolution (2005 Update)*. Gartner, Stamford, CT, 2005.

8. Powell, A., Piccoli, G., and Ives, B. Virtual teams: A review of current literature and directions for future research. *Database for Advances in Information Systems*, 35(1), 6–36, 2004.

9. Hambley, L.A., O'Neill, T., and Kline, T. Virtual team leadership: Perspectives from the field. *International Journal of E-Collaboration*, 3(1), 40–63, 2007.

10. Hackman, J.R. The design of work teams. In J.W. Lorsch, ed., *Handbook of Organizational Behavior*. Prentice Hall, Upper Saddle River, NJ, 1987.

11. McLennen, K.J. *The Virtual World of Work: How to Gain Competitive Advantage through the Virtual Workplace*. Information Age Publishing, Inc., Charlotte, NC, 2008.

12. Thompson, C. and Caputo, P. *Reality of Virtual Work: Is Your Organization Ready?* Aon Consulting, http://www.aon.com/attachments/virtual_worker_whitepa per.pdf.

13. Gibson, C.B. and Cohen, S.G. Virtual Teams that Work, http://www.communi cationcache.com/uploads/1/0/8/8/10887248/virtual_teams_that_work_creat ing_conditions_for_virtual_team_effectiveness.pdf.

14. MSG Management Study Guide. Virtual teams vs traditional teams, http:// managementstudyguide.com/virtual-teams-and-traditional-teams.html.

Section II

Classical Initial Decisions

10

Make-versus-Buy Decision

10.1 Introduction

Here is the multimillion dollar question: Should start-ups perform manufacturing operations on their own or should they buy them from an outsourcing provider? Current global competition forces companies to reevaluate their existing processes, technologies, and services in order to focus on core strategic activities.

Love it or hate it, outsourcing is now a permanent feature of business. As companies search for faster and more efficient ways of manufacturing increasingly more complex products, outsourcing noncore functions to lower-cost specialists can be an alluring prospect. Outsourcing is now increasingly used as a competitive weapon in today's economy. Outsourcing contract manufacturers can often do the job quicker, cheaper, and better.

This has resulted in an increasing awareness of the importance of the make-versus-buy decision, the dilemma start-ups face when deciding between keeping manufacturing services in-house or purchasing them from an outside provider (outsourcing contract manufacturing) [1]. Let us consider the fundamentals of outsourcing:

- Outsourcing contract manufacturing involves the transfer of the management and day-to-day execution of an entire business function to an external service provider.
- The client organization and the supplier enter into a legally binding agreement that defines the transferred services and terms.
- Under the agreement, the supplier acquires the means of production in the form of a transfer of intellectual property, know-how, people, assets, and other resources from the client.
- The client agrees to procure the services from the supplier for the term of the contract.

This chapter provides you with a make-or-buy decision process methodology that any founder can implement—whatever the size or industrial type of your organization. The make-or-buy methodology is one of your most critical strategic decisions within outsourcing contract manufacturing and should be taken in a structured and consistent manner.

A practical guide to this decision is a step-by-step guide to addressing make-or-buy decisions in a consistent and structured manner. The high-level steps are as follows:

- Evaluate whether outsourcing is right for your company.
- Determine exactly what functions to outsource and your performance expectations.
- Use a well-defined professional selection process to evaluate and select which provider(s) are right for the job.

10.2 Determining Your Core Competency

Core competency is the collection of skills and technologies that enables a company to provide a differentiated benefit to their customers. For example, Table 10.1 presents a summary of the core competencies of three well-known companies.

If the manufacturing process you are considering is a critical component of your company's business or dependent on highly valuable intellectual property, it is probably not a good candidate for outsourcing. After all, if the manufacturing process itself is your key differentiator, you'll want to maintain control of that crucial proprietary information.

On the other hand, if the manufacturing process is not a significant component of your business model today, there is probably no benefit to keeping manufacturing in-house. If your strengths are product marketing and commercialization, for example, you may want to find a contract manufacturer that can take over the manufacturing so that you can focus on what you do best—ideally, helping you save production time and costs in the process.

TABLE 10.1

Core Competencies

Company	Benefit	Core Competency
Sony	Pocketability	Miniaturization and portability
Federal Express	On-time delivery	Dependability and logistics management
Apple	Ease of use; intuitive operations; high-quality graphics; portability	Wireless communications Device mobility Cutting-edge technology

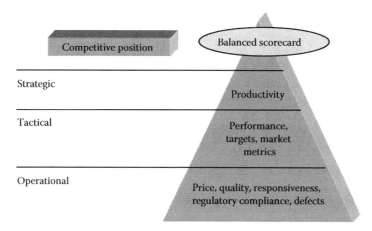

FIGURE 10.1
Outsourcing goals and objectives.

The 21st century is proving to be a crucial time for the knowledge-based industry. There has been a great deal of transformation in outsourcing caused by the continued drive of start-ups to cut commercialization time and focus on core competencies.

Logistics and supply chain management have often been among the first functions to be outsourced. This has moved beyond the warehousing and trucking functions and spread to ancillary services. Usually, companies decide to outsource some or all of their manufacturing functions in order to reduce costs, make more effective use of the working capital, and focus their energies creating differentiation and promoting revenue growth.

Your outsourcing goals and objectives are strategic, tactical, and operational, as summarized in Figure 10.1.

To maximize these goals and objectives, a review of make-or-buy decision must be one of your first initial decisions. The make-or-buy decision is the act of making a strategic choice between producing a product internally or buying it externally. Making the right choice can be the key factor in sustaining your company's competitive advantage and is one of the most important tasks of a successful management. This is the subject of subsequent paragraphs.

10.3 Deciding to Make or Buy (Outsourcing)

Sourcing is the act of transferring work from one internal party to another. *Outsourcing* is the act of transferring work to an external party. Whether or not to outsource is the fundamental decision of whether to make or buy.

How do you determine which products to outsource and which ones to manufacture in-house? Each business and owner is different, of course, but you need to answer these questions before making the decision:

- Can I better manage my available cash if I outsource? The answer here will primarily depend on how much cash you have. For example, by outsourcing the manufacturing process, you avoid the costs associated with maintaining an inventory of raw materials and hiring manufacturing employees.
- What do I do best? Because your time is finite, why spend a lot of time doing the things you don't do well when you can outsource those duties, thereby leaving you with more time to do the things you do well?
- Will the cost of the outsourcing tasks include a product whose quality is better than what I can produce myself at that same cost? The answer to this question is often yes, given the fact that the best outsourcing sources are almost always specialists in their specific areas of expertise.

The decision to make or buy extends beyond manufacturing, encompassing human resources, information technology, maintenance, regulatory requirements, and other fundamental business functions. According to Booz & Company [2], the dynamics of make-or-buy decisions is built on three key pillars—business strategy, risks, and economic factors. Table 10.2 presents the three key pillars in the make-or-buy decision.

10.3.1 Reasons for Outsourcing

Outsourcing decisions are those strategic decisions that change the operations strategy of your organization in both manufacturing and services. Your most important step in any outsourcing decision is to clearly define the

TABLE 10.2

Three Key Pillars in the Make-or-Buy Decision

Pillars	Make (In-house)	Buy (Outsource)
Business strategy	High differentiation	Suppliers willing and able to meet requirements
Risks	Few alternate sources Quick response times	Low switching costs No sensitive intellectual property involved
Economic factors	Efficacy; reliability; high quality; manufacturing expertise	Lower costs; higher quality; regulated facilities; no investment required

scope of the operations that you are considering for outsourcing. Below are some of the most important strategic decisions you will face:

Improved quality: Achieve a step change in quality through contracting out the service with a new service level agreement.

Predictability: Services will be provided via a legally binding contract with financial penalties and legal redress. This is not the case with internal services.

Specialized skill sets: If the manufacturing process demands specialized expertise or a new technology that does not currently exist within your organization, you may want to seek out an outside resource that has the skills and experience needed to make your product successful.

Production capacity: Often, the lack of sufficient production capacity is the single driver of the decision to outsource manufacturing. In those cases, making the move to contract with a partner that has the needed physical space is a no-brainer.

Ramping up: There is a potentially dramatic difference between in-house manufacturing and outsourcing when it comes to ramping up people and processes. If your staff does not currently possess the capabilities needed to manufacture the component or product, you'll need to consider the cost and time involved in integrating a new team into your organization.

Technological changes: When inevitable technology advances happen, a part becomes obsolete or feedback from the field necessitates a change in a product or component, and the company that developed the original design will be able to turn around changes more quickly. In this case, working with a contract manufacturer with design and manufacturing capabilities offers real benefits. It reduces risks when you transfer from design to manufacturing and the time and costs involved when the need for updates arises.

Operational expertise: Access to operational best practice that would be too difficult or time-consuming to develop in-house.

Knowledge: Access to intellectual property and wider experience and knowledge.

Cost savings: The lowering of the overall cost of the service to the business. This will involve reducing the scope, defining quality levels, repricing, renegotiation, and cost restructuring. Access to lower-cost economies through offshoring is generated by the wage gap between industrialized and developing nations.

Cost restructuring: Operating leverage is a measure that compares fixed costs to variable costs. Outsourcing changes the balance of this ratio by offering a move from fixed to variable cost and also by making variable costs more predictable.

Reduced time to market: The acceleration of the development or production of a product through the additional capability brought by the supplier.

Staffing issues: Access to a larger talent pool and a sustainable source of skills.

Capacity management: An improved method of capacity management of services and technology where the risk in providing the excess capacity is borne by the supplier.

Risk management: An approach to risk management for some types of risks is to partner with an outsourcer who is better able to provide the mitigation.

Catalyst for change: An organization can use an outsourcing agreement as a catalyst for major step change that cannot be achieved alone. The outsourcing partner becomes a change agent in the process.

Commodification: The trend of standardizing business processes can be served by a contract manufacturer. Outsourcing allows a wide range of businesses access to services previously only available to large corporations.

To summarize, Figure 10.2 presents a go/no-go algorithm for outsourcing your product.

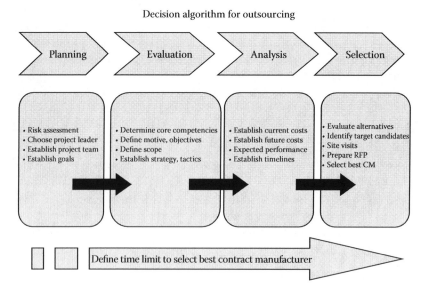

Decision algorithm for outsourcing

FIGURE 10.2
Go/no-go algorithm for outsourcing.

10.4 Partnerships with Suppliers

After you have determined the core activities of your business and laid out the necessary infrastructure, you will have to decide who will best carry out the individual stages. Activities outside the chosen focus should be assigned to third parties. Also, supporting activities within the new company need not necessarily be performed by the company. For each individual activity, the same basic question should be asked:

> "Do it ourselves or have someone else do it?"—or in business jargon: "Make or buy"?

Partnerships with suppliers, for example, often cannot be dissolved from one day to the next, and many partners are hard to replace if they drop out. When making your "make or buy" decisions, you should rely mainly on the following criteria.

10.4.1 Strategic Significance

Your ability to render a specific service better than the competition was a major factor in your decision to start a company in the first place. This service is of "strategic" significance to your company and should be kept under your strict control. A technology company would never let go of research and development (R&D), and a manufacturer of consumer goods will never hand over marketing to a third party.

10.4.2 Best Supplier

Any entrepreneurial activity requires specific skills that may not be available within the management team. Your management team must therefore consider whether, in specific instances, it makes sense for the company to carry out a particular task itself. Should the company want to acquire the necessary skills, or would it be more advantageous to assign the task to a specialized supplier? For example, a team developing some electronic equipment may have mastered the electronics, but it lacks the necessary manufacturing capability—so it would do better "buying" this task. Their experience often enables specialist higher production volume.

10.4.3 Commercial Availability

Before you can make a decision to buy, you need to find out whether the product or service is available on the market in the desired form or with the necessary specification. Whenever possible, negotiate with several suppliers: you generally end up with better terms, and you will also find out more about whatever you are purchasing. You can also often help a supplier improve an offer. If you cannot find a supplier for what you need, you may be able to find a partner who is prepared to develop the necessary skills.

10.4.4 Outsourcing Partnerships

Most companies have business relationships with other companies—as a purchaser, as a supplier, or as an equal business partner. These relationships vary in their quality and intensity, from a loose, more or less coincidental relationship (a company buys its chemical supplies from a distributor with the cheapest prices) to a strategic alliance that results in intensive cooperation and mutual dependency (e.g., Microsoft and Intel in the 1980s). Exchanging ideas and people with a partner and jointly developing products or components can prove to be very fruitful.

For any start-up company, the question of how to work together with other companies is particularly relevant. Every type of cooperation (loose or close partnership) has advantages and disadvantages as discussed below:

- Loose, casual partnerships represent no great obligation for either side. Both partners can end the partnership quickly and simply; both, however, also live in the knowledge that supply or demand can dry up quickly. Furthermore, a supplier will not take much notice of a customer's particular requirements, as he will not be able to sell individually adapted products to his other customers. Loose relationships are thus typical for mass-market products, undemanding services, and standard components, for which replacement suppliers and purchasers are easily found.

- Close partnerships are characterized by a degree of tight interdependence between the partners; they are typical for highly specialized products and services, or for large volumes. In such situations, it is usually difficult for both sides to change partners at short notice, to obtain large quantities of specialized components quickly from another supplier, or to find a market for such components. The advantage for both sides is the security of a firm relationship and the possibility of concentrating on one's own strength, while also profiting from the partner's particular strengths.

For any partnership to develop into a successful business relationship, three important elements need to be in place:

1. **"Win–win situation":** both sides must get fair shares of the advantages of the situation; without an incentive for both sides, the partnership is not viable in the long term.

2. **Balance between risks and investments:** partnerships involve risks, and often not enough attention is paid to these risks, particularly when business is good. A supplier with an exclusive contract can find himself in a difficult situation, for example, if his customer suddenly cuts back production and purchases fewer components. This is even more the case if the supplier has purchased special production tools that cannot easily be used for other customers' orders. Conversely, a customer can find himself in serious difficulties if a supplier cannot deliver (on account of bankruptcy, fire, strike, etc.). Risks and their possible financial consequences need to be taken into account in advance and, if necessary, considered in the contract.

3. **Dissolution:** just as in human relationships, tensions can arise in business relationships. Make sure that in any partnership, the conditions under which the partnership may be dissolved or one partner may withdraw are clearly defined from the start. While working on the business plan, start thinking about who you will cooperate later, and what form this cooperation will take. Partnerships offer your new company the chance to profit from the strengths of established companies and to concentrate on building up your own strengths. In this way, you can usually grow faster than you could on your own.

10.5 Contract Manufacturers in the Medical Device Industry

The global medical device contract manufacturing (outsourcing) market is expected to reach $50.37 billion by 2020, according to a new study by Grand View Research, Inc. [3]. Key findings in the report include the following:

- Class II medical device emerged as the largest application segment of the market in 2013. Presence of high sales volume coupled with relatively less stringent device approval regulations (as compared to class III medical devices) are some factors accounting for high outsourcing rates in this segment.

- North America was the leading regional market in 2013. Increasing prevalence of chronic diseases in the region and the consequent growth in demand for medical devices are some factors contributing to the region's large market share. Presence of stringent government regulations and healthcare-related cost-curbing endeavors are also expected to enhance the demand for outsourcing.

- Asia Pacific is expected to present this market with lucrative future growth opportunities. Growth of this region as a manufacturing hub offering lower labor and infrastructure costs is expected to fuel future market growth.

- The medical device outsourcing market is consolidated in nature and is marked by the presence of numerous mergers and acquisitions. Some key players of this market include Shandong Weigao Co. Ltd., Sterigenics International Inc., Hamilton Company, Shinva Medical Instruments Co., Inteprod LLC, Mitutoyo Corporation, Kinetics Climax, Inc., CFI Medical, Omnica Corporation, Infinity Plastics Group, Teleflex Medical OEM, Daiichi Jitsugyo Co. Ltd, ProMed Molded Products Inc., and GE.

According to Cirtec Medical Systems [4], contract manufacturers have played a significant role in the medical device industry for decades, and that role will be expanding in the years to come—some analysts expect the volume of devices built by contract manufacturers to double in the next 5 years. There are many reasons for using a contract manufacturer, but several stand out in today's industry:

- Downward price pressure, a continuing trend in foreign markets, and an increasing trend in the US market
- Limited venture capital funding
- Increasingly complex device designs leading to a need for increasingly complex manufacturing technologies

For a medical device start-up company, they key benefit of using a contract manufacturer is often efficient use of limited funds; with a strong manufacturing partner, a small company can minimize or even eliminate the need for direct capital investment, and the contract manufacturer can help speed the manufacturing because of their experience and expertise with Food and Drug Administration (FDA)–approved products.

For more moderate-size companies, contract manufacturing provides an opportunity for the company to focus on their core technology by outsourcing the day-to-day concerns of manufacturing, without employing large numbers of specialized technologists.

10.5.1 Medical Device Contract Manufacturing Challenges

The benefits of working with contract manufacturers are myriad, but there can also be difficulties. Some of the more common issues in the medical device industry include the following:

- Identifying a partner with a robust quality system. Some contract manufacturers have made the transition to medical devices after getting their start in telecommunications or other less regulated industries.

The quality system and quality culture may be insufficient, particularly for manufacturing FDA Class II and Class III devices.

- Finding a manufacturer with both breadth/depth in manufacturing techniques for fabrication of complex devices. The industry is seeing a surge in development of mechanically and electrically intricate, minimally invasive surgical devices, high-risk implantable devices, and miniaturized monitoring devices among other complex designs. To build these types of devices, a manufacturer must be competent in more than basic electro-mechanical assembly.

- Selecting a supplier who can support your entire product life cycle. Contract manufacturers often have a specialty—they may work primarily in a high-mix/small-volume mode or in a low-mix/high-volume mode. This may mean that as your product transitions from small development and clinical volumes to higher commercial volumes, you will need to move to a new manufacturer. This kind of change can be costly, risky, and distracting to your in-house resources, and can create regulatory delays for your product launch.

- Obtaining the right resources to support your project. Many contract manufacturers work primarily in a "build to print" mode. While this helps you achieve the primary goal of getting your device fabricated, it won't help you improve your device design for manufacturability, reduce the cost of your manufacturing process, or lean out your supply chain.

10.5.2 Selecting Your Ideal Medical Device Contract Manufacturer

How can you avoid these common pitfalls and develop a relationship that provides all the benefits that contract manufacturing can offer? There are some important steps that will help keep you on the path to contract manufacturing success:

Step 1: Understand the quality system requirements for your product and research potential suppliers to find a match.

- Determine the regulatory path and classification for your device. Look for manufacturers with experience working with devices of that class.

- Will the contract manufacturer deliver you a finished device, or will you perform final operations at your facility or a third party? If the device will be finished by the contract manufacturer, limit your search to suppliers who are appropriately registered with the FDA.

- How will your quality system mesh with the system at your supplier? Your contract manufacturer should have a robust method for documenting and executing quality system interfaces.

- How will you approach process risk management and qualification? A manufacturer with existing procedures for these activities could streamline your project.

Step 2: Identify a manufacturing partner with the right combination of capability and expertise for your device.

- Understand the key manufacturing processes required for fabricating your device. This might include extrusion, mechanical joining, plating or coating, overmolding or adhesives work, sealing, complex packaging, or other processes.

- Determine which key processes require high value capital equipment. Focus your search for a contract manufacturer on companies with the appropriate high value equipment already in place. This is particularly important for processes that should be completed in a cleanroom environment.

- Identify key processes that require customized process parameter development. Look for contract manufacturers with demonstrated expertise developing and qualifying those types of processes.

- Will your device include a power source? Seek a manufacturer with experience handling and shipping power sources safely; in some cases, the manufacturer may need to be specially certified for shipping.

- How will your device be tested for safety and functionality? Complex designs may require a variety of test techniques, including power up and power supply recharge testing, air and water ingress testing, mechanical strength testing, electrical function testing, pressure response testing, or package seal testing. The contract manufacturer you select should have sufficient expertise to help you determine which tests should be performed and implement those tests.

Step 3: Outline your product life cycle both in time and in manufacturing volumes. Use that outline to determine a suitable manufacturing partner.

- What range of volumes do you expect to build over the life of your product? Look for a supplier with the facilities and the organizational structure to support you through clinical trials, initial production, and the ramp of commercial manufacturing.

- How will you ensure continuity in the team throughout the product life cycle? An ideal contract manufacturer will have a history of customer service and will provide a consistent point of contact through your entire product life cycle.

Step 4: Determine your strategy for in-house resources and identify a contract manufacturer who will complement your team.

- A full-service contract manufacturing can provide design for manufacturability input for your product, helping to increase yields and decrease costs.

- If your product design isn't fully mature, a contract manufacturer with prototyping and design capabilities can be a tremendous asset to your team. This is particularly true for design aspects outside the core technology of your product, which may be a distraction to your in-house team.

- Will your product require custom test systems as part of the manufacturing process? If so, a supplier with test engineering capabilities could be ideal.

- How will your supply chain be managed? You may benefit from a contract manufacturer with the engineering and materials management personnel to provide supplier development and materials management. Early-stage companies may further benefit from a contract manufacturer with a strong Approved Vendor List to help build an initial supply chain.

10.6 Outsourcing in the Biopharmaceutical Industry

The biopharmaceutical industry is among the world's industrial wonders. The pharmaceutical industry is looking at an emerging market expansion and growth potential of 12% year on year, and the biologics market is expected to grow to $41 billion by 2014 [5].

However, biopharmaceutical companies are under enormous economic pressure and are facing unprecedented challenges. Current market and economic realities compel the industry to reduce fixed costs, improve efficiency, and maximize their limited resources on core competencies. Consider the following statistics:

- An anticipated loss of sales of approximately $80 billion in 2010–2015 resulting from expiring patent portfolios
- Shrinking profit margins and increasingly heavy competition
- Growing regulatory pressure owing to highly publicized exploding healthcare costs
- Recurring threats of litigation over real or perceived drug side effects

- Shifting demographic trends in both western and emerging markets, driving the demand for "smarter" pharmaceuticals to treat chronic diseases
- Growing threats to intellectual property from Third World countries
- Weak pipelines for new drugs in many of the largest firms
- Skyrocketing development and regulatory expenses

These are just some of the challenges the global pharmaceutical industry is facing today. The challenge of accelerating pharmaceutical product development while controlling costs creates a difficult balancing act for industry executives. For example, R&D spending declined in the last 4 out of 5 years, primarily attributed to the following [6]:

- Patent expirations on blockbuster drugs
- Declining R&D productivity
- Consequences of global attempts to reduce healthcare expenditures

10.6.1 Clinical Development Outsourcing

A Parexel Strategic Partnerships 2013 report included in-depth interviews with senior-level executives from global biopharmaceutical companies representing 39% of the industry's total R&D expenditure. The interviews included both quantitative and qualitative questions to better understand the current state of clinical development outsourcing and future trends in Strategic Partnerships [7].

Key findings from the Parexel report include the following:

- Industry executives who have already implemented Strategic Partnerships recognize the value, believing that these integrated relationships positively affect CRO (Contract Research Organization)–sponsor relationships as well as their operations.
- The operational efficiencies and impact seen by implementing Strategic Partnerships will continue to drive clinical development outsourcing.
- Biopharmaceutical executives most often equate Strategic Partnerships with oversight, governance, and the level of mutual partnership investment, rather than the volume of work, an important consideration for smaller and mid-sized companies.
- Executives believe that showcasing consistent value and measuring results are critical for the future success of this more integrated model.
- Strategic Partnerships will continue to evolve away from the traditional transactional model toward more integrated relationships

that drive value through increased alignment and efficiencies. The next generation of Strategic Partnerships must involve a greater alignment of commercial terms and a true collaboration of the best talent from the CRO and sponsor, according to biopharmaceutical executives.

- The hallmark of an optimized Strategic Partnerships model will be the measurable success of collaboratively bringing a compound to market faster.

10.6.2 Factors Driving Outsourcing in Biopharma

The global biopharma outsourcing market is expected to reach $40.7 billion by 2015, according to a recent report by Global Industry Analysts, Inc. [8].

There are a number of factors driving the executives' decisions to increase their investment in outsourcing. Two of the leading factors include the ability to access capabilities not found internally and the ability to reduce fixed costs and minimize utilization of internal resources. Executives felt that outsourcing provides sponsors with flexibility, helping to manage the volatility and unpredictability of the pipeline. Outsourcing allows for the sponsor to utilize internal resources more effectively while the outsourcing partner handles the peaks and troughs in activities as seen in Figure 10.3.

Biopharmaceutical manufacturers increasingly consider outsourcing as a viable option for cutting their organization's costs, especially as industry service suppliers offer a broader array of potential activities. Biopharma

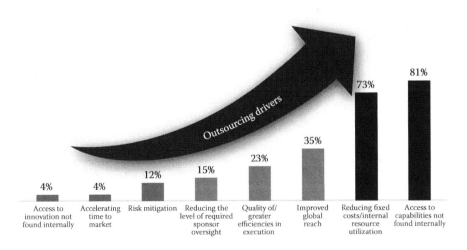

FIGURE 10.3
Outsourcing drivers in the biopharmaceutical industry. (Source: Parexel Strategic Partnerships 2013.)

companies report that they are contracting out more and different jobs and manufacturing operations in an effort to reduce costs, according to BioPlan Associates' *12th Annual Report and Survey of Biopharmaceutical Manufacturing Capacity and Production* [9].

It is worth noting that the BioPlan study is international in scope, and in years past, there have been significant geographic differences in potential destinations. In the 2014 study, for example, European companies considered China and the United States as likely destinations, whereas US companies preferred Singapore and Germany.

Preliminary data show that China is again the most attractive of the emerging destinations. In fact, many see it as a likely outsourcing destination during the next 5 years, most likely because of perceived cost advantages and expectations for developing quality initiatives. Among the BRIC countries (Brazil, Russia, India, and China), China continues to lead the pack, followed by India.

Contract Manufacturing Organizations (CMOs) and CROs based on emerging markets will continue to capture market share, albeit slowly. These CMOs continue to face domestic regulatory and legal hurdles and are far from obtaining approvals for US and EU markets. Perceived cost-effectiveness offered by CMOs in these markets may be eroding as other supply chain costs are figured in, and whatever advantages could be gained from cost-competitiveness also appear to be declining, judging by BioPlan's recent survey results that suggest that cost-effectiveness is waning as a selection attribute.

Nevertheless, the internationalization of biomanufacturing outsourcing markets can be expected to grow. BRIC and other developing countries have yet to pose a significant threat to US and European dominance. However, simply based on the weight of their emerging populations, their growing economic power, and demand for better, cheaper domestic biologics, it is likely that their growing bioprocessing competence will result in cGMP (current good manufacturing practice) production and export of biologics to US and EU markets in the future [10].

10.6.3 Performance Metrics Used in Pharma Partnerships

According to Alkermes Contract Pharma Services [11], the following initiatives are part of its service offering:

- Inspection Ready Status and Continuous Quality Improvement strategies that are reinforced by an extensive self-inspection program and a Corrective and Preventive Action database.
- Operational Excellence initiatives where a process improvement culture is enthusiastically encouraged within our manufacturing facilities, with a focus on reducing variability and eliminating waste.

- Problem solving throughout the organization is approached in a collaborative and professional manner by focusing on the specific (and often unique) needs of our partner projects, empowering employees, and optimizing existing activities in our development, scale-up, and manufacturing processes.
- A systematic training program that has created highly skilled problem solvers (black belts, green belts, and yellow belts) who can anticipate, overcome, and improve workflow challenges of partner products.
- Highly qualified chemists and scientific staff who operate in fully equipped, best-in-class facilities that include the following: raw materials, in-process and finished product release testing laboratories, microbiology laboratories, bioanalytical laboratories, stability incubators and testing facilities, method development laboratories, and method validation laboratories
- Dedicated project management staff and resources including secure intranet portal access for partners.

10.6.4 Outsourcing Drug Manufacturing

According to Taylor Wessing [12], for many pharma companies conducting preclinical and clinical development programs, it is often necessary, and usually cost-effective, to outsource manufacturing of the investigational drug to a CMO.

Outsourcing of investigational drugs gives rise to a number of commercial and legal issues that need to be carefully managed to limit the risks to the company concerned. Let us examine some of the risks, the problems that can arise, and the strategies that can be employed to minimize the potential exposure.

10.6.4.1 Contract Manufacturing Agreements

Many of the leading CMOs are major pharma companies, and they can afford to be relatively inflexible, particularly with start-up pharmaceutical or biotech companies, when negotiating the terms of their contracts.

- Limits on liability. Understandably, CMOs will normally seek to limit their obligations to their customers to producing a drug to comply with the specification and in accordance with cGMP. While CMOs will not (by law) be able to exclude their liability for death or personal injury as a result of their negligence, it is common for the CMO to exclude liability to their customers for indirect, special, or consequential losses or for any loss of profits, revenue, business opportunity, or goodwill.

- Delivery dates. Particularly in the early stages of manufacturing, or where there is any development component to the manufacturing services, CMOs will be very reluctant to agree to fixed delivery dates for finished product. This is likely to be in direct conflict with the need of the company to manage preclinical and clinical development timelines and related costs, and there are limits to how this can be addressed. Nevertheless, it is usually possible to negotiate at least some provisions in relation to flexibility on timing of slots and forecasting that can mitigate the risks.

- The impact of partnering. The limited availability of funding for start-up biotech companies means that there is a necessity to partner programs earlier and earlier in development, and outsourcing risks can be accentuated where the biotech company has partnered the relevant program with a pharmaceutical company. An increasingly common occurrence in partnering agreements is for the pharmaceutical company to provide financial support to the biotech to enable it to take forward the preclinical and clinical development of a program to a point at which an option to commercialize the drug may be exercised and the program is then transferred. It is essential when determining the level of financial contribution from the partner that there is sufficient flexibility to deal with certain additional costs that can unfortunately arise given the risks inherent in the manufacturing process.

- Adverse events. From a legal perspective, additional problems can arise if adverse events occur in a trial or the trial drug is found to have a latent defect. It may be by no means immediately clear whether the fault lies in an innate property of the drug itself, a problem with raw materials supplied to the CMO, the manufacturing of the product, the storage or transportation of the drug, or its administration. Where the biotech company is an intermediary, there will always be a risk that it becomes embroiled in the process of determining the cause, which can result in additional costs at the very least and potentially defense of any claims that are issued by or on behalf of the trial subjects or the sponsor of the trial.

- Auditing provisions. It is important that any agreement with a CMO contains strong auditing provisions, a common formulation being a right to a minimum number of audits or inspections each year as well as unlimited additional rights in the event of a quality issue. Additional rights should also be sought to attend any audit or inspection by relevant regulatory authorities relating the drug covered by the agreement where this is permitted by the regulator. A notification of inspection provision will therefore be required, and it is useful to provide that any licensee of the drug program should also be permitted to attend as this is likely to be a requirement of any partner.

- Transfer to a new manufacturer. As development progresses from preclinical studies through clinical trials to commercialization, there is often a need to scale up the manufacturing process and frequently a need to change manufacturers as a result. When a new CMO is selected, particularly in relation to biologicals, the standard form agreements of many CMOs often contain provisions that have the effect of potentially limiting the ability of the customer to transfer manufacturing to a new manufacturer. Such a need to transfer may arise for any number of reasons including a failure of the original CMO to produce drug product to specification, delays in supply, an inability of the original CMO to supply greater volumes, insolvency, a need to be able to dual source, or quite frequently the desire of a partner to bring the manufacture of the product in-house.

- Transfer of proprietary processes. CMOs have an understandable commercial imperative to retain a manufacturing and supply mandate and will frequently argue that they need to be protected against the transfer of their proprietary process to another manufacturer. This may well be reasonable if they have a patented manufacturing process or some confidential process know-how that is essential to the manufacture of the drug. Frequently, however, it is the company that is providing the process, having developed it itself or transferring it from the previous manufacturer, and in fact, it is merely that the new manufacturer does not want to share its confidential background know-how with its competitors. The consequence of this is that a barrier to transfer is potentially created and it is worth examining in some detail how such a barrier can be overcome.

- Who developed the manufacturing process? Clearly, if the company is transferring the process to the CMO, there can be no technology proprietary to the CMO that is essential to the manufacture of the drug, and it should be possible as a condition of transfer to them that they will facilitate the subsequent transfer to another manufacturer if necessary or required. Of course, if the new manufacturer is intended to contribute considerably to the scale up of the manufacturing process or has otherwise substantially contributed to the development of the process, it may seek to negotiate financial compensation in the event of its loss of the manufacturing mandate, at least in circumstances where it is not in default.

- In practice, the prospective manufacturer may be relatively relaxed about a subsequent transfer of the manufacturing process to a customer's pharma partner compared with the potential transfer of its process to a rival CMO.

- Foreground intellectual property. What intellectual property is needed by the new manufacturer? Although CMOs will generally readily assign rights in all foreground intellectual property relating to the product, or exclusively relating to the manufacture of the product, they may well wish to retain rights to other more general foreground intellectual property in relation to the manufacturing, including the manufacturing documentation, to the extent that they are applicable to the manufacture of other products, as this will also be some compensation for the potential loss of the manufacturing mandate.

  From the company's perspective, the ideal position would be to own all foreground intellectual property, which it has arguably paid for through the service fees. In practice, if this is resisted, it may be sufficient for the customer's ability to transfer manufacturing to another manufacturer to be granted an exclusive or even just a nonexclusive freedom-to-operate license in relation to the product, or closely related class of products, which it can sublicense on to the new manufacturer along with a copy of the manufacturing documentation.

- Freedom to operate. For security, however, it would also be desirable to obtain a freedom-to-operate license under the manufacturer's background process intellectual property solely to the extent necessary for the exploitation of the foreground intellectual property. While this may well not be strictly necessary, on the basis that any subsequent manufacturer is likely to have its own existing proprietary process that it would adapt for the purposes of manufacturing the product, rather than seeking to copy the basic process and equipment of the preceding manufacturer, a freedom-to-operate license in the absence of an obligation to provide details of any proprietary process know-how is nevertheless valuable as it removes the risk of a later allegation of infringement.

- It may also be essential for the licensee to obtain copies of the manufacturing documentation. Although actual copies of this documentation may not need to be passed to a subsequent manufacturer, a full understanding of the contents may be essential to an effective transfer.

- Transferability of process. How will the transfer practically take place? It is one thing to have a license of proprietary know-how and a right to a copy of documentation, but in the event that the relationship breaks down or the manufacturing agreement is terminated as a result of breach by the manufacturer or the manufacturers insolvency, it will be essential for the customer to be able to transfer the process as quickly as possible to another manufacturer in order to minimize the impact on development and commercialization. This will be much more easily achieved if any necessary proprietary know-how and documentation is placed in escrow for automatic release in the event of breach or insolvency.

10.6.4.2 Pharma Outsourcing Conclusions

Outsourcing drug manufacture is often an essential part of preclinical and clinical development programs but should not be entered into lightly, and it is always worthwhile to conduct a full investigation into, and understanding of, the capabilities, reputation, and resources of a potential CMO. The performance of the CMO is likely to be a key element in the commercialization success of a drug, and companies should consider avoiding CMOs whose conditions are advantageous in the short term, but have the effect of practically preventing the company from moving manufacturing to another manufacturer in the future.

As the development of a drug moves from preclinical development toward approval, however, the financial risks arising from problems in respect of manufacturing increase substantially, and it is essential to put in place agreements (even at the preclinical stage of manufacturing) that minimize the potential exposure. This applies both when the company is contracting with a CMO and when it is acting as an intermediary in the supply chain.

Even where a CMO insists on imposing its own terms and conditions, a company that fully understands these terms and the potential areas of risk may be able to negotiate better terms or otherwise seek to lessen those risks.

10.7 Due Diligence: Questions to Ask Any Contract Manufacturer

When you outsource the production of your product or component to a CM, you can focus on your core capabilities. That's the idea, but not all CMs were born alike. Table 10.3 presents a few questions that may help you determine whether the potential partner is right for you [13].

TABLE 10.3

Due Diligence Questions for Contract Manufacturers

Questions to Ask	Significance
Do you have best-in-class production systems in place?	A simple "yes" is not a sufficient answer. You want assurances that the CM will deliver the quality you expect, so make sure the CM has adopted quality standards and can provide documentation and test data.
	Best-in-class is not simply that you ARE measuring, but HOW you are measuring yourself to a high standard.
Do you have quality management systems in place?	• ISO 9001 certification requires a CM to focus on continuous improvement in customer service and satisfaction.
	• ISO 13485 is a specific quality management system for the design and manufacture of medical devices.
	• AS 9100 is a specific quality management system for the aerospace industry.
	The CM must have a strong record with no certification disruptions or black marks for performance.
Can you help with regulatory compliance issues?	The CM should not only understand the regulations and standards that your product needs to meet but also be willing to provide labeling guidance and manage regulatory filings that may be necessary.
Do you operate with an open book?	The CM should provide information about their production processes and costs (material, labor, and overhead) so that there are no surprises later.
What's your inventory management process?	You want to be sure that the CM can ensure that components are available when needed and that they are willing to inventory parts that may not be needed immediately.
How will you protect my intellectual property?	Your CM should have the systems in place that can ensure that your sensitive proprietary information is 100% secure.
Can you demonstrate expertise in manufacturing specifically to the technology in my device?	You should understand the specifics about the experience the CM has in working with various technologies, applications, and platforms. This means getting out on the production floor in addition to case study demonstrations and examples.

References

1. http://search.aol.com/aol/search?enabled_terms=&s_it=wscreen-smallbusiness-w&q=make+vs+buy+++pdf
2. Schwarting, D. and Weissbarth, R. Make or Buy Three Pillars of Sound Decision Making, 2011, http://www.strategyand.pwc.com/media/uploads/Strategyand-Make-or-Buy-Sound-Decision-Making.pdf.
3. http://globenewswire.com/news-release/2014/11/24/685770/10109613/en/Medical-Device-Outsourcing-Market-Worth-Is-Forecasted-To-Reach-50-37-Billion-By-2020-New-Report-By-Grand-View-Research-Inc.html

4. Cirtec White paper. Cirtec is a full service contract manufacturer of Class II and III devices, http://cirtecmed.com/wp-content/uploads/2013/11/Best-Practices -in-Medical-Device-Contract-Manufacturing.pdf.
5. KPMG. Outsourcing in the pharmaceutical industry: 2011 and beyond, https://www.kpmg.com/Ca/en/IssuesAndInsights/ArticlesPublications /Documents/Outsourcing-pharmaceutical-industry.pdf.
6. http://www.resultshealthcare.com/media/116314/20131216_results_cro_pre sentation_for_rh_website.pdf
7. https://www.parexel.com/files/5013/9420/3451/2013_Strategic_Partnerships _Report.pdf
8. http://www.strategyr.com/Pharmaceutical_Contract_Manufacturing_Market _Report.asp
9. BioPlan Associates, *12th Annual Report and Survey of Biopharmaceutical Manufacturing Capacity and Production*. Rockville, MD, April 2015.
10. Langer, E. Biomanufacturing outsourcing globalization continues. *BioPharm International*, 28(5), 2015.
11. Outsourcing in the Pharma Industry—Experience, Expertise and Enthusiasm, http://www.alkermes.com/assets/content/files/Partnership_Whitepaper _August_2012.pdf.
12. Outsourcing the manufacturing of drugs. Taylor Wessing LLP, http://www .taylorwessing.com/synapse/may13.html.
13. Should YOU Manufacture Your Product? Sparton Corporation, http://vert assets.blob.core.windows.net/download/e2e4447f/e2e4447f-f3bf-4ea3-b2ca -33e207a0dcfa/spa_14080_make_vs_buy_wp_150210_final_client_approved.pdf.

11

Patents versus Trade Secrets

11.1 Introduction

The world-famous Coca-Cola formula has been kept as a trade secret asset since 1889 because competitors cannot reverse engineer the exact Coca-Cola formula. If the inventor had patented the famous composition (and disclosed the ingredients and their exact proportions), then all intellectual property protection would have been lost forever upon the expiration of the patent. Interestingly, in May 2006, a Coke employee and two others were charged with stealing and trying to sell guarded Coke secrets to Pepsi. Pepsi quickly notified Coke of the breach and the FBI was called to investigate.

Both patents and trade secrets are part of intellectual property rights. **Intellectual property (IP)** is a legal concept that refers to "creations of the mind" for which exclusive rights are recognized [1]. In its broadest sense, intellectual property means the legal rights that result for intellectual activity in the industrial, scientific, literary, and artistic fields, and protection against unfair competition [2].

A **patent** grants an inventor exclusive right to make, use, sell, and import an invention for a 20-year period (on June 8, 1995, the new term took effect in the United States), in exchange for the public disclosure of the invention, and its practical application. An invention is a solution to a specific technological problem, which may be a product or a process. You cannot patent naturally occurring products in nature, scientific principles, laws of nature, mental processes, and mathematical formulas.

The birth of every patent starts out as a trade secret. At the time of conception, the idea or information can only be protected by keeping it secret. However, a subsequent decision needs to be made to determine whether or not to convert the trade secret asset into a patent asset. The traditional approach is based on the NUN factors: novelty, usefulness, and nonobviousness [3].

If the trade secret asset meets the patentability requirements, then the decision tree often dictates that the owner seek patent protection because a patent will provide greater protection for the duration of the patent life.

In the past, there was a great deal of variation of the term of protection afforded by patents in different countries. The members of the World Trade

Organization (formerly GATT) have now harmonized recognition of technology patents for a 20-year period that begins with the priority date.

A **trade secret** is a formula, practice, process, design, instrument, pattern, or compilation of information that is not generally known or reasonably ascertainable, by which a business can obtain an economic advantage over competitors or customers. The following are some techniques for creating and maintaining trade secrets:

- Keeping private and confidential documentation
- Restricting access to all forms of confidential information
- Establishing a security system for maintaining secrecy
- Controlling visitor's access to documents or facilities
- Requiring written employee secrecy agreements
- Conducting new hire and exit interviews emphasizing secrecy and confidentiality

11.2 Who Benefits from Intellectual Property Rights?

How can legal monopolies such as patents, trademarks, or copyrights benefit society? A monopoly that is rightfully obtained gives the owner the right to exclude others from (a) making, (b) using, or (c) selling the invention, and (d) using substantially similar "expressions." For example, a patent gives a benefit to an inventor and a benefit to the public, as shown below:

- A patent gives the public a set of detailed instructions that explain how the patent works. Thus, the inventor is teaching others and thus contributes to the promotion of national and societal progress.

- Anyone is free to use these techniques as inspiration or reference, or to make new contributions, as long as the results do not infringe the patent while it is in force.

A patent is a bargain between society and an inventor wherein the inventor discloses all inventions to the public in exchange for a time-limited monopoly. This ensures that society will be able to enjoy the full benefit of the invention after the expiration date of the patent. (A US Patent expires as of noon on the expiry date.)

11.2.1 Real Estate Analogy

Claims are considered legal property—that is, they can be bought, sold, rented, or allowed to lie fallow. Patent claims can be likened to the description of a parcel of land in a real estate deed as described in Table 11.1.

TABLE 11.1

Similarities between Patents and Real Estate Deeds

Patent Terminology	Real Estate Terminology
Claim limits	Metes and bounds that locate and define the perimeter of the property
Exclusion	No trespassing sign; building a fence; limited access
Licensing or demanding a royalty	Charging a fee for entering the property Charging rent
Cross-licensing	Providing common access for mutual benefit
Infringement	Trespassing Entering into the property without permission

Source: Modified from Maynard, J.T. and Peters, H.M. *Understanding Chemical Patents.* American Chemical Society, Washington, DC. p. 86, 1991.

11.2.2 Provisional Patents

For the entrepreneur/inventor trying to be as frugal as possible, a **Provisional Patent Application** may be your savior. Starting on June 8, 1995, the United States Patent and Trademark Office or USPTO has allowed inventors the option of filing a provisional application for **utility (mechanical, electrical, or chemical) patents**. The keyword here is "provisional." A provisional patent only gives 1 year of protection. After that, you must file for a nonprovisional patent or abandon your patent.

A provisional patent is a low-cost alternative, a *preliminary* step before filing for a regular patent that gives one additional year of protection or grace—maybe enough time to test market your invention before investing in the full cost of a regular patent. A provisional patent allows filing without any formal patent claims, oath, or declaration, or any information disclosure (prior art) statement.

- It provides the means to establish an early effective filing date in a nonprovisional patent application (also known as a docket).
- It also allows the term *Patent Pending* to be applied to your invention.

11.2.3 Time Limits

A provisional patent application can be filed up to 1 year after the date of first sale, offer for sale, public use, or publication of the invention. These prefiling disclosures, although protected in the United States, may preclude patenting in foreign countries.

Unlike a nonprovisional patent, the provisional patent is filed without any formal patent claims, oath, declaration, information disclosure, or prior art statement. What must be provided for in an application for a provisional patent is the (1) written description of the invention and (2) any drawings necessary to more fully understand the invention.

TABLE 11.2

Provisional Patents

Advantages	Disadvantages
Relatively simple and inexpensive.	A provisional application automatically
The specifications will not be examined.	becomes abandoned when its pendency
More comprehensive disclosures can be	expires 12 months after the provisional
followed at a later time.	application filing date by operation of law.
Can claim priority to multiple provisional	Provisional applications will not mature into
applications, as measured from the earliest	a granted patent without further
filed application.	submissions by the inventor.
Once docketed, the term *Patent Pending* can	If not followed by a utility filing within
be used for business purposes.	1 year, the inventor must cease using patent
	pending to avoid charges of false marking.
The effective patent term is 21 years from	Examination is delayed up to 1 year.
filing date of the provisional application.	

If either of these two items is missing or incomplete, your application will be rejected and no filing date will be given for your provisional application.

11.2.4 Advantages and Disadvantages of Provisional Patents

There are several advantages and disadvantages to a provisional patents—the reader is well advised to seek competent patent counsel. A well-written provisional patent application should satisfy all formal and substantive legal requirements of the patent law. A provisional patent application should always be as complete as possible as compared to a nonprovisional patent application; however, you will not be required to file any claims. You can conveniently use that grace year to collect additional data that may form a basis for eventual claims.

The entrepreneur/inventor must carefully balance the plusses and minuses of provisional patents, as shown in Table 11.2.

11.3 The Special Case Involving Life Sciences Patents

> Life sciences and biotechnology are widely regarded as one of the most promising frontier technologies for the coming decades [4].

Research and development (R&D) in the life sciences is extremely costly and time-consuming. The pharmaceutical industry provides a good example of the time scales (8–10 years) and funding to bring a drug or biological product to market, and most biotechnology start-ups do not have the financial resources available to them to survive for that period.

The business model of biotech firms often relies heavily on intellectual property rights, in particular patents, as they are often the most crucial asset they own in a sector that is extremely research-intensive and with low imitation costs. Investors in biotech companies are generally well aware of the centrality of patents and the survival of such companies may very well depend on their ability to convince investors that they have a solid IP strategy and that risks are reduced to a minimum [5].

Why are patents so important for companies in the biotechnology sectors? It may be difficult to understand this without understanding how the industry operates. According to Estevan Burrone, a consultant for Europe's Small and Medium Enterprises (SME) Division [6], there are five major reasons:

1. Biotechnology is probably one of the most research-intensive industries. Compared with other major industries that also rely on R&D, such as the chemical industry, where the ratio of R&D expenditure to total revenues is approximately 5%, or the pharmaceutical industry, for which the equivalent figure is generally no more than 13%, biotechnology companies generally invest between 40% and 50% of their revenues in R&D. As in any research-based industry, the protection of research results becomes a major issue.

2. There are generally exorbitant costs for the development of new products and processes, but relatively low costs of imitation. The costs of performing biotechnology research are to be considered in the context of the high risks involved in any research project. It is hard to predict at the outset whether years of research will lead to breakthrough innovations with a great market potential or may simply leave a company empty-handed with results that are unlikely to bring revenues. Given the high costs involved in R&D, the relative ease of imitation is an issue that is of great concern. According to the founders of Nordic Biotech, "the present reality in drug development (…) is that almost any technology or compound can rapidly be reverse engineered" [7]. Adequate IP protection becomes a means to ensure that biotechnology companies can appropriate their R&D results and reduce the likelihood of imitation by competitors.

3. Contrary to traditional industries, where there is a clear distinction between the basic research performed in universities and public sector R&D institutions on the one hand, and the applied R&D undertaken by private enterprises on the other, in biotechnology, basic and applied research are often profoundly interlinked. Research undertaken in academic research institutions is often the basis for the establishment of biotechnology spin-offs. Similarly, biotechnology companies are often involved in (and are actively patenting) what some consider to be basic research.

4. The biotechnology industry, in most countries, consists mainly of recently established small enterprises, an important number of which have yet to take a product to market. In many cases, biotechnology SMEs are established on the basis of one or more patents developed within, or in partnership with, public research organizations or universities.

5. Finally, a point that derives from some of the issues discussed above is that for some biotech companies, intellectual property rights are actually the *final* product. It is not uncommon, in fact, to find biotechnology companies that develop innovative inventions, patent them, and then license them to larger companies that have the resources to take the product to market. Such companies may actually never sell a product themselves in the traditional sense but base their revenues on their ability to develop, protect, and out-license their innovations.

In addition, biotechnology patents are a breed onto themselves. For example, you cannot obtain general patent protection for DNA sequences of a novel gene in a number of species if you have only sequenced a single vertebrate or invertebrate example. Description of the species usually does not allow protection for the genus in patents in the biosciences. Also, DNA sequences for which no function has been demonstrated are generally not considered patentable. There are many laws and regulations that must be met, as shown below [8].

11.3.1 Genetic Engineering Patents

Isolated DNA sequences and proteins to which functions have been attributed and other metabolites are usually viewed in patent terms as chemical compounds, much like a new organic drug molecule. The unique sequence of the nucleotides or amino acids that you have uncovered constitutes a novel biological molecule (much like a novel chemical molecule) and may thus be patentable. In addition, vectors containing your nucleotide sequence and cells containing the vector/DNA may also be patented, provided they are considered new.

11.3.2 Microbiological Sciences Patents

Genetically modified organisms used in such processes may be eligible for patent protection. In addition, new microbes that you have isolated, purified, and cultured are generally considered patentable, provided they can fulfill the usefulness patent requirements.

11.3.3 Plant and Animal Sciences Patents

According to the patent laws of several countries, you cannot obtain biotechnological patent protection for plant or animal varieties, or essentially biological processes for the production of plants or animals. The United States is the exception to this and issues so-called *plant patents*. Similarly, biotech patent claims to animals obtained by traditional breeding methods are not allowable at most patent offices, but a genetically modified animal is considered patentable in the United Kingdom, Europe, and the United States. There is currently no equivalent in the animal sciences field to the protection offered by Plant Breeders' Rights [9].

11.3.4 Pharmaceutical and Chemical Sciences Patents

Novel purified chemical or pharmaceutical compounds are patentable, as well as their pharmaceutically acceptable isomers and salts. Crude extracts in which a compound is enriched may also be patentable, depending on the level of enrichment relative to the natural, unfractionated state. Importantly, novel pharmaceutical carriers may also be patented. Patent protection may also be obtained for pharmaceutical compositions containing your novel pharmaceutical compound.

11.3.5 Medical Sciences Patents

Because of the medical patent restriction on methods of treatment, diagnosis, or surgery mentioned above, surgical techniques are specifically excluded from patent protection in these regions. However, instruments for use in surgery, diagnosis, or therapy may be patented. In addition, diagnosis based on a sample obtained from the body is allowable and should, accordingly, be limited to in vitro applications in a patent application.

11.3.6 Microorganisms and Sufficiency of Description

In the complex field of biotechnology, it is not always possible to fully describe a microorganism in terms of physical, chemical, and genetic characteristics in a patent specification. The Budapest Treaty [10] provides a solution to this patent problem—patent applicants may deposit a sample of the organism (as claimed in the patent specification) at a recognized patent depository and in doing so may overcome patent examiners' arguments as regards insufficiency of description of the microorganism in the biotech patent application. The deposit number of the sample must be reflected in the patent specification and the deposit must have been made before or at the time of filing the patent application.

11.4 Practical Advice to the Entrepreneur/Inventor

I'm not going to buy my kids an encyclopedia. Let them walk to school like I did.

Yogi Berra

Patents do not merely protect inventions against imitators; they can also be used to block a competitor's technical progress. Thus, they are an integral part in your competitive advantage armamentarium.

These exclusive rights allow owners of intellectual property to benefit from the property they have created, providing a financial incentive for the creation of an investment in intellectual property, and, in the case of patents, attract investment capital.

The founder/entrepreneur needs to be fully aware of the time required to "prosecute" a patent, as shown in Figure 11.1.

Patents enable entrepreneurs to acquire financial capital under the most favorable terms in earlier founding rounds [11]. Firms of having larger patent portfolios enjoy a greater likelihood of sourcing initial capital and of achieving liquidity through an initial public offering. Given the lengthy government certification process, it provides a reliable "due diligence" signal for investors by which the quality of their investment can be quantified [12].

Given the fundraising importance of patent protection, the entrepreneur/investor must guard against making innocent mistakes that may prevent their ability to obtain a patent. An inventor has 1 year from the date of "first public disclosure" of the invention to file a patent application in the US Patent Office. "**First public disclosures**" are many, and surprisingly they include the following:

- Disclosures at presentations and poster sessions
- Prior public uses or demonstrations
- Prior conversations with potential partners
- Prior publications or interviews
- Prior sales of prototypes at beta sites

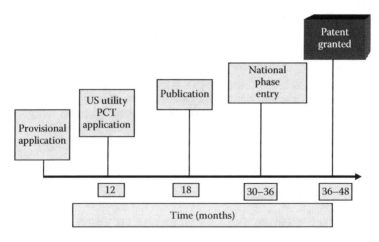

FIGURE 11.1
Patents are not a sprint; they are a marathon.

Also, keep in mind that if the US application is filed after the public disclosure, the inventor is not able to file or patent protection in many countries. There is only a 6-month "grace" period in Japan, Korea, and Russia. There is a 1-year grace period in Canada, Australia, and Mexico.

Also understand that the loss of foreign patent rights greatly diminishes the financial value of intellectual property in the eyes of investors. For that reason, and for your maximum protection, consider filing a patent application before embarking on any public disclosure.

- Is the patent in a subject area that is earning significant profits?
- Are there currently patent litigation cases in process in the subject area?
- Does the invention allow for reduced costs or increased performance?
- Are there any competitors that could directly benefit from your invention?
- Are there blocking or dominating patents in this area?
- Do you have freedom to operate?
- Do you have an inventorship/ownership policy in place?

In summary, a patent can help your company be more "investable." Fundamentally, investors will analyze the risks and potential rewards of a single investment. Owning one or more patents can reduce the risk of the company by strengthening the competitive advantage and providing an additional marketable asset.

11.5 Trade Secrets in the Start-Up Environment

Trade secrets are confidential and undisclosed business information that provides the owner with a competitive advantage. Virtually all types of information can be protected as a trade secret as long as reasonable and accepted measures are taken within the confines of the law. For example, the Uniform Trade Secrets Act, codified as Iowa Code Chapter 550, defines a trade secret as "information of nearly any kind that derives economic value from not being generally known or readily ascertainable by proper means, and is the subject of reasonable efforts to maintain its secrecy."

Examples of trade secrets include the following:

- Software, including source code
- Chemical formulations
- Customer lists

- Business plans
- Pricing models
- Marketing and sales strategies
- Manufacturing costs

A start-up needs to strongly consider whether to opt for patent protection or trade secret for certain innovations. Patent protection lasts for 20 years; a trade secret can last indefinitely unless (a) the information is no longer confidential, (b) the information has been discovered by legitimate means (such as reverse engineering), or (c) you do not maintain its confidentiality.

Thus, for certain innovations, the entrepreneur must decide a priori whether it will be economically more advantageous to seek a 20-year patent monopoly, or to maintain the information as a trade secret potentially indefinitely. Keep in mind that more than 80% of trade secrets are lost not only through employee disclosures but also through contractors, and insiders may inadvertently "spill the beans," as shown in Figure 11.2.

Unlike patents, state law governs the protection of trade secrets. Almost every state has adopted a variation of the Uniform Trade Secrets Act that generally provides protection to any formula, pattern, device, or compilation of information and provides a competitive advantage. The *"sine qua non"* of a trade secret is that the information is secret. The entrepreneur must also take reasonable steps to maintain the secrecy. However, trade secret protection does not protect the independent development of the secret [13].

11.5.1 Trade Secrets Must Be Kept Secret

The trade secret intrinsic value is generally established by showing that the secret is an advancement in the industry or offers a competitive advantage. As a practical matter, courts tend to protect information that was developed with a significant expenditure of time and money, is difficult to obtain, and is not generally known.

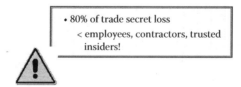

- 80% of trade secret loss
  < employees, contractors, trusted insiders!

- Departing or disgruntled employees
- Intentional (malicious)
- Inevitable (disseminated knowledge)
- Through ignorance

FIGURE 11.2
Eighty percent of trade secret loss.

Develop a trade secret protection policy

Advantages of a written policy:

– Clarity **(how to identify and protect)**
– How to reveal **(in-house or to outsiders)**
– Demonstrable commitment to protection → **important in litigation**
– Educate and train:
  • **Clear communication and repetition**
  • **Copy of policy, intranet, periodic training and audit, etc.**
  • **Make known that disclosure of a TS may result in termination and/or legal action**
– Monitor compliance, prosecute violators

FIGURE 11.3
Develop a protection policy.

Documenting steps taken to protect and develop a trade secret is accordingly crucial. Once trade secret protection is established, however, the owner should be able to prevent the following [14]:

1. Unauthorized disclosure by those formerly or presently in an express or implied confidential relationship with the owner
2. Discovery of the trade secret by improper or unethical means

Figure 11.3 summarizes ways you can develop a written trade secret protection policy.

11.5.2 Business Factors Affecting Your Decision

There are four types of intellectual property rights: patents, copyrights, trademarks, and trade secrets. Only two of these intellectual property rights protect information: patents and trade secrets. Patents protect information by dedicating the information to the public in return for a limited monopoly. Trade secrets protect information with independent competitive value derived from the secrecy of the information.

A start-up owner must weigh various factors other than just the legal scope of the different forms of protection in determining whether to maintain an invention as a trade secret or to apply for patent protection. Table 11.3 summarizes the alternatives.

11.5.3 Protecting Your Trade Secrets

As we have seen, trade secrets can include, but are not limited to, manufacturing processes, formulas, marketing and business strategies, customer lists, training programs, search algorithms, and recipes. The information

TABLE 11.3

Patents versus Trade Secrets

Factors Favoring Patent Protection	Factors Favoring Maintaining Trade Secrets
1. Patents provide a deterrent to competitors who otherwise might be tempted to make and sell similar products.	1. The expense of obtaining the patent, which does not immediately provide a revenue stream (unless licensed) and, similarly, the potential for protecting the invention in foreign jurisdictions as a trade secret without the difficulty and expense of obtaining foreign patents.
2. The protection it supplies for inventions that can be reverse-engineered.	
3. The avoidance of any need to maintain complete security for inventions to be kept as an internal trade secret.	2. The potential for product launch delay while a patent application is being filed.
4. Patents furnish value as assets potentially useful for cross-licensing technology in settlement of patent infringement (or other) litigation.	3. Disclosure in a patent provides a "roadmap" facilitating an unscrupulous competitor's copying your invention.
5. Highly attractive to investors.	4. The expense of enforcing a patent against an infringer through litigation.
6. The ability to out-license the patent and derive immediate economic value.	5. Negative know-how (what doesn't work).
7. Can apply for continuations-in-part.	6. Nonpatentable improvements.
8. Competitive advantage.	7. Attractive if patent protection is uncertain.
9. Marketing and sales tool.	
10. "Shelf life" is long.	8. No government filing.
11. Technology is easier to outsource.	9. Immediate effect.
12. Easier to enforce than trade secrets.	
13. Legal monopoly.	

can be a trade secret as long as it is of a business or technical nature and derives value from not being generally known and the information cannot be readily ascertainable by independent development or reverse engineering [15].

Finally, the owner of a trade secret must take steps to protect its confidentiality. Otherwise, it is not likely to be a secret. The following are two practical steps to ensure the maintenance of your trade secrets:

1. **Know what constitutes trade secrets.** Company leaders must examine their operations from top to bottom, documenting valuable information. As part of the trade-secret audit, companies must determine who has access to the information, where records relating to it are stored, and what the historic costs of developing it are. If an employee leaves and is believed to have taken company information, these audits place the company in a much better position to ask the courts to step in.

2. **Establish a culture of confidentiality.** After conducting an internal audit, business leaders must take an additional step: create a culture

of confidentiality. They can do this by instituting the following measures:

Confidentiality agreements—New employees who are likely to have access to trade secrets should be required to acknowledge—in writing—that they will be entrusted with such information and that they will safeguard it. This makes clear, at the beginning of the relationship, that confidentiality is something the company takes seriously.

Covenants not to compete and nonsolicitation agreements—These agreements are often combined with confidentiality agreements, but they provide additional protections to the employer. After all, what better way to ensure that an ex-employee does not use sensitive information against a former employer than preventing them from working in the same industry for some period and cutting off contact with former customers? Employers seeking to use such agreements must be careful. North Carolina law requires that covenants not to compete and nonsolicitation agreements be entered at the beginning of the employment relationship or as part of a change in duties or compensation. They also must be used to protect legitimate business interests. Courts routinely hold that the protection of trade secrets qualifies as a legitimate business interest.

Training programs—Eighteenth-century English writer Samuel Johnson said, "People need to be reminded more often than they need to be instructed." When it comes to trade secrets, regular instructions and directives from the front office serve to keep the need for confidentiality in the forefront of employees' minds.

Computer and physical security—Atlanta-based The Coca-Cola Co. does not leave its secret soft-drink formula on a table in the manufacturing room. Instead, it is locked in a vault that few people have access to. Companies should take similar measures when it comes to their secret information that competitors would love to have for themselves. Records should be segregated, and computer files should be restricted to only those with a need for them. Someone in human resources, for example, should not be able to access files that contain information regarding valuable manufacturing processes. Along these lines, companies should consider implementing computer-security measures that notify management when certain employees attach external devices to their computers or download or upload information. The number of recently filed lawsuits in which an employee, shortly before quitting, uploaded thousands of files to cloud storage or copied them to a flash drive is remarkable.

Personal devices—Work demands more of employees' time, so in an effort to provide the best service possible, employees frequently access work e-mail through a web service on their personal device, or they forward work e-mails to a personal account. "Bring Your Own Device" policies are born from the reality that more employees are conducting business on their personal devices. An employee losing his or her device, however, is a recipe for disaster. Additionally, when employees leave, company information on their phones go with them. Companies should therefore either prohibit employees from using personal devices for business purposes or mandate that employees submit to certain security measures such as password protection on the device and occasional audits of the device. Violations of these policies can be grounds for termination.

Exit interviews—When an employee who regularly had access to trade-secret information leaves, companies must take time to meet with that employee to remind him of his obligations to safeguard such information, including the duty to honor any confidentiality agreement and covenant not to compete that he signed. Companies must demand the immediate return of all their property, including not only company-issued phones, laptops, and other equipment, but work notes and other documents.

Start-up executives must understand and enforce their companies' trade secrets. To this end, executives should emphasize that trade secrets are composed of four information elements: (1) financial, (2) technical/scientific, (3) marketing, and (4) negative, as shown in Figure 11.4.

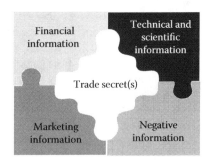

FIGURE 11.4
Trade secrets.

11.6 University Patents versus Trade Secrets Policy

Universities spend millions of dollars annually conducting basic research. The most visible rewards of this research are the host of publications, presentations, and graduate theses, which communicate these research findings to scientific colleagues throughout the world and provide the basis for educating students. Such broad dissemination of research results is unquestionably the primary goal of university research activities.

Sometimes, however, academic research also results in commercially important intellectual property that may be patentable. Intellectual property has always been an integral part of economic growth and in recent years has become critical to the US international competitiveness and industrial health. As a result, a large number of laws, as well as state and federal programs, have been developed to stimulate the inventive process and increase the rate at which valuable inventions move from the academic laboratory into the marketplace [16].

To be protected as a trade secret, the information or invention must be used in a business, and positive measures must be employed to keep it secret. Since a university's task is exactly the opposite, the dissemination of technical information, universities are seldom involved with maintaining trade secrets. This creates an inherent conflict.

11.6.1 The Academic "Research Exception"

University researchers thrive on free interchange of ideas and discoveries with scientific peers throughout the world. Why, in such an environment, would a university seek to patent the discoveries of its researchers, since a patent may be perceived as a restriction on the use of the discovery that is patented? There are four important reasons, among others:

- Traditionally, a "research exception" has been recognized as a limit on a patent's effectiveness. Generally, patents covering a technology do not limit academic research on that technology. Thus, patenting has been assumed not to prevent academic research by the inventor or by anyone else in the academic research community.

- Historical experience has shown that ideas that are not patented—which are instead "dedicated to the public"—tend not to be developed commercially. This is because few commercial businesses will invest the millions of dollars frequently required to develop a university-originated idea into a commercial product unless there is a sufficiently long period in which that investment can be recovered from a "protected" market.

- Commercial development of practical ideas has become more essential to the economic well-being of the nation and the state; the economic dominance once enjoyed by American companies continues to be eroded by nations more adept at commercializing new ideas—in many cases, new ideas that originated in the United States but were not protected through patenting.
- Ferocious competition for federal research grants has increased the importance of industrial research funding, which usually requires the resulting technology to be patent protected.

Since much state-of-the-art research is done at university laboratories, researchers within the university setting play an extremely crucial role in the technology commercialization process. However, if researchers act without regard to the patent implications of their activities, the value of this cutting-edge technology can be lost, and US opportunities to commercialize such technology can be severely compromised [17].

11.6.2 Can Academic Researchers Have Their Cake and Eat It Too?

With so many ways to lose patentability, researchers may infer that they cannot have both patents and publication freedom. THIS IS NOT NECESSARILY THE CASE. Patentability can be protected in a number of ways, while still allowing researchers to publish and collaborate. Baylor University recommends the following steps:

1. **File a Patent Application before Publication**

   Publication defeats patentability only if it occurs before filing for patent protection. Hence, one easy way of protecting patentability is to have a patent application on file before the publication, the poster session, the discussion at a scientific meeting, and so on.

   Invention Disclosure is the first step to filing a patent application. The proper Invention Disclosure form for Baylor University inventions are filed by the Office of the Vice Provost for Research. Thus, simply communicating before publication can make a significant difference. It is essential that researchers think of patentability before they publish. Given a modicum of advance notice, the Office of the Vice Provost for Research can make sure that all patent rights are protected and that publication can go forward without problem or delay.

2. **Use Confidential Disclosure Agreements**

   Publication means communication to persons with no obligation to hold the communication confidential. Thus, another way to protect patentability is to place such an obligation of confidentiality on the audience. This is unworkable with any large audience, but it is very easy with a small group—for example, a meeting with industry scientists interested in a researcher's work. Whether these scientists visit the university lab or the researcher travels to the company's labs. A simple one-page Confidential Disclosure Agreement can make the difference between retention and loss of patent rights.

Again, the Office of the Vice Provost for Research can provide these forms and assist in their use. Industrial people seldom object to the forms, since patentability ultimately helps them the most. So if a researcher is scheduling a technical meeting with people outside Baylor University, a quick call to the Office of the Vice Provost for Research is all that's needed to help protect any potential patent rights.

3. **Don't Disclose "Enabling" Information**

Since a communication must be enabling to defeat patentability, a researcher can also protect patent rights merely by giving a "tantalizing glimpse" of the technology without revealing technical details. This is not always appropriate, since a presenter at a scientific meeting is expected to answer technical questions from the audience. However, smaller or less formal meetings can easily show the results or benefits of a technology without revealing the details of how they are achieved.

As a general rule, complete technical information should not be volunteered. Abstracts or oral presentations can be "sanitized" to reveal only the general objectives and results of the work, without revealing significant, patentable details.

4. **When in Doubt, Mark "CONFIDENTIAL"**

As discussed in conjunction with research proposals to federal agencies, it never hurts to mark something as CONFIDENTIAL. It's not a guarantee, but it can help if the recipient of the information could be expected to hold information confidential on the basis of it bearing that message.

11.7 Summary

To patent or not to patent? That is the question. The answer is: it all depends on your specific circumstances. In addition to Coca-Cola, consider the following well-known cases [18]:

The Big Mac Secret Special Sauce: In 2004, McDonald's acknowledged privately that they had lost the recipe for the Big Mac special sauce. As it turns out, McDonald's changed the original special sauce recipe to cut costs and lost the original. When a returning executive wanted to return to the original special sauce, no one could find the recipe. The executive remembered the name of the California company that supplied the sauce 36 years ago. They still had the sauce in their record books, and McDonald's was able to recover the recipe.

KFC Chicken Recipe: In the entire company, only two KFC executives know the finger-lickin' recipe of 11 herbs and spices. A third executive knows the combination to the safe where the handwritten recipe resides. Less than a handful of KFC employees know the identities of the three executives, who are not allowed to travel together on the same plane or in the same car for security reasons. After being locked in a safe for 68 years, Colonel Harland Sanders' handwritten recipe was temporarily relocated to a secret-secure location as KFC modernizes its safekeeping. It was ceremoniously transported in an armored car and high-security motorcade.

WD-40 Formula: The formula for WD-40 spray lubricant and rust remover is locked in a bank vault and has only ever been taken out of the vault twice—once when they changed banks and once on the occasion of the CEOs 50th birthday. The CEO rode into Times Square on the back of a horse in a suit of armor with the formula. The company mixes WD-40 in a concentrated form in three locations—San Diego, Sydney, and London—and then sends it to aerosol manufacturing partners.

In 1953, a fledgling company called Rocket Chemical Company and its staff of three set out to create a line of rust-prevention solvents and degreasers for use in the aerospace industry. Working in a small laboratory in San Diego, California, it took them 40 attempts to get the water displacing formula worked out, but they must have been really good, because the original secret formula for WD-40—which stands for water displacement perfected on their 40th try—is still in use today [19].

Convair, an aerospace contractor, first used WD-40 to protect the outer skin of the Atlas Missile from rust and corrosion. The product actually worked so well that several employees snuck some WD-40 cans out of the plant to use at home. In 1968, as a goodwill gesture, kits containing WD-40 were sent to soldiers in Vietnam to prevent moisture damage on firearms and help keep them in good working condition.

Lena Blackburne's Baseball Rubbing Mud: There is this special baseball rubbing mud, and Major League Baseball absolutely depends on it. A brand new baseball just out of the box is slippery; so much so that a pitcher has no control when throwing one unless it's dirtied up a bit first. So, an umpire spends a lot of his time before a game rubbing mud into dozens of balls, but not just any mud works. Before the 1930s, teams tried all kinds of substances, including tobacco juice and shoe polish, but nothing really worked. Then, one day, Lena Blackburne, a no-name player turned coach, was taking a walk near his house in New Jersey when he stumbled upon some strange mud. Obviously having a "Eureka!" moment to rival Archimedes', Blackburne took some home and tried it out. Amazingly enough, it worked brilliantly.

By 1938, the American League was using Blackburn Rubbing Mud exclusively on all their balls. The National League wouldn't use it until the 1950s, mostly because Blackburn refused to sell it to them, but they've been using it ever since.

11.7.1 The Big Trade-Off

A trade secret can grant proprietary rights in perpetuity, or for as long as the owner is able to maintain the secrecy. A patent, on the other hand, has a shelf life of 20 years from the time an application is filed, and while a trade secret can remain an enigma, a patent application requires the inventor to describe exactly how his invention works [20].

Trade secrets can include an intangible process, technique, or method. A trade secret can be a quantifiable design, composition, formula, or pattern. It can be a physical device or mechanism. Chemical formulas, manufacturing processes, or business information can be considered trade secrets, and even if the ingredients in a chemical recipe like a soft-drink syrup or fried chicken batter are discovered, the exact ratios involved or the way they are combined can still remain a trade secret.

Until last year, American inventors could rely on the US Patent and Trademark Office to keep a patent application secret until it was granted. If the application was rejected, the invention remained confidential, but in 2011, the United States, following the rest of the world, initiated a new practice of publishing patent applications 18 months after the application is filed.

Anyone who makes commercial use of a trade secret and later decides to apply for a patent must do so within a year. After that, the invention is no longer eligible for a patent. An idea can, however, have a copyright and also be a trade secret. The US Copyright Office allows material to be divided so that some parts can be revealed while others are kept secret.

Since trade secrets are intellectual property, courts have ruled that software algorithms, customer lists, financial data, Wall Street formulas, names of suppliers, and even blueprints can qualify. What makes them unique as intellectual property is the economic value derived from their being kept secret, and corporations have been known to spend millions to defend them.

Or forsake millions. In the 1970s, Coca-Cola withdrew from India rather than comply with a law in that country that would have compelled the soft-drink manufacturer to transfer technology—in this case, its secret syrup formula—to an Indian-owned company.

There are disadvantages to trade secrets, compared with patents, because just about anything can be analyzed, reverse-engineered, and copied, and patents and trade secrets are not equals in a courtroom; patents are accepted as valid, whereas trade secrets must be authenticated first.

To defend a trade secret under most states' laws, the owner has to show that a reasonable effort has been made to maintain the secrecy. Companies can require employees, suppliers, and subcontractors to sign nondisclosure, confidentiality, or noncompete agreements. They can divide a process or formula among workers, making sure that no one has knowledge of the entire secret.

In most cases, the courts look at how many people inside and outside a business know about the secret, what kind of precautions the owner takes to preserve the secrecy, the value the owner gains against his competitors from holding the secret, and how much trouble and expense someone else would incur to crack the secret.

Patents, trademarks, and copyrights fall under federal law, but trade secrets are covered by state law. That practice can be traced to the 19th century, when common law protected trade secrets. Most states have adopted specific laws since then, which differ from place to place, though some still use common law. In 1996, the Economic Espionage Act made theft of trade secrets a federal crime.

Despite the increasing importance of trade secrets to world economies, there is no global law on trade secrets, or even a universal definition of a trade secret. Patents, copyrights, and trademarks are addressed in comprehensive international legal treaties; trade secrets are not included. What can be protected as a trade secret differs from country to country and, in some nations, trade secrets have no legal standing at all.

Global "harmonization" of intellectual property laws has been a top American policy priority in recent years, but trade secrets are still at a disadvantage. Germany and Japan require public trials for lawsuits, for example, and anyone seeking redress must first reveal his trade secret. In other countries, confidential data are revealed when submitted for government review of safety or effectiveness.

References

1. Raysman, R., Pisacreta, E.A., and Adler, K.A. *Intellectual Property Licensing: Forms and Analysis.* Law Journal Press, 1998–2008. ISBN 973-58852-086.
2. *WIPO Intellectual Property Handbook.* WIPO Publication No. 489(E) 2004, http://www.wipo.int/export/sites/www/about-ip/en/iprm/pdf/ch2.pdf.

3. Halligan, R.M. Trade secrets vs patents: The new calculus. *Landslide*, 2(6), July/August 2010. © 2010 by the American Bar Association, https://clients.kilpat ricktownsend.com/IPDeskReference/Documents/Trade%20Secret%20or%20 Patent%20Protection.pdf.

4. European Commission. *Life Sciences and Biotechnology—A Strategy for Europe*, 2002.

5. Burrone, E. Patents at the Core: The Biotech Business, esteban.burrone@wipo .int.

6. http://www.wipo.int/sme/en/documents/patents_biotech.htm

7. Medicon Valley Patent Guide, 2002. Medicon Valley is a Danish/Swedish organization, http://www.mva.org/media(3,1033)/Medicon Valley Patent Guide .pdf.

8. Hoffelner, C. Patents Biotech Biotechnology, http://www.svw.co.za/patents -biotech.html.

9. Wikipedia Plant Breeder's Rights, http://en.wikipedia.org/wiki/Plant_breed ers'_rights.

10. WIPO Biotechnology http://www.wipo.int/patent-law/en/developments/bio technology.html.

11. Hsu, D. and Ziedonis, R.H. Patents as Quality Signals for Entrepreneurial Ventures. Copenhagen, DRUID Summer Conference, Denmark, June 2007, http://www2.druid.dk/conferences/viewpaper.php?id=1717&cf=9.

12. Spence, M. Job market signaling. *Quarterly Journal of Economics*, 87, 355–374, 1973.

13. Toren, P.J. Patent Bar Review 2014, Patents vs trade secrets, http://www.ipwatch dog.com/2014/12/09/trade-secrets-a-viable-alternative-to-patents/id=52554/.

14. Kilpatrick Stockton Intellectual Property Desk Reference. Choosing between trade secret and patent protection, https://clients.kilpatricktownsend.com / IPDeskReference/Documents/Trade%20Secret%20or%20Patent%20 Protection.pdf.

15. Durham, J.B. Three steps business leaders must take to protect valuable information. *Business North Carolina*, 2013, http://www.poynerspruill.com/publica tions/Pages/3StepsBusLeadersTakeProtectInformation.aspx.

16. http://www.baylor.edu/research/vpr/files/inventionsandtechnologytransfer .pdf

17. http://www.baylor.edu/research/vpr/files/patentlawbasics.pdf

18. Benjamin, K. Secrets Only Two Living People Know (For Some Reason), http:// www.cracked.com/article/147_7-secrets-only-two-living-people-know-for -some-reason/.

19. http://wd40.com/cool-stuff/history

20. Chartrand, S. Patents; Many companies will forgo patents in an effort to safeguard their trade secrets. 2001, http://www.nytimes.com/2001/02/05/business /patents-many-companies-will-forgo-patents-effort-safeguard-their-trade -secrets.html.

21. Maynard, J.T. and Peters, H.M. *Understanding Chemical Patents*. American Chemical Society, Washington, DC. p. 86, 1991.

12

Strategic Alliances

12.1 Introduction

Strategic alliances are a formal relationship formed between two or more parties to pursue a set of agreed upon goals or to meet a critical business need while still remaining as independent organizations. On many occasions, strategic alliances are partnerships formed between two organizations in response to an essential threat or opportunity in their business environment.

Strategic alliances are also called join ventures, interfirm collaborations, or consortium agreements. Table 12.1 summarizes the distinguishing characteristics among the alliance types.

Joint ventures and strategic alliances allow companies with complementary skills to benefit from one another's strengths. They are common in technology, manufacturing, and commercial real estate development, and whenever a company wants to expand its sales or operations into a foreign country. In a joint venture, the companies start and invest in a new company that's jointly owned by both of the parent companies. A strategic alliance is a legal agreement between two or more companies to share access to their technology, trademarks, or other assets. A strategic alliance does not create a new company [1].

12.2 The "Big Question"

Strategic alliances represent a way for aggressive companies to pursue growth by broadening product lines, penetrating new markets, and stabilizing cyclical businesses despite limited resources, but before embarking on any strategic alliance quest, management must answer the Big Question:

> Can we create organic sales growth versus sales growth through strategic alliances or acquisitions?

The firm can grow organically (by internal investment) or inorganically (by strategic alliances, i.e., cooperative ventures, joint ventures, joint ownership,

TABLE 12.1

Distinguishing Characteristics among Strategic Alliance Types

Alliance Type	Distinguishing Characteristics
Informal cooperation	Mutual help in distribution, sharing space at industry meetings No legal formalization
Formal collaborations	Uncertainty related to specific tasks Clear need for flexibility Success without losing independence Legal documentation in place
Consortium agreements	Need for large size and technical skills Need for large geographical coverage Limited financial risk for each partner Achieving goals without loss of identity
Joint ventures	Clear business need to form relationship Specific allocation of resources Legal formalization Not tied to core technologies or geographical location Independent business entities Pooling resources to share risks, rewards, and control Commercial purpose of defined scope and duration

or mergers and acquisitions [M&A]). One theoretical way of approaching the Big Question is to look at the continuum of strategic alliance options interdependence as shown in Figure 12.1.

When two or more companies combined participate in a project, it is a **cooperative venture**. This participation can be in the form of sharing financial or technical resources for mutual benefit.

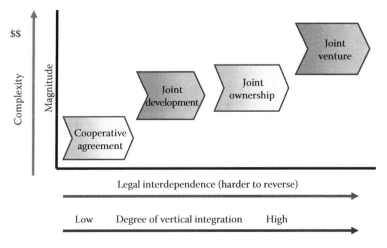

FIGURE 12.1
Strategic alliance options.

A **joint venture** (JV) creates a separate entity in which both firms invest. The JV agreement specifies investment rights, operational responsibilities, voting control, exit alternatives, and generally the allocation of risks and rewards. The entity could be a division or an entirely new business established for the venture.

In a **joint ownership** alliance, the parties agree to long-term licensing agreement, co-marketing agreements, co-development agreements, joint purchasing agreements, and long-term supply or toll agreements, with each party owning 50% of the intellectual property (IP) plus other nontangible assets.

Strategic alliances can be characterized as follows [2]:

- Relative bargaining power and ownership
- Degree of interfirm cooperation
- Individual contribution to the value chain
- Geographical reach
- Acceptable economic risk
- Legal interdependence (ability to walk away)

12.3 Advantages of Strategic Alliances

Strategic alliances represent an alluring means for start-ups to pursue high-growth strategies despite limited resources. The underlying rationale is that one plus one equals three. Alliances promise to provide the partners greater likelihood of success in a competitive context than if they were to go alone. If you are contemplating a strategic alliance, ask yourself the following preliminary questions:

- Why do you want to form a strategic alliance in the first place?
- What outcomes (benefits) do you envision from the alliance?
- Do you have other (or better) ways of achieving your goals?
- What makes the other party an attractive partner to you?
- Are your goals compatible with those of your potential partner?
- Are you and your potential partner a good match in terms of culture, background, experience organizational values, and strategic goals?

Traditionally, inorganic growth can be achieved by the judicious use of strategic alliances. In a strategic alliance, both risks and rewards are shared

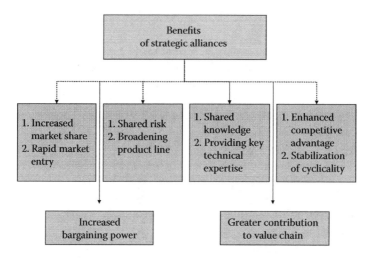

FIGURE 12.2
Benefits of strategic alliances.

and typically lead to long-term strategic benefits for both partners, as summarized below:

- Adding value to products
- Improving market access
- Strengthening operations
- Adding technological strength
- Enhancing strategic growth
- Enhancing organizational skills
- Building financial strength

In addition, strategic alliances display other advantages, such as those seen in Figure 12.2.

12.4 Pitfalls of Strategic Alliances

Although a properly planned and implemented strategic alliance can undoubtedly boost the growth and profitability of the participating partners, the route to a successful partnership is not without pitfalls.

One of the most common occurs when there is a substantial difference in the sizes of the two partner organizations. Such a disparity can easily

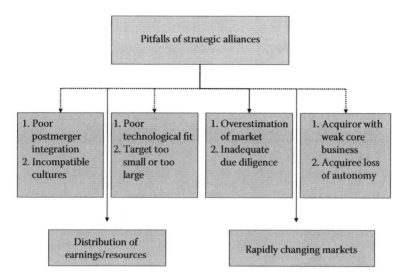

FIGURE 12.3
Pitfalls of strategic alliances.

generate conflict and misunderstanding [3]. Conflict does not have to be a roadblock to a successful alliance if you and your partnering alliance members are willing to resolve the conflict at the core level, in a timely manner. In fact, the resolved conflict can lead to a stronger relationship through improved communication. Unfortunately, conflict that is left unresolved will lead to fatal flaws that will erode the relationship [4].

Just because you're working with a company of integrity, it doesn't mean they will look out for you. Even in a partnering relationship, you are still accountable for your own success and well-being. Make sure your bottom-line expectations take into account that servicing the partnering agreement is going to require extra resources. Be certain of everybody's alliance partnering goals. Some of the more common areas of conflict in alliance relationships are shown in Figure 12.3.

12.5 Best Practices

Three are two schools of thought regarding strategic alliances. Practitioners of the first school argue that transactions are accomplished by the hubris of the two respective executives, with details negotiated at a later time by the respective company specialists. The second school of thought recognizes the intricacies of the transaction and develops a systematic methodology, thus increasing the likelihood of long-term success.

TABLE 12.2

Best Practices for M&A Negotiations

Common Mistakes	Common Solutions
Unrealistic timetables and expectations	Select an acquisitions team experienced in cost/benefit time allocation
Inexperienced M&A negotiation team	Establish an acquisitions team with defined responsibilities and authority
Lack of structured transaction process	Clearly define team member roles Be prepared to "walk away" from a bad deal
Disproportionate time spent on minor issues	Focus on outcomes, not activities Set "drop dead" dates
Incomplete or irrelevant information	Obtain corroborating data
Inadequate or nonexistent due diligence	Engage industry experts
Inadequate sensitivity analysis	Perform financial and commercial sensitivity analyses Set minimums
Overlooking integration issues	Thoroughly assess the impact of "culture clashes" Can value be created?
Poor negotiating techniques	Preplan negotiation strategies, tactics, and strategic objectives
Naïve and inexperienced negotiators	Decide on deal breakers ahead of time
No meeting transcriptions or minutes	Include a "secretary" as note taker
Communications failures	Debrief other party on issues discussed and agreements reached
Long time to reach a Term Sheet agreement Deals have a life. A lengthy negotiation for a Term Sheet is an early warning sign of impending impasse	This is the most significant document in the early stages. It should list price, form of payment, deal structure, and management issues. The Letter of Intent will follow the overall principles contained in the Term Sheet
Overreliance on a Letter of Intent by seller It is merely "An agreement to agree"	Understanding that a Letter of Intent is a nonbinding agreement. While it is crucially important, an agreement to agree is not an agreement

The establishment of a methodology for analyzing a potential M&A is the difference between an amateur and an experienced buyer. Table 12.2 presents a summary of best practices to be followed.

12.6 Strategic International Alliances

Strategic international alliances (SIAs) are sought as a way to shore up weaknesses and increase competitive strengths. Opportunities for rapid expansion into new markets, access to new technology, more efficient production and marketing costs, and additional sources of capital are all motives for engaging in SIAs [5].

An SIA is a business relationship established by two or more companies to cooperate out of mutual need and to share risk in achieving a common objective. An SIA implies (1) that there is a common objective; (2) that one partner's weakness is offset by the other's strength; (3) that reaching the objective alone would be too costly, take too much time, or be too risky; and (4) that together their respective strengths make possible what otherwise would be unattainable. In short, an SIA is a synergistic relationship established to achieve a common goal where both parties benefit.

Opportunities abound the world over but, to benefit, firms must be current in new technology, have the ability to keep abreast of technological change, have distribution systems to capitalize on global demand, have cost-effective manufacturing, and have capital to build new systems as necessary. Other reasons to enter into strategic alliances include the following:

1. Acquiring needed current market bases
2. Acquiring needed technological bases
3. Utilizing excess manufacturing capacity
4. Reducing new market risk and entry costs
5. Accelerating product introductions demanded by rapid technological changes and shorter product life cycles
6. Achieving economies of scale in production, research and development (R&D), or marketing
7. Overcoming cultural and trade barriers
8. Extending the existing scope of operations

The scope of what a company needs to do and what it can do is at a point where even the largest firms engage in alliances to maintain their competitiveness.

A company enters a strategic alliance to acquire the skills necessary to achieve its objectives more effectively, and at a lower cost or with less risk than if it acted alone.

For example, a company strong in R&D skills and weak in the ability or capital to successfully market a product will seek an alliance to offset its weakness—one partner to provide marketing skills and capital and the other to provide technology and a product. The majority of alliances today are designed to exploit markets and technology.

Of course, not all SIAs are successful; some fail and others are dissolved after reaching their goals. Failures can be attributed to a variety of reasons, but all revolve around lack of perceived benefits to one or more of the partners. Benefits may never have been realized in some cases, and different goals and management styles have caused dissatisfaction in other alliances.

12.7 Strategic Alliances and Partnerships

In an increasingly challenging marketplace, where mergers have failed to deliver R&D productivity gains, the importance of alliances has increased significantly [6]. In fact, research suggests that products co-developed by a pharmaceutical and biotech company are more likely to be commercialized than those that are developed by a single entity [7].

Demonstrating the growing importance of strategic alliances, "the 20 biggest pharmaceutical firms formed nearly 1,500 alliances with biotech companies between 1997 and 2002" [8]. In the highly competitive drug industry, effective alliance strategies have provided an opportunity to proactively manage risk.

12.7.1 International Alliances Examples

An interesting example of a successful alliance strategy may be the giant pharmaceutical company Merck, which has undergone a dramatic business development transformation. Long regarded as the pharmaceutical industry's best at internal R&D and admired for its ability to rely on its internal capability, Merck has changed corporate course and now aggressively pursues external licensing and alliance opportunities to feed its pipeline. Merck's partnership transactions have risen by almost 80%. In addition, Merck is actively engaging in co-promotion. In the past few years, three of four drug launches were co-promoted [9].

For example, the partnership between Roche and Genentech is often cited as the most successful strategic alliance to date in the industry. In 1990, Roche bought 10% of Genentech for $490 million, giving them a 60% stake and control. The agreement gave Roche a much-coveted access to Genentech's data after the completion of Phase II trials, with the option to decide if they wanted to commercialize the tested product.

While Genentech maintained its independence, Roche obtained ownership of a growing entrepreneurial company without fear of stifling innovation. Roche also gained access to a pipeline it could market outside the United States. The deal benefited Genentech by providing much needed funding and by freeing up management to focus on the core business rather than raising capital. In two separate deals, Roche's total investment in Genentech was approximately $7.7 billion. Overall, Roche raised about "$8 billion in cash after the IPO and they still own 54 percent of Genentech worth about $28 billion" [10].

In 2015, Roche maintained its strategic alliance momentum by partnering with US diagnostics firm GeneWEAVE BioSciences "superbug" diagnostics firm for up to $425 million. Roche planned to pay shareholders in the privately held Californian company $190 million upfront and up to a further $235 million depending on the future success of its products [11].

The deal gives Roche access to GeneWEAVE's "Smarticles" technology, which allows for the rapid identification of multidrug-resistant organisms direct from clinical samples, without the need for traditional preparation processes. Better testing is seen as central to fighting drug-resistant bacteria. It should allow doctors to make faster and more accurate diagnoses and give patients the appropriate drug to kill their particular infection. Roche has been building up its presence in antibacterial research since buying Switzerland's Polyphor, a developer of new medicines for resistant bacteria, in November 2013. Although Roche pioneered some of the more modern antibiotics, like many large drug-makers, it wound down its research at the end of the 1990s, given the poor returns in the antibiotics field compared to other therapy areas such as cancer.

12.8 Joint Technology Development Alliances

There is an increasing trend in business today toward the joint development of technology by two or more corporate partners. Whether these arrangements are called joint development agreements, joint ventures, corporate partnering, alliances, or other names, there are some basic legal considerations that must be considered when a joint development of technology is employed [12].

Typically, the motivating factor for a joint-development arrangement is that each of the parties brings a needed piece of the technology puzzle to the table. For example, one company may have excellent basic research, but not the practical development expertise needed to launch a successful product. Another common situation involves the joint adaptation of an existing product to a new market.

The joint-development arrangement is usually embodied in a written contract between two or more partners. The contract is the framework on which the relationship is built and must be negotiated and drafted carefully and completely in order to be effective. The contract may govern the relationship of the parties for many years and may be referred to when conflicts or other issues arise. Thus, it is important to raise and negotiate the major points at minimum of the contract in order to avoid uncertainty and potential time-consuming and expensive litigation.

One example of a possible resolution of the technology ownership question would be to determine that those inventions that are created as a result of work on the contract solely by an employee or employees of partner A are owned by partner A; inventions that are conceived during the term of the contract solely by an employee or employees of partner B are owned by partner B. In the case of inventions conceived jointly by an employee or employees of both partners, the invention can be owned in joint, undivided interests by partner A and partner B, meaning that either partner can practice the invention without accounting to the other.

12.9 Strategic Partnership Licensing

Licensing implies a legally binding agreement between parties who receive and exchange approximately equal benefits and value. A voluntary license must be a win–win arrangement in order to be successful [13]. Successful partnership licensing depends on five fundamental principles.

1. **Technology licensing only occurs when one of the parties owns valuable intangible assets, such as IP.** A license is a consent by the owner to the use of IP in exchange for money or something else of value. Technology licensing does not occur when there is no commercially viable IP.

2. **There are three different kinds of technology licenses.** Licenses may be for certain IP rights only (e.g., a license to practice an identified patent or to copy and distribute a certain work of authorship). Licenses may be for *all the IP rights of any kind* that are necessary to reproduce, make, use, market, and sell products based on a type of technology (e.g., a license to develop a new software product that is protected by patent, copyright, trademark, and trade secret law). A license may also be for all the IP rights necessary in order to create and market a product that complies with a technical standard or specification (e.g., a group of enterprises has agreed on a technical standard to ensure interoperability of devices—the group agrees to pool their IP rights and license to each other all rights each will need to manufacture and sell the product).

3. **Technology licensing occurs in the context of a business relationship in which other agreements are often important.** These agreements are interrelated, whether they are in distinct documents or integrated in one big document.

4. **Technology licensing negotiations, like all negotiations, have sides (parties) whose interests are different, but must coincide in some ways.** It is difficult to successfully negotiate a license where you wish to obtain the rights to technology if you have little to offer in return. Ideally, both sides to the negotiation will have different elements of value to offer, including, for example, skilled employees, a market that can be commercially exploited, know-how, research facilities and commitments, and some form of IP.

5. **Technology licensing involves reaching agreement on a complex set of terms, and advance preparation is essential.** In advance of the negotiation, before the other party has been approached, a party may spend many months defining business objectives, assessing leverage, researching the other party, deciding positions on key terms, preparing documentation, and protecting IP, among other tasks.

12.10 IP Joint Ownership in Strategic Alliances

An issue that arises in any joint-development arrangement is the contribution of each partner to the project. In the written contract, each partner's contribution can be set forth in a list or table that is either part of the main contract or an appendix to it. This can include the scope of the work, where the work is to be performed, a schedule for the completion of various tasks, and which partner will perform each portion of the work. An important consideration is the so-called background technology. Often, one or more partners will own patents or trade secrets that must be used if the joint development is to be a success. In this case, licenses may have to be granted under the contract, or if a new entity is formed for the joint development (such as a joint venture company), licenses may have to be granted to that new entity. As with any legal document, the more specific the listings of each partner's contribution, the better the contract.

Joint ownership often arises in connection with collaborative innovation, joint ventures, and more generally to any research project involving the co-development of IP [14]. Generally speaking, joint ownership, also called co-ownership, refers to a situation in which two or more persons have proprietary shares of an asset: they co-own a property.

Joint ownership of IP, in particular, frequently arises in collaborative projects. In most cases, one or both partners contribute IP rights to the project—usually called *background technology*. As the partners begin to work cooperatively, when the results—usually called *foreground technology*—have been jointly generated by the collaboration partners, the share of work is not easily ascertainable.

In this context, background technology means all confidential information and IP rights that are owned by a Party other than Foreground and that have contributed to the strategic alliance. Foreground technology means any inventions, improvements, and other innovations relating to the technology, developed by either party in connection with the collaboration project, plus all the related confidential information and IP rights. Table 12.3 clarifies what is being contributed by each partner.

TABLE 12.3

What Is Being Contributed?

- Intellectual property
- Patents, trade secrets, trademarks
- Background IP
- Foreground IP
- Available capital
- Capabilities (testing, access to technical expertise, manufacturing)
- Marketing expertise
- Sales and sales channels
- Related products outside core technology

TABLE 12.4

Roles Each Partner May Play in IP Co-Ownership

Joint Inventor	Executor
Originally conceived the idea	Describes a hypothesis for proof of concept
Materially (technical, financial) contributes to the invention development	Follows instructions
Provides solutions to problems as they arise	Performs standard procedures
Provides the background innovation	Executes necessary P–O–C testing

Even more precisely, for a work to be considered jointly owned, two basic requirements are needed:

1. **Originality**, in the sense that one partner's contribution could be considered as its own personal creation
2. **Indivisibility**, in the sense that one partner's contribution is not easily discernible from the other's contribution

Table 12.4 clarifies the roles each partner may play in IP co-ownership.

Many people confuse the concepts of the ownership of IP and the inventorship or authorship of creations, or sometimes they are simply not aware of their different nature. Yet, it is crucial to understand how to manage these rights as their improper handling could cause real problems, such as the validity of IP rights granted or the risks of legal disputes [15].

12.11 The Complex Issue of Modifications to the Background Technology

A very important, but often overlooked aspect of a joint-development arrangement is the ownership of any IP rights arising out of the development work. For example, during the term of the contract, if an employee of partner A and an employee of partner B jointly create an invention, who owns the resulting technology? There are a number of ways of resolving technology-ownership issues. The key point is that the issues must be raised in negotiations and that the resolutions are reflected in the language of the contract.

Of particular importance is the definition of modifications to the background. It is not always easy to draw a distinction between derivative work and new work made under collaborative effort. Once the parties have defined the joint IP expected to be generated as "project results," a clear mention about the ownership of the background modifications should be included within the contract.

As far as the jointly owned IP is concerned, there are several ways to apportion it. Normally, this should be in line with the scope of the project. Because the background technology is needed to achieve results through the partners' collaborating efforts, one of the most common structures is the equal share of foreground ownership between collaboration partners. A particularly common agreement is shown below:

- Each Party retains exclusive property of its own background.
- The modifications to or derivative works of the parties' background shall be the sole property of the contributing party.
- Foreground developed in connection with the collaboration project hereof shall be jointly owned in equal shares by parties.

12.12 Rights of Exploitation

Through joint ownership contractual arrangements, parties are able to define the terms by which each co-owner can assign, license, and in general exploit jointly owned foreground. Such activities can be done with or without the consent of the other parties, depending on the partners' interests.

One important issue to be agreed from the outset is the compensation that the other partners will have in respect of the exploitation of the joint foreground made by one party, as described below:

RIGHT OF EXPLOITATION—first option [consent required]

1. A Party shall not pledge, assign, sell, or otherwise dispose of its interest in the foreground to third parties without the other Party's prior written consent.
2. Licensing of foreground to third parties shall require written agreement between the Parties, setting out their respective rights and obligations, including but not limited to, the distribution of licensing costs and income.

RIGHT OF EXPLOITATION—second option [consent not required]

1. Each Party shall have the right to pledge, assign, or otherwise dispose of its interest in the foreground to third parties as they may desire notifying its intention to the other Party [...] days before the activity concerned.

2. Each Party shall have the right to grant [type of licenses] on the foreground to third parties as they may desire without accounting to the other Party.

3. The total income after deducting costs as derived from the licensing of the foreground shall be distributed [...%] to Party [...] and [...%] to Party [...]. According to the type of license granted, said distribution *ratio* may be adjusted upon written agreement by the Parties.

12.13 Management of the Jointly Owned IP

Management of the jointly owned IP refers to the protection, maintenance, and defense of the foreground generated under the collaboration project. That is to say, contractual rules should set forth how confidential information, IP rights filing, prosecution, and infringement should be dealt with by the co-owners.

12.13.1 IP Rights Prosecution

Starting with the assumption that the IP rights protection and maintenance costs can be equally shared between joint owners, parties may also establish the following:

- Who will decide to protect the IP generated or keep it as a trade secret
- Who will follow the procedures to register the IP rights
- Who will bear the costs of the IP rights prosecution and maintenance

Where the designated party might fail to, or decide not to, file an application for the granting of IP rights, contractual provision should allow other parties to take steps in place of the unfulfilling party.

A further consideration is territory for ownership of the invention. In some cases, one partner may want ownership of all inventions in a specific country created during the term of the contract, whether created by their company, the other company, or jointly. Finally, the contract may also specify that although one partner may own the invention, the other may have a license to use or practice the invention either for a royalty payment or royalty-free. The license can be either exclusive or nonexclusive.

Ancillary to the ownership issue is the responsibility of the partners to file, prosecute, and maintain patent applications on the inventions. Usually, the

TABLE 12.5

IP Applications Filing, Prosecution, and Costs

First option [shared management]. Sample clauses

1. The Parties shall decide, by mutual agreement, whether to file, prosecute, and maintain IP rights protection of the foreground. The Parties shall equally bear all costs resulting from these activities.
2. The Parties shall agree which Party shall conduct the activities thereof in the names of and on behalf of the Parties. The elected Party shall provide a copy of relevant documents relating to the activities thereof for the other Parties examination.
3. If a Party declines to bear its share of the costs associated with the activities thereof, the other Parties may conduct such activities in their own name and at their own expense. The declining Party shall retain its rights of use, but shall lose its rights of ownership and exploitation in respect of foreground.

Second option [single management]

1. Party [...] hereto agrees to file, prosecute, and maintain IP rights applications of the foreground in a timely manner and at its own expense and after consultation with the other Parties.
2. Within [...] days of receipt of filing, Party [...] shall provide the other Parties with copies of the IP rights applications and all documents received from or filed with the relevant IP office in connection with the prosecution of such applications, for the other Parties' examination.
3. If Party [...] elects not to file IP rights applications, it so informs the other Parties [...] days before the expiration of any applicable filing deadline, priority period, or other statutory date, so that such other parties may elect to file and prosecute IP rights applications at their own expense. The declining Party shall retain its rights of use, but shall lose its rights of ownership and exploitation in respect of foreground.

owner of the invention is given the first right to file, prosecute, and maintain (as well as pay for) patents throughout the world. In the event of joint ownership, the partners may share in the costs of the patents. If the first right is not exercised, the contract usually requires that notice be provided to the other partner or partners, and the notified partner or partners then have the right to file, prosecute, and maintain the patents. In that case, it is conventional that the partner who undertakes the expense of filing, prosecuting, and maintaining the patents will assume ownership of them, as shown in Table 12.5.

12.13.2 IP Rights Infringement

Of extreme importance are also the defense of the IP rights and the consequent handling of infringement claims. Hence, joint owners should agree which of the parties will be responsible for monitoring and policing the joint IP and pay the expenses for any infringement in connection with it. The latter can arise either because the jointly owned IP infringes third-party IP rights or because it is the third party who infringes the co-owned IP, as shown below:

INFRINGEMENT CLAIMS. Sample clauses

1. Each Party shall be responsible for monitoring and defending the joint IP. Each Party will, however, notify the other Parties promptly if it has a reasonable basis for believing that the joint IP has been infringed by a third party or if the joint IP would infringe any IP right of a third party.
2. The Parties shall equally bear any costs in connection with the law prosecution of third-parties' infringement of the joint IP. Any accorded awards will be shared in equal parts.
3. The Parties shall equally bear any costs in connection with claims that the joint IP infringes third parties' IP rights.

12.13.3 Termination Clauses

Another major issue is termination. This issue is often avoided because it is akin to discussing with your future spouse what happens if you get divorced. Unpleasant as it may seem, full discussion concerning how a contract is to be terminated and the ramifications of such termination will avoid many later problems that can lead to costly and time-consuming litigation. Termination clauses must be drafted carefully and completely because it is those clauses that are the most carefully reviewed once a relationship starts to go wrong.

Termination clauses should specify how and when one partner can end the relationship. Often, the contract can be terminated only by breach of contract by the other partner, subject to a period (usually 30 days) to remedy the breach. The termination clause should set forth detailed procedures regarding how notices (preferably in writing) should be made to the other partners and, importantly, the effective date of the notice (i.e., effective upon sending the notice or effective when the other party receives the notice). There should also be clear provisions as to ownership of the tangible assets (e.g., pilot and laboratory equipment) brought to the arrangement. Furthermore, any continuing rights to use the background technology or technology developed during the term of the contract should be spelled out.

12.14 Summary Questions

Now that you have explored the intricacies of strategic alliances, you are in a better position to answer the following questions:

- Is your interest in the venture/alliance primarily strategic or financial in nature?
- What consequences would stem from a sale of your interests in the venture/alliance?
- Why does it make sense for you to partner on this project rather than go it alone?
- What opportunities will you forgo by entering into the venture/alliance?
- What is the scope of the noncompetition and exclusivity provisions that are envisioned?
- What are the strengths that each party brings to the table?
- What are the parties' bargaining powers, both up front and over time?
- How much money do you wish to invest in the venture, both up front and over time?
- What are the expected exit strategies and do all parties have a shared view of the likely exit scenarios?
- Have you adequately considered all that could go wrong with the venture/alliance and how to adequately protect its interests in such various downside scenarios?

References

1. Marzec, E. http://smallbusiness.chron.com/difference-between-joint-venture -strategic-alliance-11922.html.
2. Root, F. *Entry Strategies for International Markets*. Lexington Books, 1987, http:// teaching.ust.hk/~mgto650p/meyer/readings/9c/Root.pdf.
3. Irwin, T. http://www.tcii.co.uk/2013/04/04/avoiding-the-pitfalls-of-strategic -alliances/.
4. Rigsbee, E. The Pitfalls to Successful Strategic Alliances, http://www.rigsbee .com/ps5.htm.
5. International market entry strategies, http://highered.mheducation.com/sites /dl/free/0077122852/823243/gha22852_Ch11.pdf.
6. Cohen, J., Gangi, W., Lineen, J., and Manard, A. Strategic Alternatives in the Pharmaceutical Industry. Kellogg School of Management, https://www.kellogg .northwestern.edu/research/biotech/faculty/articles/strategic_alternatives .pdf.
7. Shalo, S. *The Art of the Deal*. BioPartnerships—A Pharmaceutical Executive and Biopharm International Supplement, October 2004, pp. 8–16.
8. Lam, M.D. Dangerous liaisons. *Pharmaceutical Executive*, 24(5), 72, May 2004.

9. Bernard, S. *Back to the Pharma Future*. BioPartnerships—A Pharmaceutical Executive and Biopharm International Supplement, October 2004, pp. 6–7.
10. Mills, L. Great science not all that matters developing treatments. *Financial Times*. 11/10/2004, p. 5.
11. http://www.reuters.com/article/2015/08/13/us-roche-diagnostics-bacteria -idUSKCN0QI0OA20150813.
12. Radack, D. Joint technology development arrangements. *JOM*, 49(2), 68, 1997. A publication of The Minerals, Metals & Materials Society, http://tms.org/pubs /journals/JOM/matters/matters-9702.html.
13. WIPO. Successful technology licensing, http://www.wipo.int/edocs/pubdocs /en/licensing/903/wipo_pub_903.pdf.
14. IP joint ownership. European IP Helpdesk. 2013, https://www.iprhelpdesk.eu /sites/default/files/newsdocuments/IP_joint_ownership_updated.pdf.
15. https://www.iprhelpdesk.eu/sites/default/files/newsdocuments/Inventorship _Authorship_Ownership_final_1.pdf.

13

Deciding to Be Acquired

13.1 Introduction

As a start-up, you may decide to be acquired by an established strategic partner before launching your knowledge-based product. Many entrepreneurs no longer build companies for the long term; they build companies for the short term, hoping to sell their company for quicker exits.

When we use the term *merger*, we are referring to the merging of two companies where one new company will continue to exist. The term *acquisition* refers to the acquisition of assets by one company from another company. In an acquisition, both companies may continue to exist. However, throughout this chapter, we will loosely refer to mergers and acquisitions (M&A) as a business transaction where one company acquires another company. The acquiring company (the buyer, acquiror, or acquirer) remains in business and retains its corporate name. The acquired company (the seller, target) will be integrated into the acquiring company and, thus, the acquired company ceases to exist after the merger.

Every M&A deal has its own unique reasons why the combining of two companies is a good business decision. The underlying principle behind M&A is deceptively simple: 2 + 2 = 5. The joining or merging of the two companies should theoretically create economic value that we call "synergy" value. Synergy value can take three forms [1]:

1. **Expenses:** By combining the two companies, you will realize lower expenses than if the two companies operate separately. Thus, the hugely expensive launch of your first product can be better absorbed by the combination of the two companies.

2. **Revenues:** By combining the two companies, you will realize higher revenues than if the two companies were to operate separately.

3. **Cost of capital:** By combining the two companies, you will experience a lower overall cost of capital. Thus, the combined companies will have a stronger balance sheet.

Strategic M&A alliances allow money-hungry start-ups to pursue their individual strategies despite limited financial resources. These alliances allow the entrepreneur to pursue product launches with greater likelihood of commercial success.

13.2 Mergers and Acquisitions

Mergers and acquisitions are an aspect of corporate strategy, corporate finance, and management dealing with the buying, selling, dividing, and combining of different companies and similar entities that can help an enterprise grow rapidly in its sector or location of origin, or a new field or new location, without creating a subsidiary or another child entity or using a joint venture [2].

13.2.1 Mergers

Theoretically, a **merger** happens when two firms agree to go forward as a single new company rather than remain separately owned and operated. This kind of action is more precisely referred to as a "merger of equals." In practice, however, actual mergers of equals don't happen very often. Usually, one company will buy another and, as part of the deal's terms, simply allow the acquired firm to proclaim that the action is a merger of equals, even if it is technically an acquisition [2].

13.2.2 Acquisitions

Practically speaking, an **acquisition** is the process through which one company completely takes over the controlling interest of another company. Such controlling interest may be 100%, or nearly 100%, of the assets or ownership equity of the acquired entity. An "acquisition" usually refers to a purchase of a smaller firm by a larger one.

13.3 The Acquisition Courtship by Motivated Strategic Buyers

You have developed your initial idea into a knowledge-based product. It has taken a lot of sweat and hard work, and you have experienced and overcome many technical challenges. Strategic buyers are now taking note of your development and making inquiries.

A strategic buyer is a type of buyer in an acquisition that has a very specific reason for wanting to purchase the company. Strategic buyers look for companies that will create a synergy with their existing businesses [3].

Because strategic buyers (also known as synergistic buyers) may actually get more value out of an acquisition than the intrinsic value of the company being acquired, strategic buyers will usually be willing to pay a premium price in order to have the deal go through. You have arrived!! Right? Well, not quite.

According to Lior Zorea of startupPerColator [4], the potential acquisition courtship that starts with these preliminary conversations will be lengthy, complex, and potentially very disruptive to your business. It will take away significant management attention from the day-to-day operations, and leaks can affect your ability to retain your employees and, potentially, your customers.

Since deals have a life span, the longer the process takes, the greater the potential for a transaction to fall through. While the acquisition process is generally well established, time is not on your side. When the acquisition call comes in, you want to be ready. You have limited resources, but by focusing on a few key areas, you can make a big difference in accelerating the process and the likelihood of a successful transaction.

1. **Maintain good records on an ongoing basis.** Strategic buyers, particularly serial acquirers, have professional corporate development and/or acquisition teams. They have been through the process many times and approach it in a very systematic and serious fashion. You want to be ready to handle the detailed, lengthy, and invasive due diligence process. The pace can be overwhelming at times, but you can alleviate that dynamic by getting your records "due-diligence ready." Consult your legal and financial advisors to find a solution that is most appropriate for you.

2. **Maintain your credibility.** Acquirers do not expect start-ups to be perfectly oiled organizations, but they will nevertheless demand perfection, as if you are a multibillion dollar organization. As you well know, problems and issues come up with your business on a regular basis and acquirers know that. Some are less important and some are serious. You may have a disgruntled former co-founder, you may have imperfections or gaps in your IP title, you may have accounting or tax issues—whatever it is, own up to it.

   Acquirers with professional M&A teams will ultimately dig up these issues during due diligence. When they do and, particularly, when it is at the tail end of a lengthy transaction, it can be harmful to the relationship, potentially causing the acquirer to revalue your business or, if serious enough, kill the deal.

3. **Lean on your advisors.** Your key advisors in an M&A transaction are your legal and financial advisory teams. The process can be daunting and complex and you may not have the benefit of having venture capitalists or other professional board members with significant M&A experience. Talk to your advisors and educate yourself about the process. Set realistic expectations for how long the process will take. Your financial advisor's job is to create market interest for your business and, ultimately, to maximize your valuation. Both your bankers and lawyers are experts in structuring transactions— broadly speaking, bankers will focus on economics and lawyers on terms and post-closing liabilities. Work with each to maximize your understanding of the process and the deal structure that is optimal *for you and your team.*

4. **Maintain control of the process.** There are lots of players and each has its own set of interests. The key players are the executives driving the deal at the acquirer and members of your management team, but there are many other players, including the acquirer's finance, legal and M&A teams, the bankers, the lawyers, and the accountants. In most deals, a working group list is put together at the beginning of the process to allow for good communication among the parties. With all these players contributing to the process, sometimes deals, particularly larger deals, tend to gain a momentum of their own. It is a natural and welcomed result of the process.

   As the target-company chief executive officer (CEO), you may find it difficult to run your business and maintain firm control of the process. Lots of decisions are made in the negotiation process, some which you may not even be aware of. To assist you in the process, identify the key executives and advisors who will be your core M&A execution team and meet with them on a regular basis to make sure that the transaction is progressing in a manner you are comfortable.

5. **The devil is in the details.** When selling the business, the parties typically focus on the aggregate purchase price. However, hidden value or hidden costs can be buried in the deal terms and can have a significant impact on the bottom line economics. For example, is the portion of the purchase price that is paid in stock subject to vesting after closing? If so, under what conditions can stock be forfeited? Are the indemnification provisions for the benefit of the acquirer outside market norms, and do they expose the equity holders to potentially outsized clawbacks of the purchase price?

6. **Pigs get fat, and hogs get slaughtered.** Be thoughtful and aggressive (but realistic) in positioning your business in the marketplace and crafting your value proposition to potential acquirers [5]. Accordingly, private companies need to think long before dismissing overtures from strategically motivated suitors. Listen carefully

to your advisors (and follow their advice). They know the market well, and when an acquirer has a number of potential competing targets to choose from, you want to take reasonable action in light of all the facts available to you. If your acquirer turns negative on the deal and instead decides to buy one of your competitors and if at the same time other potential acquirers have also acquired certain of your competitors, your position as a viable acquisition target may diminish significantly.

13.4 The Enduring Questions

Before consummation of the transaction, the buyer and the seller find themselves in an adversarial position. Table 13.1 lists the 10 most frequently asked questions in buying or selling a business. Paradoxically, although the questions look similar, the answers are not.

The list below presents the 10 biggest risks/challenges faced by start-ups when contemplating being acquired by a strategic acquirer:

1. Amount of funding available to execute the product launch
2. Overcoming weak market acceptance
3. Successful integration of the cultures

TABLE 13.1

The Ten Most Frequently Asked Questions

Seller ("Target")	Buyer ("Acquirer")
Why is their offering price so low?	Why is their asking price so high?
Are they bottom fishing?	Are they serious about selling?
Is it OK for us to shop around?	This should be a no-shop negotiation.
Why are they interested in us?	What do we really know about them?
Do we really need money now?	What will they do with our money?
Is this transaction for cash or shares?	What are their future financial demands?
Who should be part of our negotiation team?	Are we really negotiating with the decision-makers?
How much independence do we retain post-transaction?	How do we integrate them into our winning culture?
Could we do better on our own?	Do we really need them?
What happens if the deal collapses? How vulnerable do we remain?	What if we find deal-killers during due diligence?
What happens if our CEO is run over by the mythical train during negotiations?	How indispensable is their CEO? Do they have a succession strategy?

4. Purchase price gap between target and acquirer
5. Possible turnover of key personnel
6. Technology transfer hurdles
7. Consolidation and integration of manufacturing
8. Credibility of technical and marketing forecasts
9. Competitive response to the contemplated merger
10. Tax implications and shareholder's reply

13.5 The Due Diligence Process

There is a common thread that runs throughout much of the M&A process. It is called due diligence. Due means "appropriate" or "warranted," and diligence means "careful assessment" or "detailed analysis."

Due diligence is a comprehensive and extensive evaluation of the proposed transaction. An overriding question is, "Will this merger work?" In order to answer this question, we must determine what kind of "fit" exists between the two companies. This includes the following:

- **Investment Fit**—What financial resources will be required, what level of risk fits with the new organization, and so on?
- **Strategic Fit**—What management strengths are brought together through this M&A? Both sides must bring something unique to the table to create synergies.
- **Marketing Fit**—How will products and services complement one another between the two companies? How well do various components of marketing fit together—promotion programs, brand names, distribution channels, customer mix, and so on?
- **Operating Fit**—How well do the different business units and production facilities fit together? How do operating elements fit together—labor force, technologies, production capacities, and so on?
- **Management Fit**—What expertise and talents do both companies bring to the merger? How well do these elements mesh together—leadership styles, strategic thinking, ability to change, and so on?
- **Financial Fit**—How well do financial elements fit together—sales, profitability, return on capital, cash flow, and so on?

13.6 Cultural Issues in M&A

The business world seems littered with integrated companies that have lost value for shareholders. The question that inevitably arises is, "What forces are powerful enough to counteract the value-creating energy of economies of scale or global market presence?" [6].

Culture has emerged as one of the dominant barriers to effective integrations. In one study, culture was found to be the cause of 30% of failed integrations [7]. Companies with different cultures find it difficult, if not often impossible, to make decisions quickly and correctly or to operate effectively.

13.6.1 What Is Corporate "Culture"?

In plain English, culture is "how we do things around here." Deal and Kennedy [8] created a model of culture that is based on four different types of organizations. They each focus on how quickly the organization receives feedback, the way members are rewarded, and the level of risks taken:

1. **Work-hard, play-hard culture:** This has rapid feedback/reward and low risk resulting in the following: Stress coming from quantity of work rather than uncertainty. High-speed action leading to high-speed recreation. Examples: restaurants, software companies, and ladies' shoe manufacturers.

2. **Tough-guy macho culture:** This has rapid feedback/reward and high risk, resulting in the following: Stress coming from high risk and potential loss/gain of reward. Focus on the present rather than the longer-term future. Examples: police, surgeons, politicians, and sports figures.

3. **Process culture:** This has slow feedback/reward and low risk, resulting in the following: Low stress, plodding work, comfort, and security; stress that comes from internal politics and stupidity of the system; and development of bureaucracies and other ways of maintaining the status quo. Focus on security of the past and of the future. Examples: banks, insurance companies, teaching hospitals, and universities.

4. **You-bet-your-company culture:** This has slow feedback/reward and high risk, resulting in the following: Stress coming from high risk and delay before knowing if actions have paid off. The long view is taken, but then much work is put into making sure things happen as planned. Examples: aircraft manufacturers, oil companies, and start-ups.

Culture consists of the long-standing, largely implicit shared values, beliefs, and historical assumptions that influence behavior, attitudes, and meaning in a company (or society). This definition has three important implications:

1. **Culture is implicit.** People who share in a culture find their culture challenging to recognize. The most insightful cultural observers often are outsiders, because cultural givens are not implicit to them.
2. **Culture influences how people behave and how people understand their own actions.** As a result, culturally influenced beliefs and actions feel right to people, even while their implicit underpinnings make it difficult for those people to understand why they act the way they do or why other ways of acting might also be appropriate.
3. **Culture is resilient and enduring.** Its elements are long-standing, not a matter of fads. The resilience of culture is supported by culture being implicit. It is difficult for people to recognize their own culture and how it exerts an influence on them. The staying power of culture is that it feels right to people; new cultural values that are imposed on people seldom replace their underlying values and beliefs in the long run.

According to Larry Senn [9], M&As are a fact of life in today's highly competitive global business environment. Unfortunately, statistics indicate that up to one-third of mergers fail within 5 years, and as many as 80% never live up to their full expectations. Deals go bad because of the reasons shown in Table 13.2.

A great deal of evidence indicates that the ultimate success of M&A and the amount of time it takes to get them on track is determined by how well the cultural aspects of the transition are managed. Best practices show how to systematically and consciously avoid cultural clash and gain the most synergy from any merger or acquisition.

M&As are a key part of many organizations' strategies. Often, billions of dollars are at stake as well as the very future of the organizations and the executives who are coordinating the merger. Unfortunately, more often than not, the benefits of mergers or acquisitions fail to materialize or fall short of expectations.

Learning to systematically and consciously avoid cultural clash is a necessary skill because mergers are a fact of life in business. One reason is the continuing consolidation of industries. Phone companies, cellular companies,

TABLE 13.2

Deals Can Go Bad Because...

Cultural clashes and incompatibilities	50%
Incompatible strategic rationale	20%
Business model change	20%
Synergies did not materialize	10%

utilities, oil companies, financial services companies, insurance companies, healthcare organizations, retailers, defense and electronic companies, and dozens of others are a part of this consolidation trend.

13.6.2 The Importance of Addressing the Cultural Clash

Since the human factor is so critical, it is important to understand the role of this phenomenon and to address it in each phase of the merger or acquisition process.

Over a period, organizations, like people, develop distinctive and unique personalities. This personality of the organization has been referred to most often as corporate culture. An individual's personality is made up of one's habits, beliefs, values, and behavioral traits. A company's culture is also made up of its habits, values system, customs, and norms that govern behavior within the organization. The culture reflects the unwritten ground rules of behavior, or simply "the way we do things around here."

As a result of all the personality conflicts, the term *cultural clash* has been coined to describe what happens when two companies' philosophies, styles, values, and habits are in conflict. That may, in fact, be the most dangerous factor when two companies decide to combine.

The "corporate culture" is frequently seen in the larger, better established buyer, and the "entrepreneurial (innovation) culture" is seen in the start-up seller, as explained in Table 13.3.

TABLE 13.3

A Clash of Cultures

Corporate Culture "Buyer"	Entrepreneurial (Innovation) Culture "Seller"
Rewards ultraconservative decisions	Trial and error "You will miss 100% of the shots you don't take"
Demands to wait for instructions "It usually takes 3 weeks to prepare a good impromptu speech"	Rewards quick actions "Don't punish failure; reward success"
Expects "no surprises"	Encourages new approaches that may fail "Starting up is hard to do"
Collects information "Paralysis of the analysis"	Expects decisions even under imperfect information "Take risks, not chances"
Controls information "Information is power"	Encourages open discussion "Gentlemen do read each other's mail"
Structured decision-making process	Make decisions quickly "Decide first, then repent"
Market centric	Technology centric
Bureaucratic	Democratic

13.6.3 Key Human Problem Areas to Avoid

1. **Loss of key people.** Whenever acquiring an organization, remember that "the natives have the maps." Even if you need to downsize, if not handled right, the wrong people will leave and the venture can be jeopardized. A number of studies document the high exit rate from acquired companies. One survey indicated that only 42% of the managers remained with the acquired company for as long as 5 years ("Merging Human Resources," *Merger and Acquisition Magazine*).

   SBC's acquisition of Pacific Bell is an example of an exodus of senior talent. It was heralded as a merger of equals when the two chairmen announced the historic coupling. It didn't turn out that way. "Within months all six top officers were gone, having either retired or quit. Of its 35 corporate officers, just six remained," reported the article "Executive Exodus" in the *San Francisco Business Times*. Most of this was attributed to a clash in cultures and no attempt to bring the cultures together.

2. **Winners versus losers—"we" versus "they."** When companies are acquired or combined, people almost immediately start to focus on the differences in the companies. They also quickly begin to "keep score" on who are the winners and losers. It is typical in an acquisition for the acquiring company to see themselves as the winners and the acquired company as the losers. Typically, the controlling company wants to impose changes and views those in the acquired company as highly resistant to change.

   On the other hand, the most frequent complaint from employees of companies that are being acquired is that the new owners don't appreciate them. They often feel that they don't get any credit for what they've done well and what is working and that their new leaders only want to point out how the new way is better.

   In a newly merged or acquired company, the appointment of people to positions is closely watched. This is a specific area in which people immediately keep score, tallying which side won or lost on each issue or appointment.

3. **Judgment versus respect for differences.** There is a tendency for each group to be judgmental about the way things are handled by the other. Rather than respecting and building on differences, people frequently enter into right and wrong judgments.

4. **Fear of the unknown—insecurity is the enemy.** Uncertainty and insecurity are associated with almost all mergers or acquisitions. As a merger is announced, fears and anxieties are fueled by uncertainty about what the changes will bring. There is typically a feeling of personal vulnerability and loss of control. People often spend time updating their resumes and exploring their options. People fear the

unknown. It might be more accurately called "fear of the imagined," since people have a tendency to fill in the blanks of what they don't know by imagining the worst.

Whether a merger is for the better or worse, it throws relationships, norms, work behavior and support systems out of balance. If these psychological losses are not addressed early on, chronic problems in attitude and behavior can result.

5. **Loss of organizational effectiveness.** The uncertainty surrounding the change often causes the employees to lose enthusiasm about their work and their organization, and a drop in morale and organizational pride follows the merger. Countless hours are spent feeding the rumor mill, and large numbers of people adopt a wait-and-see attitude. Results usually suffer and customers are lost.

13.7 Guidelines for Creating a Successful Merger

The dustbin of business history is loaded with the stories of ill-conceived M&A, but while there are no magical solutions or silver bullets that ensure success, a process that is co-designed by the buyer and seller from the beginning will make the transaction appear seamless and fluid, with a high degree of positive, engaged energy throughout the organization [10]. To that end, below are nine specific recommendations:

1. **Retain your key leaders.** It is essential to identify those people critical to continued success and initiate a plan to ensure that these key people stay and remain engaged and aligned.

2. **Communicate your vision.** The sooner that some semblance of certainty about the future can be communicated, the sooner people will settle down. Once a new vision for the organization is created, new future targets are set, and new teams are connected and aligned, people can refocus their energy in a forward direction.

3. **Address the new organizational structure as early as possible.** Failed mergers are characterized by a tendency to have unclear reporting relationships and frequent changes in the reporting structure. In one study of merger successes and failures, it was found that 81% of the failures were characterized by frequent changes in the reporting relationship after the merger. Successful acquisitions were characterized by clear reporting relationships that were established early on and not changed ("Merging Human Resources," *Merger and Acquisition Magazine*).

4. **As the leader of an acquiring company, go out of your way to acknowledge as many positive aspects of the acquired company as possible.** At the same time, set clear expectations and create an environment in which there is a high level of openness to change.

5. **Avoid throwing out the baby with the bathwater by identifying which cultural factors have historically made an organization great.** For example, if a company had historically been successful based on its culture of service and quality, rapid and insensitive cost-cutting could begin to destroy what made that organization great in the first place. One example is the acquisition of a smaller, highly entrepreneurial company by a larger, more formalized one. That combination poses cultural challenges because it is hard to provide direction and additional structure. However, this must be done without killing the entrepreneurial goose that lays the golden eggs.

6. **Be clear about the nature of the union and be willing to talk about it.** Is it a true merger of equals, an acquisition that attempts to use the best of both, a stand-alone holding company, or just a stand-alone assimilation?

7. **Clearly communicate your mutual benefits.** Most people understand that M&A take place for business reasons. It is important at the outset to communicate the benefits of the merger. People may not like it, but if they see that it has a legitimate purpose, and the benefits are obvious, there is less resentment and employees are more likely to accept it.

8. **Make sure the acquiring company's leaders communicate in person as much as possible.** It is easier to be resentful toward an unknown, invisible giant than it is to be resentful about a person you have personally experienced as being real, rational, and concerned. Successful mergers only happen when senior managers make themselves visible and accessible to all employees affected by the merger and promote the benefits at all levels. Employees at all levels need to experience the buy-in and support of their leaders for the merger or acquisition.

9. **Create an integration plan.** Perform adequate due diligence on the cultures both before and after the merger. Create a specific cultural integration plan led by the CEO and the senior team, not just delegated to the HR team, or to chance.

13.7.1 Variations in the Human Nature of M&A

Specific steps needed to deal with the human side of the merger or acquisition are greatly influenced by the basis for the merger as well as the cultures of the organizations. For example, in a merger where the acquiring company is interested only in the physical and financial assets of a target company and expects to lay off most managers and employees, major efforts to manage culture are unnecessary. However, when a true "marriage of two equals" is the end goal, attention to the management of culture becomes critical and detailed planning is most crucial. The varying goals for merger outcomes are shown below in their most common forms.

1. **Autonomy or semi-autonomy.** In the "hands-off" scenario, the goal is to create mutual support and synergy without necessarily changing the nature of the organizations. It is unrealistic to assume that the acquiring company will not want some modifications. For example, there may be a desire to shift one or more qualities, such as innovation, bias for action, and a higher level of expectations. This is graphically shown in Figure 13.1.

   However, when the basis for the acquisition is autonomy or semi-autonomy, it is important to respect the reasons for the differences in culture and to proceed slowly with integration activities.

2. **Absorb and assimilate.** If the goal is to completely absorb and assimilate the acquired company, then the primary need is to educate the acquired employees in the rules of the new corporate culture. Edgar Schein [11] provides us with a working definition of the corporate culture: "a pattern of shared basic assumptions that the group learned as it solved its problems of external adaptation and internal integration, that has worked well enough to be considered valid and therefore, to be taught to new members as the correct way to perceive, think, and feel in relation to those problems."

   It should be remembered that they have been playing a different game under a different set of unwritten as well as written ground rules. Orientation to the new organization should include

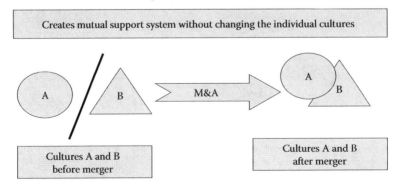

FIGURE 13.1
Autonomous M&A.

letting them know about the vision and values of their new organization. It is also important to focus on how the new game is going to be different and not on judging the past or telling them why what they were doing was wrong. This is graphically shown in Figure 13.2.

3. **Co-create a new entity (integrated cultures).** While avoiding cultural clash is always important, the greatest attention should be paid to successful cultural integration when a true marriage of equals is intended (see Figure 13.3).

The acquiring company must capture the full value of the merger by integrating carefully each element of both organizations. The development of an integrated culture is one of the critical factors for M&A success. The initial challenge for all organizations that consider a merger or acquisition is to

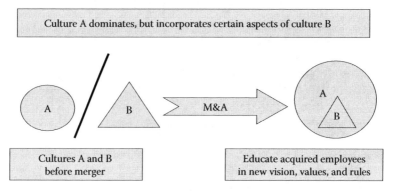

FIGURE 13.2
Absorb and assimilate.

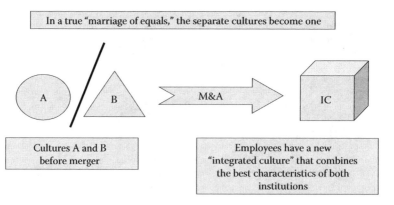

FIGURE 13.3
Integrated cultures.

understand that the culture has deep roots that cannot be easily pulled out, examined, and reprogrammed to create a new shared culture. As Beaudan and Smith admonish: creating an integrated culture involves careful discovery, inventing, reseeding, and letting go [12].

13.8 How to Successfully Integrate Cultures

This is easier said than done. To successfully integrate the two cultures, savvy acquirers first define the cultural objective in broad terms. This is invariably a job for the chief executives—and the CEO of the buying company as well as the founder of the target company must be willing to sustain their commitment until the objective is realized [13]. Integrating cultures can be achieved by adhering to the following activities:

1. **Integrate teams and shape culture.** Whenever new leaders or new teams at any level are put in place, processes to align those teams around the greater vision and direction are vital. Companies can no longer afford to take months to get acquainted and work out differences.

   Off-site sessions with the top leaders are vital as part of a process to begin reshaping the culture to a desired new state. This brings new teams together in a relaxed and collaborative environment to focus their energy in the same direction.

   Use of a more formal, customized culture-shaping process is often skipped owing to the demand of business. This leads to unintended loss of people and slow starts for teams, and wastes time and energy.

   A "cultural clash" is not hypothetical. It is real and it happens among people who have not taken the time to develop openness and trust. Think of a team of newly drafted ball players trying to play in the major leagues with no practice, no commonly understood signals, and no time to learn to play well together. It wouldn't matter how good the individual players were; they probably wouldn't succeed. A customized process can be used to embed the new values and shape the culture through values and guiding behaviors.

2. **Inspire and align people around vision, mission, and shared values.** During a merger or acquisition, people need to be inspired to move toward new goals and visions. In the absence of a compelling purpose for a new organization, people tend to stay locked in the past and to unhealthy speculation.

13.8.1 Role of the Senior Team

In a merger designed to create a new combined entity, the senior teams of each organization need to work together to clarify the new mission and the shared values, or behavioral ground rules by which they are all going to play.

In acquisitions that are assimilations, the acquiring company needs to have a clear vision and set of values and guiding behaviors and a process to orient employees of the acquired company. If the company is not clear about these things themselves, it is very confusing and disruptive.

Academic studies on culture point to a powerful phenomenon called the "Shadow of the Leaders." As leaders go, so goes the company and the merger. If leaders show up unaligned, the two merging companies will be unaligned. If they fight over turf, so will all those who look to them. That is why the leaders need to spend time coming together as "one team" and aligning vision and strategy.

The shadow leaders cast across the organization are a powerful form of communication. For that reason, it is critical that the new senior team be the first team to come together (beyond the transition planning team). Members should spend time in a series of well-designed off-site sessions. The alignment process described earlier can be used by the senior team not only to build the team but also to come together around the shared values and guiding behaviors for the merged entity. Because of its importance, this process is best handled with assistance from skilled and experienced outside facilitators.

The senior team can ease the clash of cultures by

- Recognizing there are culture differences between buyer and seller
- Expecting a clash to occur, and taking steps to ameliorate the disagreement
- Sensitizing staff to the culture clash dynamics
- Proposing mechanisms for learning about each company's culture
- Emphasizing the development of a new common culture

13.8.2 The Emotional Cycle of Change

The integration process should be entered into realistically with full knowledge of the obstacles that may be encountered. Most acquisitions considered to be successful follow a pattern described as the "merger emotion syndrome" or "merger syndrome" [14]. The syndrome encompasses executives' stressful reactions and the development of a "crisis management" atmosphere, as shown in Figure 13.4.

As shown in the chart, phase 1 is unbridled optimism, when people are excited about the new venture and have not as yet faced the challenges and complications. Phase 2 is informed pessimism when all of the issues, rumors,

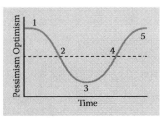

- Phase 1 unbridled optimism
- Phase 2 informed pessimism
- Phase 3 realistic outlook
- Informed optimism
- Rewarded completion

The merger emotion syndrome is a phenomenon that illustrates employees' predictable reactions after the announcement of an unexpected M&A deal

FIGURE 13.4
Merger emotion syndrome.

and disruptions are being faced. It can take one of two courses. Without a systematic plan, pessimism and rebellion can become a long-lasting reality.

In phase 3, realism sets in. The issues and challenges are understood and success requires determination. However, with a plan in place and continued commitment, the tide will begin to turn to phase 4, or informed optimism. In phase 5, rewarded completion, the benefits of the transaction start to become a reality.

The target company CEO can minimize the emotional cycle of change by taking the following proactive steps:

- Establish a transition team.
- Prepare your staff for a period of intense high-level activity.
- Rally the troops with your vision for a better and stronger organization.
- Operate in a way that says: "We are all in this together."
- Acknowledge everyone's uncertainty and concerns.
- Communicate, communicate, and communicate.
- Tell all you can, and always tell the truth.
- Orchestrate a master plan of priorities, problem areas, and synergies.
- Involve everyone in managing the transition.
- Empower teams with information, influence, guidance, and authority.
- Emphasize the benefits that each person will enjoy after transaction.

13.8.3 Merger Emotions Management

In the typical M&A transaction, many employees undergo a psychological trauma period that results in negative consequences for the organizations. Since the employees of the acquired company are more affected by the big changes, they are deeply shaken and respond with shock and strong emotional reactions.

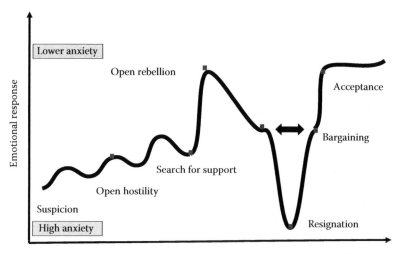

Time since unexpected M&A announcement

FIGURE 13.5
Nervousness Index.

The employees of the acquired company ask themselves many questions: "Would I still have a job?" "Will my job demands change unreasonably?" "How do I adapt to the new team?" "Do I still belong?" "Will I survive the changes?"

The predictable response can be called the "Nervousness Index," and is graphically shown in Figure 13.5. Anxieties, aggressions, and high stress levels may be managed by maintaining positive emotions [15].

Figure 13.5 depicts the seven "grieving" stages experienced by many employees of the acquired company, although it is also seen in those high-level executives of the acquirer who are not part of the decision-making group. The merger emotions of management can be summarized as follows:

- Fair and understandable personnel selection process
- Transparency of transition process
- Periodic communication of M&A status and goals
- Evoking and maintaining trust in the leadership
- Making senior management highly accessible
- Encouraging employee participation at all levels

13.8.4 Benefits of a Systematic Integration Process

One of the benefits that can come from systematically dealing with specific cultural aspects of mergers is that team members operate more quickly and effectively in their new or newly revised organization without loss of momentum. This is summarized in Table 13.4.

TABLE 13.4

Benefits of a Systematic Integration Process

Cultural Aspects	Benefits
There are fewer defections. Usually the best people leave immediately.	People don't move on because of uncertainty or imagined concerns and issues.
Negative impact on morale is lessened or eliminated.	People don't waste countless hours on speculation or on feeling victimized.
Focus on the customer is not lost and customer disruptions are minimized.	All the planned synergies, such as cross-selling, are captured.
Consolidation of functions is done faster and more smoothly and the cost benefits of consolidation are better captured.	This leads to improved productivity and profitability in a shorter period.
The process of creating a vision, mission, and shared values creates excitement, inspiration, and commitment.	All people now working for a new future goal as opposed to living in the past.
A sense of community is created sooner among all individual stakeholders.	Shared vision and values link individuals to the organization and bind people together.

13.9 What Are You Worth to an Acquirer?

> Acquirers have deep pockets, but short arms.

Every founder believes in his heart of hearts that their venture is truly worth a fortune, and it will get funded appropriately. From the founder's perspective, it should be obvious to every acquirer what an outstanding opportunity is being offered. After all, you are at the threshold of introducing a world-beating innovative product. So why don't acquirers write a big check?

A business valuation is the process used by acquirers to determine the financial worth of a closely held (private) company. For our purposes, a closely held business is an organization owned and operated by a relatively small number of owners.

The valuation process begins with an understanding of your company, following a series of generally accepted valuation techniques, such as the following:

- Determining which business valuation(s) are most applicable to your company
- Analyzing the company's financial statements and pro-forma statements
- Assessing comparative and market statistical information
- Determining appropriate discounts and premiums
- Calculating current company valuation

13.9.1 Putting Lipstick on Your Pig: Value versus Price

Some men know the price of everything and the value of nothing.

Oscar Wilde

The **value** of your start-up is an economic theoretical concept. It is an estimate of the likely price at a given point in time. **Price** is the precise amount of money asked in exchange for something. In your case, you are asking Angels to invest X amount of money into your start-up company in exchange for Y percentage of ownership (based on shares).

Since traditional company values are based on objective measures, such as gross revenues, net profits, cash flows, net assets, increased sales, and so on, valuing a pre-revenue company is highly subjective. Complicating matters is the known "founder's syndrome," which is overvaluing their baby. It all comes down to deciding if you will be satisfied with a slice of a rapidly expanding pie (Figure 13.6).

Valuation is a particularly thorny problem for innovation-focused tech acquisitions [16]. It is nearly impossible to apply traditional valuation techniques to companies in their early stages of development, when operating histories are brief and there's little or no historical or predictable future cash flow. Acquirers therefore must resort to other measurements to build the case for a particular investment.

Their executives typically consult internal research and development and product teams to determine the cost—in terms of both time and money—of building a product or service internally. Very often, the acquirer has the necessary capability, but the lead time to build the product or service is prohibitive, and an acquisition can significantly improve speed to market. Very often, the acquirer has the necessary capability, but the lead time to build the product or service is prohibitive, and an acquisition can significantly improve speed to market.

Value	Price
• Dynamic figure	• Static figure
• Nothing precise	• Precise number
• Subjective	• Objective
• Based on fundamentals	• Based on negotiations
• Based on economic benefits	• Based on intrinsic benefits
• Predictability, stability	• If can't get champagne, get wine

The method of payment for a transaction is frequently the decisive factor for both parties. Is it cash, equity, or a combination of both?

FIGURE 13.6
Value versus price.

13.9.2 Maximizing Your Value to Strategic Buyers

When it comes to valuation, it's easy to focus on the consideration a buyer is paying instead of what the buyer is hoping to gain from the purchase. Understanding what the potential buyer is seeking from the transaction can help the seller better assess a potential transaction's impact on valuation [17]. We will discuss capabilities and geographic footprint as two important components of your company's valuation in the eyes of a potential strategic acquirer.

1. **Capabilities.** Certain strategic acquirers may want to purchase a firm to build a broader corporate capability or enter a new line of business. These buyers are usually in a related business and want to "buy instead of build."

   They may use cash flow as a buying method, but could put a relative premium on a valuation if your unique strength is valuable enough. This type of buyer often exclusively seeks out start-ups with knowledge-based products, unique capabilities, and exceptional human capital.

2. **Geographic footprint.** A buyer may consider a firm simply to enter a new market and leverage the firm's network and existing clients. This is another "buy versus build" strategy and can be an attractive point of entry for a buyer. *Potential impact on valuation:* "If your location is ideal for whatever the buyer's 'concept' is, you may command a premium."

   For example, is your pharma firm located in Cambridge, Massachusetts, more valuable than a firm in the rural Midwest? Since your location gives you quick access to world-class hospitals, does it command a premium? Perhaps, but there are plenty of "successful firms" in remote locations.

   When it comes to valuation, you may want to think about the reasons a buyer may be attracted to a firm and the subsequent implications for the "sale planning" process: The multiyear process to improve the value of your business in preparation to sell.

13.9.3 What Your Business Is Worth Depends on the Buyer

There is an old saying: your business is worth what a buyer is willing pay. Of course, the first step in placing a value on your business is identifying the "right buyer" [18]. The range of values that different buyers may be willing to pay is staggering. Buyers pay for opportunity. The buyer who perceives the greatest opportunity is the buyer willing to pay the most for your business. This is shown in Figure 13.7.

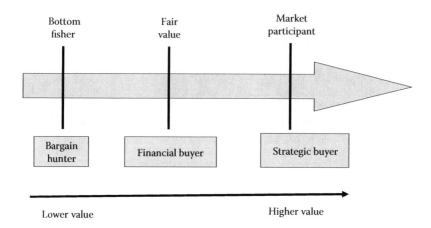

FIGURE 13.7
The value continuum and buyer types.

Identifying the right buyer requires understanding the four main classifications of buyers.

1. **The Strategic Buyer.** These are the very best buyers. They almost always pay cash and buy at a premium. Typically, public or very large private companies' decision to buy usually revolves around considerations of economies of scale, new channels of distribution, new innovative technologies, or other integration considerations. To be attractive to a strategic acquirer, your company should fit most, if not all, of the following criteria:
   - Sales in excess of $10 million
   - Proprietary product or process
   - Unique market presence or share
   - Synergistic fit with the acquirer
   - Suitable management willing to stay

2. **The Financial Buyer.** Financial buyers include private equity firms (also known as "financial sponsors"), venture capital firms, hedge funds, family investment offices, and ultra high net worth individuals. These firms and executives are in the business of making investments in companies and realizing a return on their investments. Their goal is to identify private companies with attractive future growth opportunities and durable competitive advantages, invest capital, and realize a return on their investment with a sale or an initial public offering [19].

Because these buyers have fundamentally different goals, the way they will approach your business in an M&A sale process can differ in many material ways.

While this might seem obvious, strategic buyers usually are more "up to speed" on your industry, its competitive landscape, and current trends. As such, they will spend less time deciding on the attractiveness of the overall industry and more time on how your business fits in with their corporate strategy. Conversely, financial buyers are typically going to spend a lot of time building a comprehensive macro view of the industry and a micro view of your company within the industry. It is not uncommon for financial buyers to hire outside consulting firms to assist in this analysis.

With this analysis, financial buyers might ultimately determine that they do not want to invest in any company in a given industry. Presumably, this risk is not present with a strategic buyer if they are already operating in the industry. As the seller, the risk of having a sale process fail owing to "industry attractiveness" factors is reduced by ensuring that you are soliciting strategic buyers.

13.10 M&A in Healthcare

In the healthcare field, Medtronic acquired Covidien in a $42 billion transaction. The combined Medtronic/Covidien organization is the largest medical device company in the world. Anthem's acquisition of WellPoint made it the largest healthcare management company in America. The question in each case is, "Can merging companies achieve the necessary synergy, or will their cultures clash?"

An article in the *Los Angeles Times* entitled "After Back-Slapping Wanes, Mega-Mergers Often Fail" concluded that "Perhaps more than anything else, senior management stumbles over cultural issues." They noted that: "The most important issue is **trust**. Along with cultivating trust, the keys to success in pulling together companies are crafting a shared vision, developing a precise transition plan, which includes more than structure and processes and avoiding the common pitfall of focusing so much on the merger details that customers (and employees) are neglected."

While it is clear that successful M&As must be based primarily on strategic, financial, and other objective criteria, ignoring a potential clash of cultures can lead to financial failure. Far too often, cultural and leadership style differences are not considered seriously enough or systematically addressed. Many acquisitions that looked very promising from a strategic or financial viewpoint ultimately fail and require major surgery or extensive subsequent hand-holding because these "soft" issues were neglected.

References

1. Evans, M.H. Course 7: Mergers and Acquisitions (Part 1), http://www.exinfm .com/training/pdfiles/course07-1.pdf.
2. http://en.wikipedia.org/wiki/Mergers_and_acquisitions
3. Investopedia on Facebook: Strategic Buyer Definition | Investopedia, http:// www.investopedia.com/terms/s/strategic-buyer.asp#ixzz3k8rO6Dqm.
4. Zorea., L. M&A Tips for the Bootstrapped and Early-Stage Technology Startup, PerkinsCoie, 2015, http://www.startuppercolator.com/ma-tips-for-the-boot strapped-and-early-stage-technology-startup/?format=pdf.
5. Crafting your value proposition, MaRS Discovery District, November 2012, http://www.marsdd.com/wp-content/uploads/2012/12/Crafting-Your-Value -Proposition-WorkbookGuide.pdf.
6. Cultural issues in mergers and acquisitions. Leading through transition: Perspectives on the people side of M&A Deloitte Consulting LLP, 2009, http:// www2.deloitte.com/content/dam/Deloitte/us/Documents/mergers-acqisitions /us-ma-consulting-cultural-issues-in-ma-010710.pdf.
7. Dixon, I. Culture Management and Mergers and Acquisitions, Society for Human Resource Management case study, March 2005.
8. Deal, T.E., Kennedy, A.A. *Corporate Cultures.* Perseus Book Publishing LLC, HarperCollins Publishing, New York, 1982.
9. Cultural clash in mergers and acquisitions. Senn Delaney, 2004, http://knowledge .senndelaney.com/docs/thought_papers/pdf/SennDelaney_cultureclash_UK.pdf.
10. http://iveybusinessjournal.com/publication/seven-steps-to-merger-excellence/
11. Schein, E.H. *Organizational Culture and Leadership.* Jossey-Bass Inc., San Francisco, pp. 16–17, 1992.
12. Beaudan, E. and Smith, G. Corporate culture: Asset or liability. *Ivey Business Journal*, March 2000.
13. http://www.bain.com/publications/articles/integrating-cultures-after-a -merger.aspx
14. Marks, M.L. and Toder, F. When your company is acquired: The human aspect. *The Business Journal*, October 22, 1999, http://www.managementcontinuity .com/images/When_Your_Company_Is_Acquired_-_Fran.pdf.
15. Kusstatscher, V. Cultivating positive emotions in mergers and acquisitions. *Advances in Mergers and Acquisitions*, 5, 91–103, 2006, https://karhen.home .xs4all.nl/Papers/5/Cultivating%20positive%20emotions%20in%20mergers%20 and%20acquisitions.pdf.
16. Acquiring innovation strategic deal-making to create value through M&A. PWC, March 2014, http://www.pwc.com/en_US/us/advisory/business-strategy -consulting/assets/acquiring-innovation.pdf.

17. Taking steps to help maximize the value of your firm. Fidelity, https://fiws .fidelity.com/app/literature/log?literatureURL=9857852.pdf.
18. How much is my business worth? Vanguard Resource Group, http://vrgsandiego .com/how-much-is-my-business-worth.
19. Boyle, C. 5 Differences between Financial and Strategic Buyers, February 2014, http://www.axial.net/forum/5-differences-financial-strategic-buyers/.

Section III

Product Launch

14

Pricing Strategies

14.1 Introduction

Setting the "right" price for the launch of your innovative product is one of the most crucial marketing decisions you will ever face. Too high a price and it will not sell; too low a price and you will be out of business. Meeting the price of existing products is the easiest pricing goal to implement, but how do you price an innovative product, since, by definition, it does not currently exist in the market?

Pricing must be thought of in terms of the product and adoption life cycle. Keep in mind that pricing is the only part of the marketing mix that produces revenues; all the other elements produce costs [1]. Your selected pricing strategy will

- Define your product
- Help segment the market
- Incentivize customer adoption
- Signal your quality intentions to your competition
- Establish the gold standard

Figure 14.1 summarizes the recommended six steps in setting your product launch pricing policy.

14.2 Establishing Your Pricing Tactics

Some people know the price of everything, and the value of nothing.

Your pricing tactics should accurately reflect your strategic goals. As an innovative start-up, you should be thinking in terms of value, not just pricing. Value in new product pricing ensures that customers receive fair

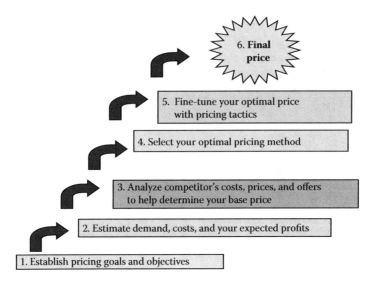

FIGURE 14.1
Setting your launch pricing policy.

value-based pricing, while enabling the entrepreneur to reach an industry price equilibrium that provides adequate revenue returns [2].

Value is the difference between what the customer gains from owning a product minus the costs of obtaining the product. **Quality** is the characteristics of a product/service that satisfy stated or implied customer needs. Value-based new product offerings can best be seen in terms of a price-quality continuum, as shown in Figure 14.2.

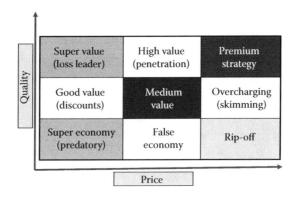

FIGURE 14.2
Value-based new products: the price–quality continuum.

14.3 The Complex Sale

Focus on success, not failure avoidance.

The complex sale is a type of selling (a) where a number of people must give their approval or input before the buying decision can be made and (b) that requires long and involved cell cycles [3]. The complex sales are primarily focused on business-to-business and business-to-government transactions, and can range from a few weeks to years [4].

Most innovative start-ups will face the challenge of the complex sale. The current business environment is characterized by four interrelated phenomena: (1) escalating customer requirements with increased complexity, (2) rapid commoditization leading to price erosion, (3) relentless competitive forces, and (4) need to respond within a tight window of opportunity. Commoditization is the pressure exerted by the customer to equalize the differences between suppliers, thus reducing their decision-making to the lowest common denominator: the selling price. This leads to the great margin squeeze as depicted in Figure 14.3.

The length of time that an innovation enjoys the advantage of being first in the market is getting shorter and shorter. For a start-up, the key to success is to differentiate your innovative offering. Differentiation allows for more profitable, preemptive, and effective product introductions.

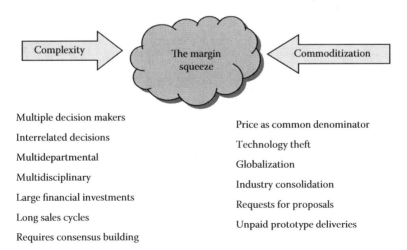

FIGURE 14.3
The great margin squeeze.

14.4 Sales Talking Points

If you are launching a knowledge-intensive product, you are inevitably faced with the intricacies of the complex sale. Sales talking points are a means of selecting best practices and communicating them to your salespeople. Sales talking points should concisely describe what the salesperson should do in different situations they might encounter in the field.

Sales talking points should be customized to a company's specific situation. A sales playbook for a company selling $5000 solutions over the phone will be very different from one for companies selling $5 million solutions in complex request for proposal (RFP) or request for quotation (RFQ) situations. Below are examples to illustrate the crucial differences.

14.4.1 Short Sales Cycles, Low Solution Prices

The sales talking points for a company selling a low-priced solution via a marketing campaign targeted at a specific customer segment with the goal of selling a specific solution might include the following:

- The e-mail campaign
- Titles mailed to specific groups
- Phone and e-mail scripts to use to follow-up
- Specific calls to action to move the prospect to the next stage (including sales tools such as case studies, analyst reports, etc.)
- Quick reference sheets for competitors
- Specific data updates based on call outcomes

The expectation is that these campaigns will be high volume and highly scripted. The sales talking points may outline the sales process from initial prospect engagement through close of sales by a purchase order.

14.4.2 Longer Sales Cycles, Higher Solution Prices

At the other end of the spectrum, salespeople selling higher-priced, more complex solutions (complex sales) generally follow a less scripted sequence. A salesperson in situations like this might have five phases of the sales process:

1. Prepare via external research how to approach companies in your prospect list.
2. Network within companies in your prospect list to locate a group within that company likely to have problems that make them great candidates for one of the solutions you sell.

3. Confirm for a specific group which problem they have and which of your solutions can overcome their problems.

4. For a group with a specific problem, move them from interest to active consideration, and then close the sale.

5. Do not sell products; sell solutions.

14.4.3 Preparation Steps for Your Sales Talking Points

Before embarking on your sales talking points, you should have completed these steps:

- Segment your market by different needs and priorities.
- Select the market segments that best match your differentiators with their needs.
- Study your competition—which segments they concentrate on and what their strengths and weaknesses are for those segments.
- Note key differentiators.
- Create qualification criteria for ideal prospects.
- Identify buyers' roles and typical titles encountered by role.
- Outline the sales process (sequence of steps, order in which roles are approached if relevant).
- Identify impediments to selling and sales strategies and processes to overcome them.
- Map out what supporting sales tools you need by sales stage, role, and segment.

14.4.4 What Maximum Price Can You Command?

Do not price to sell; sell the price.

With your positioning, you have decided how you will differentiate your product against the competition—this includes pricing. Specifically, you should answer the following questions:

- What maximum price can you ask?
- What pricing strategy will you adopt for optimum sales volume?

The price you can ask is the price (value) the customer is prepared to pay. This contradicts the widespread opinion that price is determined directly by cost. Of course, cost is a factor, but the cost/price ratio only becomes critical when the price that can be asked does not cover the costs.

This, by definition, means that the business is unattractive. Cost naturally also plays a role because the difference between cost and price defines the profit—and the ultimate goal of any commercial enterprise is to maximize profit.

The price you can ask depends entirely on how much the *benefit* of your product or service is worth to the customer. You have defined, and perhaps also quantified, the customer benefit in your business idea or product description.

14.5 What Pricing Strategy Will You Adopt?

Your pricing strategy depends on your goal: do you want to penetrate the market quickly with a low price ("penetration" strategy), or do you want to get the highest possible return right from the start ("skimming" strategy)?

New standard: When Netscape, for instance, distributed its Internet browser for free, it was able to set a new standard. Apple, on the other hand, followed a skimming strategy with the Macintosh, and thus missed the opportunity of establishing it as a standard.

System-related: Businesses with high fixed costs must find a large number of customers very quickly if they are to be profitable. FedEx is the classic example: air transport and sorting offices require similar investments, whether the company moves thousands or millions of letters.

Competition: Low-entry barriers make strong competition likely. A penetration strategy is the best way of securing a large market share more quickly than the competition. However, this raises the question as to whether a business of this sort is appropriate at all for a start-up company.

Penetration: Unlike a skimming strategy, a penetration strategy generally requires high initial investments to produce supply that is adequate to meet the high demand. Whenever possible, start-ups prefer to avoid this additional investment risk and adopt a skimming strategy, retaining the option to adopt a more aggressive approach when appropriate.

Skimming strategies: There are usually good reasons for new companies to pursue skimming strategies: The new product is generally positioned as "better," "more effective," "quicker," and so on; hence, its price can also be correspondingly higher.

Higher prices generally produce higher margins, thus enabling the new company to finance its growth itself. New investment can be financed out of profit, and there is no need for additional outside investors.

14.6 Typical Gross Margins

Gross margin is the difference between net revenue and cost of goods sold, or COGS, divided by revenue, and is expressed as a percentage. Generally, it is calculated as the selling price of an item, less the cost of goods sold (production or acquisition costs, essentially). Gross margin is often used interchangeably with gross profit, but the terms are different.

When speaking about a dollar amount, it is technically correct to use the term *gross profit*; when referring to a percentage or ratio, it is correct to use *gross margin*. In other words, gross margin is a % value, while gross profit is a $ value [5]. The purpose of margins is "to determine the value of incremental sales, and to guide pricing and promotion decisions" [6].

Gross margins vary widely from business to business, and they depend on various factors:

- The competitive situation in the market (strong competition produces low margins)
- The entrepreneur's business efficiency (improves the margins)
- The complexity of the product (increases margins), the quantity, throughput time, and stock levels (the higher the number of units and the shorter the throughput time, the lower the margins)

14.6.1 Gross Margins in Different Industries

Table 14.1 lists the average gross margins expected in different industries [7].

TABLE 14.1

Gross Margins Expected in Different Industries

Industry	Average Gross Margins (%)
Legal	93
Healthcare	91
Banking	91
Telecom	87
Publishing	77
Computer design	71
Research and development	64

14.6.2 Your Pricing Strategy Checklist

A business can use a variety of pricing strategies when selling a product or service. The price can be set to maximize profitability for each unit sold or from the market overall. It can be used to defend an existing market from new entrants, to increase market share within a market, or to enter a new market. Businesses may benefit from lowering or raising prices, depending on the needs and behaviors of customers and clients in your particular market niche. Finding your right pricing strategy is a crucial element in launching your product and running a successful and profitable business [8,9].

So how did you arrive at your pricing policy? Did you

- Determine the costs involved?
- Set prices for selling and profit?
- Fit pricing into sales forecast for cash flow projections?
- Consider clients' perception of value?
- Consider internal marketing strategies (the image you wish to project)?

Did you include the following factors into your pricing policy?

- Costs (Material + Labor + Overhead)
- Competition
- The competitive pricing strategy
- Ability to adjust pricing
- Ceiling prices
- Customers' buying behavior
- Your anticipated return on investment (profit margin)

Did you factor in any of the following overhead expenses into your pricing?

- Fixed expenses:
  - Rent
  - Vehicle
  - Bank charges
  - Insurance
  - Lease
  - Utilities
  - Salaries
  - Other
- Variable expenses:
  - Labor
  - Overhead
  - Materials

- Inventory
- Commissions   - Professional fees
- Vehicle Costs   - Materials
- Other

Did you perform a break-even analysis using the following formula?

- Units Break-Even = Annual Fixed Costs
- Unit Selling Price – Unit Variable Costs
- Sales Break-Even = (# Units to Break-Even) × (Selling price/unit)

14.7 Pricing High-Tech Products

The term *high technology* is a catchall category that includes any product manufactured with some type of an advanced technology, from computer electronics or wireless devices, to medical telemetry, to long-range missiles. However, there is no specific class of technology that is high tech—the definition shifts over time—so products hyped as high tech in the past may now be considered to have everyday or dated technology [10].

Every developer would like to set a high price for its high-technology products to cover their investments in research and development (R&D) or to prove the high quality of their innovative products, but there are some internal and external factors that put pressure on prices [11].

Forces affecting the price are varied and very strong: volatile short life cycle of the product, the rapidly changing market, big investments in R&D, compatibility with existing products, the Internet, competition, external networks, the cost of the first produced unit, price/performance ratio, and consumers' perception of the cost/benefits ratio for new technologies.

A key feature of advanced technology is the rapid changing rhythm that leads to a shortened product life cycle and the need for frequent rapid decisions. Pressures on the price/performance ratio are explained in a clear manner by Moore's law [12]: "Every 18 months, technology improvements double the product performance without a price increase." In other words, this type of improvement reduces the price by half for the same level of performance [13].

"Moore's law" is the observation that the number of transistors in a dense integrated circuit has doubled approximately every 2 years. The observation is named after Gordon E. Moore, the co-founder of Intel and Fairchild Semiconductor, whose 1965 paper described a doubling every year in the number of components per integrated circuit and projected that this rate of growth would continue for at least another decade [14].

His prediction proved accurate for several decades, and the law was used in the semiconductor industry to guide long-term planning and to set targets for R&D. Advancements in digital electronics are strongly linked to Moore's law: quality-adjusted microprocessor prices, memory capacity, sensors, and even the number and size of pixels in digital cameras

14.7.1 Skimming or Penetration Pricing?

According to Spann, Fischer, and Tellis, a skimming strategy is more profitable than a penetration strategy at the camera level. However, a strategy mix appears to be preferable at the portfolio level after taking into account demand and cost interdependencies between products [15].

The current market environment, especially for high-tech categories, is characterized with rapid introductions of new products. In this environment, the pricing of new products is a difficult and important task affecting the financial success of any company. On the one hand, if the price is set too low, a company not only gives up potential revenues but also sets a low value position for this new product, which can make future price increases difficult [16].

Conversely, a price set too high might harm the diffusion of the new product [17], limit gains from experience effects [18], or inhibit the product from reaching its critical mass for success [19]. The literature suggests two basic dynamic pricing strategies for new products, *skimming* and *penetration* strategy [20,21].

A skimming strategy ("cream rises to the top to be skimmed") involves charging a high introduction price, which may be subsequently lowered [22]. The rationale for this strategy is to *skim* surplus from customers early in the product life cycle in order to exploit a momentary monopolistic position or a low price sensitivity of innovators.

A penetration strategy involves charging a low price to rapidly *infiltrate* the market. The strategy works on the expectation that customers will switch to the new brand because of the lower price. Penetration pricing aims at exploiting economies of scale or experience. Further, if word-of-mouth is important in the market, then achieving large early sales increases word-of-mouth and enables rapid market penetration [23,24].

Penetration pricing is most commonly associated with marketing objectives of enlarging market share and exploiting economies of scale or experience [25,26]. The chief disadvantage, however, is that the increase in sales volume may not necessarily lead to a profit if prices are kept too low. Also, if the price is only an introductory campaign, customers may leave the brand once prices begin to rise to levels more in line with rivals [27].

The choice of the pricing strategy is particularly important for high-tech products such as digital cameras where new products are frequently introduced and life cycles are short. Differentiation by features leads to a proliferation of products in each price tier. Textbooks recommend a skimming strategy for differentiated products where companies have some additional source of competitive protection.

However, many textbooks also recommend a penetration strategy for price-sensitive markets where new products usually face strong competition soon after introduction [28], which is the case for digital cameras. Hence, while the normative literature on dynamic pricing strategy provides plausible guidelines under what conditions to choose which strategy, it falls short of offering guidance in markets where conditions favor both strategy types.

Unfortunately, many if not most markets for modern consumer durables (e.g., computers, mobile phones, TV sets, and digital cameras) present the same dilemma: extensive feature differentiation supporting a skimming strategy concomitant with strong competition supporting a penetration strategy. Moreover, popular examples support the success of either strategy.

In contrast, in the automotive industry, Lexus has been successfully competing with Mercedes and BMW in the US premium *luxury car* market with its penetration pricing strategy relative to these two brands.

14.8 Determining Your Price Parameters

The price of your high-tech product always fluctuates between two points: the price ceiling and the bottom price (see Figure 14.4). The market segment being addressed will ultimately determine the price ceiling; no customer will buy above this level, and this price ceiling will be translated into a zero market share [29].

The bottom (lowest) price is established by the cost structure of a product; below this price, the company loses money on every product sold, which leads to a negative return. With the specifications of high-tech products, a marketing manager must evaluate these two limits by analyzing the price elasticity of demand of your targeted market segments and by the costs' learning curve.

	Price pointers	Actions	Pricing policies
Ceiling price	Market segment acceptance	Demand elasticity of price	Pricing to value
	Current market pricing	Competitor's list prices	Lowest bidding price
Bottom price	Product cost structure	Determine life cycle of product and learning cost	Your break-even price

FIGURE 14.4
From bottom price to ceiling price.

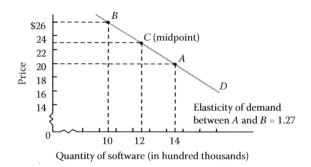

FIGURE 14.5
Elasticity of demand. This is an example of new software pricing versus expected demand.

14.8.1 Evaluating Your Price Elasticity of Demand

The price elasticity of demand in relation to price measures the variation of customer purchases according to price changes. Thus, if elasticity is high, demand for a product is heavily influenced by its price. Understanding demand elasticity for a product allows you to determine which products drive market penetration and thus require a low penetration price, and which products can be priced at a premium, like in the case of smart cellphones or broadband subscriptions. Figure 14.5 is a classical depiction of elasticity of demand for a new software product entry, showing that as price decreases, demand will increase.

Usually, innovative high-tech products have low elasticity. This means that high variation in price, an increase as well as a decrease, does not significantly modify demand. These high-tech products have few substitutes, meaning that the costs to switch to another product are high. Additionally, at the first stage of the technology, buyers—either innovators or forerunners—are less sensitive to price than to additional performance; they often have deep pockets or are ready to spend more for a new innovative and outstanding product (often referred to as early adopters). Furthermore, the high price of these products is often perceived as a sign of quality and reinforces a customer's confidence in the company.

14.8.2 Estimating Your Learning Curve Costs

Successful high-tech firms are constantly monitoring costs in order to keep these costs down. To show a profit that encourages future investments, a company must at least cover its variable costs that are linked to production volume and its fixed costs (salaries, rent, administration, and R&D) that are necessary to manufacture its product. Identifying and controlling these costs allow you to measure your learning curve.

This learning curve effect corresponds to the company's improved know-how as its production increases during the growth stage of the product life cycle:

- Purchasing optimization
- Design simplification for manufacturing purposes
- Output increase for production facilities
- Improvement of sales force
- Selection of distributors
- Increased performance of sales promotion campaigns

All these gains in productivity lead to a decrease in the average manufacturing unit cost. This decrease in cost could be passed on to the price in order to react to a competitor's actions or to increase price-sensitive demand.

The learning curve is valid for high-tech products because of the high level of R&D costs required by these products. Because the product life cycles are fairly short, these expenses must be written off very quickly (e.g., in 1 year for computers and in 2 years for robotics), and these R&D costs inflate the average unit cost at the beginning of the product's life, before decreasing very quickly. This unit cost variation is reflected in the changing unit price.

14.9 Pricing Pharmaceutical Global Launches

Pharmaceutical companies pursuing global product launches are faced with a choice between minimizing the time to market and maximizing prices. Limited intellectual property protection and stockholder expectations (among other factors) often suggest that the best product launch strategy is one that provides the fastest commercialization [30].

This strategy is appropriate in those countries where manufacturers are free to set innovator product price; however, in countries that require price negotiations before launch, such acceleration to enter the market risks sacrificing significant revenues over the product life cycle.

Of course, this choice is merely the first of many hurdles faced by manufacturers pursuing global product launches. Others include price maintenance, unilateral regulatory price changes, managing price negotiations, and sequential launch timing.

A successful global launch strategy includes far more than determining price. Typical launch issues, including product positioning, price determination, and reimbursement negotiations, must include an evaluation of all the factors that affect the launch and life cycle of the new therapy.

For example, a profitable global launch strategy must

- Demonstrate the clinical attributes of the therapy against products
- Protect against the possibility of a generic or new competitive entry
- Incorporate each country's healthcare system and physician prescribing patterns
- Comply with country-specific regulatory environments while successfully negotiating suitable prices

14.9.1 Practical Pharma Pricing Tips

Price is the amount of money charged for a product or service, or the sum of the values that consumers exchange for the benefits of having or using the product or service. Economic theory contends that the market price converges at a point where the forces of supply and demand meet [31].

Regardless of theoretical economic theories, price is one of the most controversial topics in pharmaceutical marketing, and is a frequent topic of media discussion. How much should you charge for a new pharmaceutical product? Charge too much and you will not sell—a problem that can be fixed relatively easily by reducing your price. Charging too little is far more dangerous: a company not only forgoes significant revenues and profits but also fixes the product's market value position at a low level, and as companies have repeatedly found, once prices hit the market, it is difficult, even impossible, to raise them [32].

Internal factors affecting pricing include the company's marketing objectives, marketing mix strategy, costs, and organizational considerations. External factors that affect pricing decisions include the nature of the market and demand, competition, and other environmental elements. Besides, a company may amortize its R&D cost over a period, which becomes an additional cost component [33].

In view of the peculiar characteristics of pharmaceutical industry, the different approaches applicable and practiced in the industry are as follows:

- Cost-plus pricing
- Break-even pricing
- Value-based pricing
- Competition-based pricing
- Economy pricing

14.9.2 Cost-Plus Pricing

Cost-plus pricing is a method for setting retail prices of medicines by taking into account the production cost of a medicine together with allowances for promotional expenses, manufacturer's profit margins, and charges and profit margins in the supply chain.

The manufacturing cost structure forms the basis of this type of pricing. The required profit margin is added to the cost of the product to arrive at the ex-factory price and then the trade price and market retail price. This type of pricing is usually done for old molecules where the market is very crowded, and a higher price cannot sustain the required market share. The objective of a company in such scenario is to either get some additional volume for their manufacturing facility or complement their existing product range.

14.9.3 Break-Even Pricing

Break-even pricing strategies are normally adopted for products specifically manufactured for government tenders and for institutional buyers. The objective is not profit, but either to (1) get volumes or (2) to gain entry into large hospital pharmacies so that the positive impact may come from out-of-hospital practice of the doctors who have to prescribe their brand in hospital because of inclusion in pharmacy. Normally, this type of pricing policies are never adopted for research-based high-profile molecules, so that there may not be a negative impact on their high in-market price.

14.9.4 Value-Based Pricing

This approach for pricing is most commonly used by multinational companies, especially in case of new chemical entities [34]. There are countless examples where the cost of product has no relevance whatsoever and the company has priced a product as per the perceived medical/therapeutic value.

14.9.5 Competition-Based Pricing

This is what most marketing-oriented companies attempt to do these days. They take into account not only the perceived value but also the value being offered by the competition and then arrive at a reasonable price, giving them good margin as well as keeping them competitive in the long run. It is extremely important to take into account not only current competitors but also expected competitors, which come with a much lower price and snatch the market share.

14.9.6 Economy Pricing

There are some companies that focus only on offering brands of established molecules at the lowest possible price. They base their price on cost and keep the margins to bare minimum. The reason this is being discussed separately is that the molecules selected have no impact whatsoever on the pricing strategy. They may even pick up a molecule where there is just one leading brand and price their "bioequivalent" at 75% lower price.

14.9.7 External Reference Pricing

External reference pricing (also known as international reference pricing) refers to the practice of using the price of a pharmaceutical product (generally ex-manufacturer price or other common point within the distribution chain) in one or several countries to derive a benchmark or reference price for the purposes of setting or negotiating the price of the product in a given country. Reference may be made to single-source or multisource supply products.

14.10 Differential Pricing in the Pharma Industry

Adapting drug prices to the purchasing power of consumers in different geographical or socioeconomic segments could potentially be a very effective way to improve access to medicines for people living in low- and middle-income countries [35].

Recent trends, however, are prompting the pharmaceutical industry to pay more attention to differential pricing, such as economic and demographic growth in some low- and middle-income markets, which has increased the potential market size of many low- and middle-income countries; greater recognition by the pharmaceutical manufacturers and their investors of the social responsibilities; stronger global advocacy for access to medicines; and growing competition from generic manufacturers in emerging markets.

Differential pricing allows pharmaceutical companies to signal that their pricing policies are socially responsible and consistent with their obligations to society and not just geared toward maximizing profits. In addition, differential pricing on select drugs opens opportunities to serve low- and middle-income markets and creates economies of scope for pharmaceutical companies

It is important to note that differential pricing is not a panacea to ensuring access. For patients with affordability levels lower than the marginal cost of manufacturing, donor subsidies and government support will continue to be required. Despite some evidence that differential pricing of pharmaceuticals can benefit manufacturers and poor countries without adversely affecting higher-income countries, the widespread and systematic use of such pricing has been limited to vaccines, contraceptives, and antiretrovirals mostly in low-income countries.

14.11 Regulatory Role in Pharma Pricing

The final responsibility of allowing a particular price resides with the regulatory bodies of each country. The objective of regulatory bodies is two pronged; on one hand, they have to ensure the protection of patients' rights and provision of quality healthcare of masses, and on the other hand, they have to allow companies to make reasonable profit so that they keep developing and manufacturing the medicines needed for the people.

The process of pricing at the company level goes through the same steps as it goes in case of any other product, but the matter becomes totally different when an application is filed with the regulatory bodies for allowing a specific price.

In most countries, the perceived potential for manufacturers to exploit a monopoly position when facing relatively inelastic demand for medicines has led many countries to regulate prices for at least some portion of the pharmaceutical market. Two countries with pluralistic coverage schemes—Canada and Mexico—have established price regulation for on-patent pharmaceuticals intended to assure that prices paid by any part of the population, insured or not, are not excessive [36].

Regulatory authorities use a common set of tools to limit the prices charged by pharmaceutical firms. The most commonly used methods involve comparing proposed prices for new products against those prices paid by other payers, a practice known as external price referencing, or against those prices already paid for products judged to be similar, a practice known as internal price referencing.

Pharmaco-economic assessment is used by some schemes as a means of making a formal judgment as to the value provided, in terms of benefits and costs. There are a limited number of other approaches used, including profit controls, which serve as an indirect form of price regulation. Pricing policies are not limited in focus to the payment received by pharmaceutical firms; regulation of the distribution chain is undertaken in many systems.

With the possible exception of profit controls, public and private payers and purchasers of pharmaceuticals use the very same approaches to define the acceptable payment or reimbursement price. In the context of reimbursement, so-called reference price systems are often used to set common reimbursement amounts for products judged to be equivalent or similar, leaving patients to pay any price difference out-of-pocket.

14.12 Medical Technology Industry

The medical technology industry is central to the development of medical devices and diagnostics that will provide the lifesaving and life-enhancing treatments of the future. Patient access to advanced medical technology generates efficiencies and cost savings for the health care system and improves the quality of patient care. Between 1980 and 2010, advanced medical technology helped cut the number of days people spent in hospitals by more than half and add 5 years to US life expectancy while reducing fatalities from heart disease and stroke by more than half. The industry is also an engine of economic growth for the United States, generating high wage manufacturing jobs and a favorable balance of payments [37].

The medical technology industry is composed of companies that develop and manufacture medical devices and diagnostics. These products are diverse, running the gamut from tongue depressors to the most complicated molecular diagnostic tests, advanced imaging machines, and cardiac implants.

Structurally, small firms are a key part of the medical technology industry. A 2007 study by the US International Trade Commission found a total of 7000 medical technology firms in the United States [38]. The US Department of Commerce estimated that 62% of medical technology firms had fewer than 20 employees and only 2% had more than 500 employees.

Small firms, often funded by venture capital, are particularly critical to the future of US scientific and technology leadership because they are the source of a disproportionate number of the breakthrough implantable technologies that drive medical practice and industry growth [39].

Whether created by large or small firms, medical technologies are characterized by a rapid innovation cycle. The typical medical device is replaced by an improved version every 18–24 months. To fuel innovation, the medical device industry is research intensive. US medical technology firms spend over twice the US average on R&D. Medical device companies specializing in the most complex and technologically advanced products devote upward of 20% of revenue to R&D [38].

In no small measure as the result of the diagnostics, treatments, and medical tools developed by the medical technology industry, the health advances of recent years have been breathtaking. According to the National Center for Health Statistics [40], between 1980 and 2010, medical advancements helped add 5 years to US life expectancy. Fatalities from heart disease were cut by 57%; deaths from stroke were reduced by 59%; mortality from breast cancer was cut by 31%; and disability rates declined by 25% [41]. Moreover, the pace of positive change has quickened. Between 2000 and 2010, life expectancy increased by nearly 2 years. Fatalities from heart disease were cut by 30%; deaths from stroke were reduced by 36%; and mortality from breast cancer was cut by 18%.

The dramatic improvements in health have gone beyond reduced mortality to improved quality of life. The proportion of the elderly with a functional limitation has declined and the years of disability-free life expectancy have increased [42]. To cite one example of technology's impact, patients who received total hip or total knee replacements typically transitioned away from disability within 1 year. Their risk of dying was cut in half and their risk of a new diagnosis of heart failure or depression was significantly reduced [43].

14.12.1 Medical Device Prices

The medical technology industry is highly competitive. A study of medical device prices from 1989 to 2009 found that they increased, on average, only one-fifth as fast as other medical prices and less than one-half as fast as the regular Consumer Price Index (CPI) [44]. Because the highly competitive market kept prices low, medical devices and diagnostics accounted for a relatively constant 6% of national health expenditures throughout the 20-year period despite a flood of new products that profoundly changed medical practice.

The US medical technology industry is also a source of economic growth and good jobs. The industry employs more than 420,000 people in the United States. It generates an additional four jobs in suppliers, component manufacturers, and other companies providing services to the industry and its employees, for every direct job—for a total of more than 2 million jobs nationwide [45].

14.12.2 Downward Pressure on Prices

If medical device manufacturers wish to avoid additional downward pressure on prices, the challenge for medical devices companies is to ensure that spending on medical technologies is seen not as a cost but as an investment, both in terms of patient outcomes and in terms of treatment times [46].

The medical devices (or medtech) industry, following the path of the pharma industry, is adapting to a healthcare ecosystem that increasingly values better health outcomes and effective cost-containment. It is no longer enough for medtech companies to rely on their traditional market access models, which tended to be focused on commercial or sales and marketing functions. To gain access and obtain optimum price reimbursement, medtech companies need to showcase innovations that can clearly demonstrate evidence of better health *outcomes* at reasonable costs [47].

14.12.3 Average Prices for Implantable Medical Devices

Bereft of the effective monopolies created by pharma patent protection, medical device companies have been far more exposed to the competition created by globalization and the rise of developing market producers. The rapid product cycle in the industry—akin to that in the smartphone or software sectors—has also made competition more intense.

Average prices for implantable medical devices paid by hospitals have declined substantially in recent years on an inflation-adjusted basis [48]. Table 14.2 reports the change in the average selling price for each category of device relative to the 2007 average price and after adjusting for inflation. The average selling price for each device category declined in real terms between 2007 and 2011. The size of this decline ranges from a 17% decline for artificial knees to a 34% decline for drug-eluting stents (corresponding to an average annual rate of decline of −4.6% and −10.5%, respectively).

TABLE 14.2

Price Decline in Inflation-Adjusted Prices

Device Name	2007	2011	Total Percent Change
Cardiac resynchronization therapy defibrillators	100%	74%	−26
Implantable cardioverter defibrillator	100%	76%	−24
Cardiac pacemakers	100%	74%	−26
Artificial hips	100%	77%	−23
Artificial knees	100%	83%	−17
Drug-eluting stents	100%	66%	−34
Bare metal stents (not medicated)	100%	73%	−27

14.12.4 Practical Pricing Tips

According to HBS Consulting, pricing strategies need to balance the demands of the market, that is, what the customer needs and wants, with the needs of the company. Pricing objectives need to be closely linked with organizational and marketing objectives, as well as taking account of cash flow requirements, profit objectives, and return on investment. In addition, they must take into account the market's price sensitivity, which is defined as the relative importance of price in a purchasing decision. In view of the complexities involved in pricing, obtaining an efficient pricing strategy is an important issue for all medical device and diagnostic companies.

In HBS's 2006 publication [49], they argue that medtech companies should first recognize that there are few truly innovative, lifesaving devices being developed—most are developments on an existing technology and thus competition is high. Therefore, persuading a customer to purchase one technology in favor of another can be a difficult process.

The second reason is that most of the major medical device companies in the market have been established for generations, and rather than their pricing systems evolving smoothly, new processes have been built on top of old ones to create a highly complex mesh that hinders communication between the various processes. These systems are often put to the test when negotiating discounts and the addition of other products and services (bundling) to the deal in order to entice the customer to make a purchase, and they frequently break down.

Medtech companies need to establish a clear pricing policy based on the price influencers, as shown in Table 14.3.

14.12.5 Assessing Your Market "Pain"

Innovative medical devices with a high medical need (market pain) can frequently command privileged prices, especially in its launch phase. Table 14.4 illustrates the critical questions a company should ask in order to evaluate

TABLE 14.3

Price Influencers

Pressures Influencing Pricing	Your Competitive Differentiators
Competitor's technology	Is your technology more effective?
Existing price structure	Should you match or exceed prices?
Reimbursement schemes	Is your product approved for reimbursement?
Procurement methods	What are your sales channels?
Global pricing trends	Falling or rising?
Customer identification	Who is your customer? The hospital? The patient? The healthcare provider?
Product brand strength	Can your brand protect your price?
Economic/medical value	Can you command a premium?
Company's financial strength	Can you afford to promote heavily? Can you afford to undercut?

TABLE 14.4

Device Therapy Value and Its Price Result

Therapeutic Value/Utility	Expected Price Result
Will severity of the disorder or the symptoms affect price sensitivity? Is the disorder disabling?	Disorder severity can either make price sensitivity high or low.
What is the position of the disease in the payer, provider, or the public's perception?	A high profile can either make the payer prepared to pay a premium or feel that price should be lowered to make the therapy widely available.
What does this disorder cost the health care system and society (direct, indirect, quality of life)? Can society afford the cost?	The more the disorder costs the health system (or society), the higher can be the price sought for the device.
What is the potential to reduce the healthcare cost with your product?	The greater the potential to reduce the cost, the greater the potential to increase the price, as long as the price doesn't exceed the ceiling of the decreased cost.
What information will be needed to document and demonstrate any savings? Are clinical trials necessary, or are published papers sufficient?	This can be information from clinical trials against competitive technologies combined with economic data using prices of the technologies and cost savings on patient care.
Is the product likely to be used as mono- or combination device? Combination problems require longer regulatory development time.	The whole of the cost of the therapeutic process needs to be considered and the prices combined if it is a combination device.
Will the value of the product be different for different potential indications? Are all stents born equal?	For example: Will a stent placed in a carotid artery have the same perceived value as a coronary artery stent? Is the brain more important than the heart?

the medical need for its medical device and the effect this may have on its proposed price.

The answers to these questions are not always clear-cut. Ultimately, many companies find themselves in a position where they gather this information and then combine their marketing research and current market conditions to make a final pricing decision.

References

1. Kotler P. *Marketing Management*. Simon & Schuster Company, Englewood Cliffs, NJ, 1994.
2. Bernstein, J. and Macias, D. Engineering new product success: The new product pricing process at Emerson. *Industrial Marketing Management*, 31, 51–64, 2002.
3. http://en.wikipedia.org/wiki/Complex_sales
4. Thull, J. *Mastering the Complex Sale*. John Wiley & Sons, Inc., 2000.
5. https://en.wikipedia.org/wiki/Gross_margin
6. Farris, P.W., Bendle, N.T., Pfeifer, P.E., and Reibstein, D.J. *Marketing Metrics: The Definitive Guide to Measuring Marketing Performance*. Pearson Education, Inc., Upper Saddle River, NJ, 2010. ISBN 0-13-705829-2.
7. http://research.financial-projections.com/IndustryStats-GrossMargin.shtml
8. https://en.wikipedia.org/wiki/Pricing_strategies
9. http://www.mindofmarketing.net/2008/10/your-pricing-should-be-influenced -by-your-customers-reference-point/
10. https://en.wikipedia.org/wiki/High_tech
11. Dovleac, L. Pricing policy and strategies for consumer high-tech products. Transylvania University of Braşov, http://webbut.unitbv.ro/bulletin/Series %20V/BULETIN%20V%20PDF/05_DOVLEAC%20L.pdf.
12. Moore, G.E. Cramming more components onto integrated circuits. *Proceedings of the IEEE*, 86(1), 1998.
13. Mohr, J., Sengupta, S., and Slater, S. *Marketing of High-Technology Products and Innovations* (3rd ed.). Prentice Hall, 358–366, 2010.
14. https://en.wikipedia.org/wiki/Moore%27s_law
15. Spann, M., Fischer, M., and Tellis, G.J. Skimming or penetration? Strategic dynamic pricing for new products, https://business.ualberta.ca//media/business /departments/mbel/documents/marketingseminars/2008-09/strategicdynamic pricingpaper.pdf.
16. Marn, M.V., Roegner, E.V., and Zawada, C.C. Pricing new products. *The McKinsey Quarterly*, 3(July), 40–49, 2003.
17. Golder, P.N. and Tellis, G.J. Pioneer advantage: Marketing logic or marketing legend? *Journal of Marketing Research*, 30(May), 158–170, 1993.
18. Tellis, G.J. Beyond the many faces of price: An integration of pricing strategies, *Journal of Marketing*, 50(October), 146–160, 1986.
19. Dhebar, A. and Oren, S.S. Optimal dynamic pricing for expanding networks. *Marketing Science*, 4(4), 336–351, 1985.

20. Kotler, P. and Armstrong, G. *Principles of Marketing*. Prentice Hall, Upper Saddle River, 2005.
21. Nagle, T.T. and Hogan, J.E. *The Strategy and Tactics of Pricing: A Guide to Growing More Profitably*. Prentice Hall, Upper Saddle River, NJ, 2006.
22. Dean, J. Pricing policies for new products, *Harvard Business Review*, 54(Nov–Dec), 141–153, 1976.
23. Clarke, F.H., Darrough, M.N., and Heineke, J.M. Optimal pricing policy in the presence of experience effects. *Journal of Business*, 55(4), 517–530, 1982.
24. Robinson, B. and Lakhani, C. Dynamic price models for new product planning. *Management Science*, 21(10), 1113–1122, 1975.
25. https://en.wikipedia.org/wiki/Penetration_pricing
26. Tellis, G.J. Beyond the many faces of price: An integration of pricing strategies. *Journal of Marketing*, 50(October), 146–160, 1986.
27. http://www.investopedia.com/terms/p/penetration-pricing.asp#axzz2ETtC9 KCQ
28. Monroe, K.B. *Pricing—Making Profitable Decisions*. McGraw-Hill, New York, 2003.
29. Viardot, E. *Successful Marketing for High-Tech Firms*. Third Edition. Artech House, Norwood, MA, 2004, http://www.kolegjifama.eu/materialet/Biblioteka%20 Elektronike/Artech_House_Successful_Marketing_Strategy_for_High-Tech _Firms_3rd.pdf.
30. Rankin, P.J., Bell, G.K., and Wilsdon, T. Global pricing strategies for pharmaceutical product launches. Chapter 2 of *The Pharmaceutical Pricing Compendium*, http://www.crai.com/sites/default/files/publications/Global-Pricing -Strategies-for-Pharmaceutical-Product-Launches.pdf.
31. http://www.investopedia.com/terms/m/market-price.asp
32. http://www.mckinsey.com/insights/marketing_sales/pricing_new_products
33. Khoso, I., Ahmed, R.R., and Ahmed. J. Pricing strategies in pharmaceutical marketing. *The Pharma Innovation Journal*, 3(7), 13–17, 2014, http://thepharmajournal .com/vol3Issue7/Issue_september_2014/14.1.pdf.
34. http://www.forbes.com/sites/forbesinsights/2012/06/11/value-based-health -care-fad-or-future/#29da073473ca
35. Yadav, P. Differential pricing for pharmaceuticals. U.K. Department for International Development (DFID). Review of current knowledge, new findings and ideas for action, https://www.gov.uk/government/uploads/system/uploads /attachment_data/file/67672/diff-pcing-pharma.pdf.
36. Pharmaceutical Pricing Policies in a Global Market. OECD Health Policy Studies. 2008, http://apps.who.int/medicinedocs/documents/s19834en/s19834en .pdf.
37. AdvaMed's Innovation Agenda: Background and Detail, http://advamed.org/res .download/839.
38. United States International Trade Commission. Medical Devices and Equipment: Competitive Conditions Affecting U.S. Trade in Japan and Other Principal Foreign Markets, March 2007, http://www.usitc.gov/publications/332/pub3909.pdf.
39. Platzer, M. *Patient Capital: How Venture Capital Investment Drives Revolutionary Medical Innovation*, 2007, http://www.contentfirst.com/past/Patientcapital/NVCA PatientCapital.pdf.
40. National Center for Health Statistics. *Health, United States, 2012: With Special Feature on Emergency Care*. Hyattsville, MD, 2013.

41. The Value of Investment in Health Care: Better Care, Better Lives. Report compiled for The Value Group by MedTap International, 2004. Data cited on disability rates is limited to 1982–2000.

42. Federal Interagency Forum on Aging-Related Statistics. Older Americans 2012: Key Indicators of Well-Being. Federal Interagency Forum on Aging-Related Statistics. Washington, DC: U.S. Government Printing Office, June 2012; D. Cutler, K. Ghosh, and M. Landrum. Evidence for Significant Compression of Morbidity in the Elderly U.S. Population. National Bureau of Economic Research, July 2013.

43. Medscape Medical News (by Kathleen Louden), http://www.medscape.com /viewarticle/781620.

44. Long, G. et al. Recent Average Price Trends for Implantable Medical Devices, 2007–2011, the Analysis Group, February 2013.

45. The Lewin Group. State Economic Impact of the Medical Technology Industry, June 7, 2010, and February 2007, http://www.socalbio.org/studies /MTI_Lewin_2010.pdf.

46. Value-based healthcare. Strategies for medtech, http://pages.eiu.com/rs/eiu2 /images/MEDTEC%20Value based%20healthcare%20WEB.pdf.

47. Value-based healthcare. White paper from The Economist Intelligence Unit Healthcare, 2014, http://pages.eiu.com/rs/eiu2/images/MEDTEC%20 Value-based%20healthcare%20WEB.pdf.

48. Long, G., Mortimer, R., and Sanzenbacher, G. Recent average price trends for implantable medical devices, 2007–2011 Advamed, 2013, http://advamed.org /res.download/365.

49. Pricing Strategies—The Outlook for Medical Devices and Diagnostic Companies. HBS Consulting, 2006, http://hbs-consulting.com/HBSStrategyReviews/Pricing .pdf.

15

Product Launch Risk Analysis

15.1 Introduction

All start-up businesses entail huge risks; therefore, systematically analyzing your product launch risks will prepare you for the challenges you will face during your early years. Including a critical risk analysis is crucial because acknowledging inherent risks will allow you to establish a plan to overcome these risks.

Furthermore, having a plan to navigate around these critical risks will provide you will gain credibility, since you have not yet demonstrated your ability to survive in the fierce competitive knowledge-based environment. By understanding your critical start-up risks, you can offer creative and effective solutions to those risks if and when they occur, and thereby minimize their impact.

15.2 Critical Risk Analysis

Professor Michael Goldsby of Ball State University likens critical risk analysis to a flight simulator for pilots. It is a "what if" scenario for addressing the competitive dynamics of your chosen industry. It will prepare you for likely eventualities and provide a roadmap to counteract business adversities. A well-known "flight simulator" is Porter's forces of competition, a subject we will discuss in the following paragraphs.

In 1979, a *Harvard Business Review* article entitled "How Competitive Forces Shape Strategy" was published by industrial economist Michael E. Porter. Porter started a revolution in the field of strategic critical risk analysis and industry profitability. It provided a framework for anticipating and influencing competition and profitability over time. Porter argued that a healthy industry structure is as much of a competitive concern to strategists as their company's own position. This technique became known as "Porter's 5 forces analysis." (Since then, a sixth force has been added, namely, regulatory threats.)

TABLE 15.1

Modified Porter's Force Analysis

"An Industry's Profit Potential is Largely Determined by
  the Intensity of Competitive Rivalry within That Industry"

1. Competitive rivalry within the industry
2. Threats of new entrants
3. Threats of substitutes products
4. Bargaining power of customers
5. Bargaining power of suppliers
6. Public authorities: Regulatory threats

Porter's "Five Forces of Competition" framework describes how the structural features of an industry influences the distribution of value created by firms within that industry.

- Ideally, firms in an industry would like to capture most or all of the economic value that they create.
- However, competitive forces operate to push that value "forward" to customers (in the form of lower prices) or, in some cases, "backward" to suppliers.

The classical Porter's 5 forces analysis represents the competitive environment of the firm. It is a strategic foresight to avoid putting the competitive edge at risk and ensure the profitability of products on a long term. For the company, this vision is quite important because the firm is able to direct its innovations in terms of choice of strategies and investments. The profitability of businesses within the industrial structure depends on the six forces, as seen in Table 15.1.

This is visually summarized in Figure 15.1.

15.2.1 The Competitive Rivalry within Your Industry

The competition between firms determines the attractiveness of your selected sector. Your competitors change based on sector development, diversity, and the existence of barriers to enter. In addition, it is an analysis of the number of competitors, products, brands, strengths and weaknesses, strategies, and market shares.

15.2.2 The Threat of New Entrants

It is in your company's interest to create barriers to prevent its competitors to enter the market. Your competitors are either new companies or companies that intend to diversify. These barriers can be legal (patent regulations) or industrial (products or single brands). The arrival of new entrants also

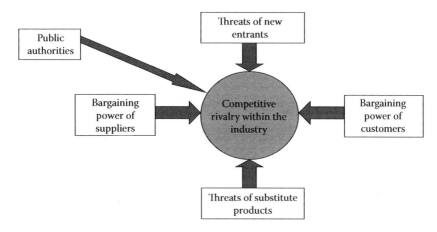

FIGURE 15.1
Modified Porter's force analysis.

depends on the size of the market (economy of scale), the reputation of a company already established, the cost of entry, access to raw materials, technical standards, or cultural barriers.

15.2.3 The Threat of Substitute Products

The substitute products can be considered as an alternative compared to supply on the market. Substitute products are attributed to changes in the state of technology or to the innovation. The companies see their products be replaced by different products. Substitute products often have a better price/ quality report and come from sectors with higher profits. These substitute products can be dangerous and your company should anticipate coping with this threat.

15.2.4 The Bargaining Power of Suppliers

The bargaining power of suppliers is very important in a market. Powerful suppliers can impose their conditions in terms of price, quality, and quantity. On the other hand, if there are a lot of suppliers, their influence is weaker. One has to analyze the number of realized orders, the cost of changing the supplier, and the presence of raw materials.

15.2.5 The Bargaining Power of Customers

If the bargaining power of customers is high, they influence the profitability of the market by imposing their requirements in terms of price, service, or quality. Choosing clients is crucial because a firm should avoid being in a situation of dependence. The level of concentration of customers gives them more or less power. Generally, their bargaining power tends to be inversely proportional to that of the suppliers.

15.2.6 Public Authorities: Regulatory Threats

In many industries, government rules and regulations present a formidable barrier to commercialization. Regulatory agencies such as the US Food and Drug Administration (FDA) and the US Environmental Protection Agency present huge challenges, especially to start-ups. The cost of meeting FDA requirements can be overwhelming to undercapitalized start-ups. In the medical/pharmaceutical fields, the inability to obtain FDA approval is one of the main causes of bankruptcies.

15.3 Knowledge-Based Enterprises

The knowledge-based enterprise process encompasses the complete life-span of the enterprise and the career of the entrepreneur. Entrepreneurial knowledge-based ventures mimic the familiar pattern of life on earth in that there is a beginning and there is an end. Businesses open and sooner or later they close. The only question is how long they will survive—at least in their initial form.

Individuals undertake entrepreneurial ventures at different stages of their lives and careers. There is also a cycle of entrepreneurship that relates to what the entrepreneur is doing—which may not coincide with what is happening to your enterprise.

At one extreme, an enterprise may be thriving, but the founding entrepreneur may wish to leave it for a variety of possible reasons; at the other end of the spectrum, the business may fail and close but the founder remains an entrepreneur by starting a new venture.

15.3.1 Knowledge-Based Start-Up Classification

Hisrich and Peters [1] divided knowledge-based start-ups into three groups: lifestyle, foundation, and high-potential:

1. A **lifestyle firm** that exists primarily to support the owners. Privately owned, it achieves modest growth because of the nature of the business and the motives of the entrepreneur. These are typically micro-business with up to 10 employees.
2. A **foundation company** is created from research and development (R&D) and lays the foundation of a new industry. Its innovation changes the nature of an entire sector, for example, Apple

Corporation founded by Steven Jobs and Stephen Wozniak that turned computing from a specialized technology into a mass market.

3. A **high-potential venture** achieves rapid growth because of its innovative product/service in a large market and also receives greatest investment and public interest. For example, Boston Scientific changed the minimally invasive surgical world and became a multi-billion-dollar company.

15.3.2 Which Start-Ups Close and When?

The data on business closures indicate that there are two groups of start-ups that are most vulnerable to closure. Smaller enterprises—the very small microfirms are most likely to close as closure rates are lower among medium-sized and larger firms. The largest numerical segment of small and medium-sized enterprises—microenterprises—are most at risk of closure. This indicates that standing still and staying small are not a good survival strategy even though many business owners do not want to grow.

The next most vulnerable start-ups are young enterprises—the chances of survival improve as the business ages so that the most vulnerable are the very young, relatively new enterprises. The message to the founding entrepreneur is clear: the longer you can keep going and the more you can grow your business, the greater chance you will have of survival.

Drucker [2] made one of the earliest summaries of what is required to keep an enterprise going through the various stages of its life cycle and it stills seems valid today. He proposed that the four key factors, in chronological order, were likely to be as follows:

1. Focus on the market
2. Financial foresight, especially planning cash needs
3. Building a management team—before it is needed
4. Finding an appropriate role for the founding entrepreneur in a developed enterprise

15.3.3 The Entrepreneurship Process

The entrepreneurship process encompasses the complete life-span of a start-up and the career of an entrepreneur. This chapter will consider what happens to businesses as they grow and decline, as well as what happens to entrepreneurs as they enter into and exit from an enterprise. Life cycle models of an enterprise from start to finish typically describe five stages:

1. Product development/concept/test stage
2. Introduction (product launch)

3. Growth

4. Maturity

5. Decline or regrowth

These five stages in the conceptual life cycle of a start-up are depicted in Figure 15.2.

Such conceptual life cycle models have limitations as growth is rarely smooth and does not necessarily take place in the order of the model. Many enterprises reach steady state and never grow out of the introduction (product launch) phase. If the product is successfully launched, then the growth phase will be influenced by

- The founders—their motivation, previous management experience, demographics (age and education), and the number of entrepreneurs involved in the enterprise
- The enterprise—the legal form, age, and size of the business
- The management strategy—the market position, introduction of new products, devolution of management to non-owning managers, and sharing of equity
- The external business environment—the market sector or industry, competitive forces, and location

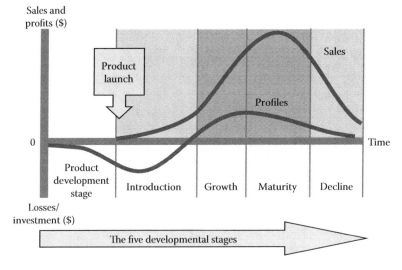

FIGURE 15.2
The entrepreneurship life cycle.

15.4 Why Do Most Product Launches Fail?

According to Schneider and Hall [3], the biggest problem they encounter is lack of preparation: Companies are so focused on designing and manufacturing new products that they postpone the hard work of getting ready to market them until too late in the game. Below is a list of the most common product launch mistakes:

15.4.1 Prelaunch Mistakes

- No prior market research on the product
- Budget used to develop product; little left for product launch or promotion
- Technically interesting but lacks market need
- Few key differentiators
- Needs extensive customer education
- Undefined target audience
- Product lacks sufficient testing to support claims

15.4.2 Launch Phase Mistakes

- Product lacks reliability
- Product aimed at wrong target audience
- Insufficient inventory to satisfy orders
- Claims cannot be verified
- A regulatory body orders the product withdrawn for market
- No "influencers" to promote product
- Product design is confusing to customers
- Product priced too high
- Poor product quality and reliability
- Product not yet ready to market and falls short of expectations
- Product revolutionary but there is no market demand

15.5 Approaches to Product Launch

A successful product launch depends on careful planning and preparation. It is the final stage in the product development process, which represents a significant investment in future revenue and profit for your small business. A successful product launch can take you into new markets or give you access to new customers, as well as increasing business with existing customers [4]. It's important to look at a product launch not as a single event but as a process, as shown below:

Step 1. Set measurable objectives for the launch. Prepare a comprehensive launch plan and allocate a budget to cover launch expenditure. Appoint a senior manager to coordinate launch activities. Identify risk and success factors in the launch and prioritize critical tasks that could affect success. A high proportion of product launches fail because of poor planning, according to pragmatic marketing.

Step 2. Complete the final product review. Ensure that the project team has evaluated product performance in line with market requirements. Check that the product meets all certifications and complies with any relevant product legislation. Complete the production of product documentation. Operate a test market before the launch. Ask selected retailers or distributors to stock the product and run a local promotional campaign. Evaluate test market results and feedback, and make any necessary adjustments to the launch program.

Step 3. Set up training programs for sales representatives. Brief the sales force thoroughly on the product, the target market, and the benefits of the product. Provide a comprehensive sales guide and a quick-reference guide to follow up the training. Hold a launch event to build enthusiasm and commitment to the launch. Set revenue targets for the launch period and offer incentives related to the launch targets.

Step 4. Thoroughly brief the distribution network on the timing and scope of the launch. Hold training programs or provide product guides for the network. Supply promotional material for local outlets.

Step 5. Establish a support infrastructure. Train technical service staff to teach, install, and maintain the product. Produce any essential customer support documentation. Set up a help desk (telecommunications) to handle support requests and queries during the initial launch phase.

Step 6. Prepare and distribute press releases to consumer and trade publications that serve your market. Invite journalists from important publications to a press briefing to improve coverage. Plan a launch advertising or direct marketing campaign in line with available budgets. Inform existing customers about the new product via the sales force or other direct communications. Your press release should contain the following information:

- What are you going to produce
- Name of your product

- What market will you serve with what features/benefits
- Why does the market need this product (push–pull)
- Who are the first adopters that will benefit the most
- How will you produce the product. Domestic or off-shore?
- Your launch team, and who to call to get answers

Some product launches are steeped in a philosophy called "If I build it, they will come." Many start-ups find themselves building a market solution that is based on one or two customer experiences. The reality is… without the proper market research, even the best launch plans can fail. To avoid this mistake, adequate research needs to be completed to ensure that your go-to-market plan is based on facts and substance [5].

It is imperative that you validate that there is a market out there. Does the market have a business need? Who are your best customers? Are there enough to sustain growth? How does this solution tie into the bigger growth picture for a business? Your product launch should proceed in two predictable phases: (1) planning phase and (2) execution phase, as shown in Figure 15.3.

15.5.1 High-Tech Industry Risk Profile

The high-technology industry is vast, feverishly paced, and extremely competitive. For high-tech companies, one thing is certain—today's new product is tomorrow's commodity. That is the main risk of a high-tech venture, and that is only one of the challenges of a high-tech enterprise.

High-tech entrepreneurs must face that risk and that challenge with imagination, innovation, and insight, but unfortunately, many do not—and cannot—bring the same creativity and competence to the management of their companies' business affairs.

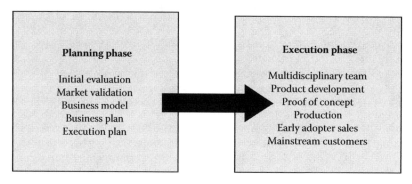

FIGURE 15.3
Start-up product launch.

As a result, promising high-tech companies often fail—not for lack of ideas, but for some very common reasons: lack of capital when they need it most, a naive understanding of the marketplace, poor forecasts of development and production costs, a botched product launch, and mismanaged rapid growth.

15.6 Keeping a Watchful Eye on Your Market

After you assembled the market analysis for your business plan, you identified your market and potential customer base and defined an initial launch strategy. Now, you need to refine that market analysis and select specific distribution channels and focus on specific key customers.

By the launch phase, you have developed and implemented a comprehensive marketing plan to guide you on an annual and a long-term basis. A thorough market analysis can assist you in your current development effort and help you position competitively for the future.

15.6.1 Monitoring Changes in the Marketplace

Prelaunch, you should monitor the market continually to assess the impact of changing competitive strategies. Keep a close eye on the functions, specifications, and features that the marketplace expects. Establish and maintain contact with your intended customers to get their feedback: what do they need? Be sensitive to how the market is changing, and incorporate those changes into your plans. It is important to keep your finger on the pulse of the marketplace to avoid the disaster of going to market with a nearly obsolete product.

However, beware of delaying your product to keep it absolutely state of the art: the way technology changes today, that might keep you out of the marketplace forever! To avoid that dilemma, you'll have to develop a strategy for future products and product enhancements, even before your current product hits the marketplace.

15.6.2 Selecting Your Optimal Marketing Channels

Analyze various marketing channels to determine which is best, for now and for later. Which channels are the most readily available, the most practical, the most cost-effective to use? Will you use a company sales force, contract with well-established manufacturers' representatives, or use some other channel to get your product to market? What is the predominant industry practice today?

15.6.3 Selling Strategies and Methodology

Long before you begin to ship, you need to determine your selling strategies and methodology. Think about

- Conditions and terms of sales.
- Forms of customer contracts.
- Policies and procedures for product warranty, credit and collection, and returns and allowances.
- Refining your product-service strategy. Who will service your customers? Your customers want to know this *before* they buy.
- How you intend to promote your product.
- What kinds of advertising, public relations, and other forms of marketing-support communications should be implemented to generate market awareness.

15.6.4 Production and Marketing Ramp Up

Now, you need to focus on setting up production facilities while you penetrate the market and consummate customer contacts. During this stage, you evolve from an engineering-oriented company to a market-driven one. You need to hire additional employees, particularly in the middle-management ranks.

You may need additional rounds of financing to support rising salaries for these extra layers of management, as well as to provide working capital for inventory and receivables.

During this stage, plan to address these important action items:

- Focus your marketing strategy.
- Plan and ramp up your production.
- Implement a strategy for future products.
- Manage the rapid growth of your company.
- Identify your information needs and develop accounting and management information systems to accommodate them.
- Begin to explore foreign markets.

15.7 Postlaunch Marketing Strategy and Approach

During this stage, marketing is key to your success and survival. The more focused your marketing strategy and the more proactive your approach to the changing market, the higher your chances of success.

A sound marketing strategy helps you use available resources in the best ways possible, because it gives you a good grasp of your opportunities and limitations. During this stage, you should return to your original marketing plan(s) developed in previous stages and complete the definition of your distribution channels. Remember that marketing plans constantly evolve.

15.7.1 Refine Pricing Policies

Refine your policies for pricing, terms, warranty, returns, credit, and collection. You already may have set a price for your product and established some initial benchmarks, but only when you are actually in the marketplace selling and servicing your product do these policies begin to work as an interactive process. Now, take a closer look at your initial policies in view of actual market conditions; they may need adjustment.

15.7.2 Refine Product-Service Strategy

Refine your product-service strategy. Decide how to service your product—through your own network, through your distributor's service capability, or through a third-party servicing organization.

Awareness of customer needs and satisfaction should be heightened. You should establish a mechanism for feedback from your distributors, service representatives, and customers. This information will help keep you abreast of product problems that may require you to modify your product, replace a component, or take other action. It will also keep you apprised of desirable product enhancements and changes that can improve your competitive position.

15.7.3 Actual Sales Performance

In the market description section of your business plan, you made initial sales forecasts. Now, you can develop and refine your methodology for creating realistic interactive sales forecasts. Your initial forecast was based on a somewhat idealized view of your environment, but now you can see the real market forces in action. This perspective will help you to formulate a methodology that can realistically capture the marketplace environment.

15.7.4 Production Processes and Facilities

Clearly, it is now time to concentrate on developing an efficient production process and facility. First, you should hire an operations executive, as well as other key production personnel, to round out your management team. In earlier stages, your concern was to set up an initial management framework and then to fill in the voids in the financial arena. Now, you need to fill out your employee roster with personnel who possess expertise in operations and production.

You should consider outside consultants to help determine the optimal facilities layout for efficient flow of the production process and for storage and movement of incoming materials and outgoing products. Your management consultant can scrutinize the process for unnecessary steps and inefficiencies that may raise your costs and help you design a smooth and efficient process. Study your production capacity and the capabilities and costs of expansion and contraction—next year and in the long term—taking into consideration your anticipated growth.

15.7.5 Inventory Management

Establish and implement procedures, policies, and systems to control your inventory, both of raw materials and of finished products. Establish policies that control engineering change orders. To achieve Just-in-Time production efficiency, you need to minimize inventory on hand, yet be able to supply your customers' needs promptly.

Adopt a policy for accounting for "field spares," plug-in components that will be replaced in the field and repaired back in the plant. Financial and tax accounting for inventory can be tricky and early planning can maximize tax benefits.

Revise and expand the sales forecast of your business plan, and use it as a strategic planning tool to help you monitor and adjust the production required to achieve those sales forecasts. This will also help forecast your material and labor requirements and procurement.

15.8 Balancing Limited Resources

As products change, the marketplace changes. You must refine your market strategy to keep your product apace with or ahead of marketplace dynamics. Then, you must reallocate resources to implement that strategy. Determine what financial, material, and human resources you will need to implement future product development, and balance that projection with current production needs. *Balancing is the key to success.*

15.8.1 Managing Rapid Growth

During this stage of your company's life cycle, you are beginning to grow rapidly. Growth is obviously good, but unmanaged growth can be disastrous. Your business organization is becoming increasingly complex and sophisticated; you may feel overextended and out of control of some aspects of the organization. The key concept here is to monitor: to put systems, policies, and procedures in place to *monitor* and help you manage, among other things, financial resources, sales, production, and your employees and their productivity.

15.8.2 Written Systems and Procedures

Establish sound accounting policies, and maintain good systems and financial controls. During this stage, you should continue to refine your financial-reporting methods: review your monthly budget-to-actual reporting of financial results and monthly financial statements, and implement strict spending authorization and revenue-recognition policies.

Does management have the key information it needs to evaluate current and future production? Identify all key accounting policies and procedures, write them up in a procedures manual, and make sure that your policy objectives are communicated to the appropriate members of your management team, as described below:

- Implement procedures to monitor and control financial performance.
- Inventories and production costs, and other service parts.
- Credit and collections.
- Service requests and calls.
- Quality control, both production and service.
- Sales returns and warranty problems.

15.8.3 Rapid Growth Risks and Pitfalls

As your growth accelerates and your business organization becomes more complex, it is crucial to resist making hair-trigger decisions or to react to immediate pressures without giving due consideration to the long-term consequences. Later, you may regret decisions made now without forethought or adequate information. If each action plan is not addressed thoroughly, you may encounter the following difficulties during this stage:

- Delays in initial product shipments
- Incomplete marketing and distribution-channel development
- Production bottlenecks: poor labor know-how; inefficient shop-floor layout
- Failure to develop timely product enhancements as dictated by the market
- Inadequate management information systems
- Chronic cash shortages
- Poor credit and collection procedures

- Improper accounting policies, particularly revenue recognition and inventory accounting
- Inadequate control over inventory and purchasing, leading to problems with vendor lead times; too much or too little key raw materials; or excess inventory
- Excessive sales returns and warranty claims
- Unrealistic shipping expectations
- Poor communication, leading to overlapping of tasks or neglect of crucial business needs
- Battles between sales and production departments

15.8.4 Managing Exponential Growth

By now, your company is truly taking off. Your products are well received and your venture is highly successful. You have good accounting systems, budgets, and continually updated business and marketing plans. To manage your burgeoning company, you must continue to use that plan as a guide.

Congratulations. You are experiencing the exponential growth phase and you may be considering branching out into new markets, new facilities, new development, and new products. You need considerable financing to expand into exciting new directions.

If you got off the ground at an earlier stage with seed capital, your investors may wish to realize some return on their investment, and you may be ready, as well, to reap some of the financial rewards of your labors.

During this exponential growth stage, your focus is *controlled* expansion. To avoid false starts and retain control, you should attend to these critical action points:

- Maintain your organizational effectiveness and ensure the attentive management of your business during the capital-raising process.
- Analyze your capital sources and determine the best for your company.
- Continue your R&D efforts to enhance existing products and develop future generations of products.
- Refine your marketing strategies and implement international expansion.
- Implement broad-based compensation plans to attract and retain employees.

By now, the financial rewards are considerable and you have ample management talent in place. Your financial environment is probably stable, well financed, and strong, and you have ready access to outside financing through credit lines, bank loans, and debt structures.

The emphasis of your compensation plan probably has moved to cash-oriented benefit plans or to sweeten existing cash-oriented plans.

In short, you *have arrived*. Now, your objectives are sustained growth and continued development of new products and expanded product lines. To achieve these objectives, you need to

- Reevaluate the direction of your organization
- Identify new directions for growth
- Improve cash flow and profitability
- Continue to attract, motivate, and retain key employees

These action items are not unique to knowledge-based companies but are common to most businesses that have reached this stage in the life cycle. They are essential to maintaining the strength of any business enterprise.

15.8.5 Continuing R&D

No matter how successful your initial products and marketing efforts may be, or how rapidly your sales may grow, you need to keep the R&D fires burning to enhance your existing products and develop future generations. In the high-tech market, it is very risky to be a "one-product" company.

The life expectancy of technology-based products can be extremely short, and you can be sure that the competition is always close behind. Multiple enhancements and fresh, marketable ideas will give your company staying power. From an R&D standpoint, you should continue to promote and reward creativity and innovation. From a tax standpoint, you should be on the lookout for R&D tax credit opportunities.

Particularly in knowledge-based industries, a business enterprise needs continual "tweaking" to respond to ever-changing markets and ever-increasing competition. Sound organizational planning is vital to help you identify problems and maximize the overall profits of your company in the early stages of your product launch.

Last, Figure 15.4 summarizes the five lessons you should follow to enhance your product launch success odds.

- Identify your key driving milestones
- Hit your milestones
- Time is more valuable than money
  - Your competition is hungry
  - Market changes on a dime
  - Knowledge-based technology moves at the speed of light
- Money is a commodity; brains are real value
- An idea is worth one dollar; execution of an idea is worth a million dollars

FIGURE 15.4
Lessons to be followed.

References

1. Hisrich, R.D. and Peters, M.P. *Entrepreneurship: Starting, Developing and Managing a New Enterprise*, 3rd edition, Irwin Inc., Boston, 1995.
2. Drucker, P.F. *Innovation and Entrepreneurship*, Heinemann, London, 1985.
3. Schneider, J. and Hall, J. Why most product launches fail. HBR, April 2011, https://hbr.org/2011/04/why-most-product-launches-fail&cm_sp=Article -_-Links-_-Top%20of%20Page%20Recirculation.
4. Sun, L. Planning a Successful Product Launch, http://www.businessdictionary .com/article/257/planning-a-successful-product-launch/.
5. Grant, J. 7 Reasons Why a Great Product Launch Can Fail and How to Avoid It .Global Strategy and Analyst Relations, Telesian Technology Inc., http://www .massmac.org/newsline/0508/article02.htm.

16

Commercializing Pharmaceutical Products

16.1 Introduction

The Economist Intelligence Unit projects that the US pharmaceutical market, the world's largest at $396 billion in 2011, will increase by 6.4% annually through 2016. Demographics and disease trends are expected to boost overall drug consumption. The expansion of insurance coverage to millions of uninsured Americans under the Affordable Healthcare Act (ACA) via health insurance exchanges and Medicaid expansion is forecast to increase revenue for drug makers. However, ACA-related pharmaceutical sector fees, a new medical device tax, and lower government drug prices could negatively affect growth.

To sustain their expected rates of growth, pharmaceutical companies have historically relied on successfully launching new drugs periodically. This pressure is only likely to increase, since many patents are expiring and product pipelines are shrinking. However, legislated austerity measures in many countries are increasing local and national hurdles for market access, and at the same time, launches are becoming more numerous, smaller, and more competitive.

Yet the drug launch track record is sobering at best. About two-thirds of new drugs fail to meet prelaunch consensus sales expectations for their first year on the market, and those that fall short typically continue to underdeliver. Improving that record requires pharmaceutical companies to recognize that the world has changed dramatically and adjust their drug launch strategy accordingly.

The August 17, 2015, issue of *Forbes* magazine [1] stated that expectations in the drug business have been getting extremely high. Hepatitis C drugs are generating some of the biggest annual sales ever. New medicines from Merck and Bristol-Myers Squibb that harness the immune system to fight tumors are stimulating new discoveries and opening new therapeutic and market avenues.

For a quick sense of what is possible in the pharmaceutical industry, the top drug multibillion-dollar launches, as compiled by pharma analysts at investment bank Evercore ISI [2], were Lipitor, Humira, Plavix, Enbrel, Advair, and Remicade. Included was the debut of Sovaldi, Gilead's hepatitis C medication, which hit $10 billion in sales its first year on the market—the fastest growth out of the gate of any pharmaceutical ever.

16.2 Idiosyncrasies of Pharmaceutical Products Approval

Pharmaceuticals are subjected to the strictest and most rigorous approval process of any product in the world. Because of regulatory requirements, it costs between $900 million to $1 billion (in year 2000 dollars) [3], and over 12 years of development to bring one pharmaceutical from discovery in a laboratory to the patient. For every one medicine that reaches the marketable stage, between 10,000 and 30,000 compounds must be screened, and the majority are discarded [4].

The complexity and cost of the regulatory approval process can be gleaned from Figure 16.1. The entire process typically takes 10–14 years, depending on the drug/disease matrix complexity [4].

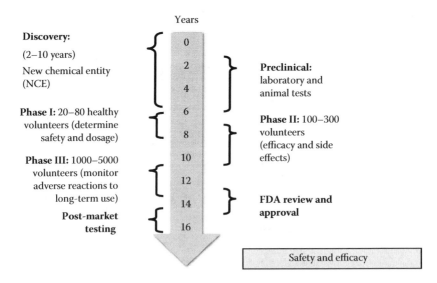

FIGURE 16.1
Pharma approval is risky and costly.

16.3 Pharmaceuticals and Biotechnology

Pharmaceutical companies develop synthetically derived chemical compounds, as well as plant-extracted products, to make medicines that cure or manage diseases, and protect us from infection [5]. The term *pharmaceuticals* is a catch-all category that includes many diverse products that together comprise the category. While many firms also produce animal health products, livestock feed supplements, vitamins, and a host of other products, we will focus solely on their drug products used to treat human illness.

Pharmaceutical companies deal in generic or brand medications and medical devices. They are subject to a bewildering variety of laws and regulations that govern the patenting, testing, safety, efficacy, and marketing of drugs [6]. The pharmaceutical industry is one of the most heavily regulated industries in the world.

16.3.1 Biotechnology Sector

Biotechnology is the applied knowledge of biology. It seeks to duplicate or change the function of a living cell to work in a more predictable and controllable way. The biotechnology industry uses advances in genetics research to develop products for human diseases and conditions. Several biotech companies also use genetic technology to other ends, like the manipulation of crops.

The biotechnology segment had a total revenue of $233 billion in 2012, representing an increase of 9.6% over the previous year. Focus therapeutic areas include oncology, autoimmune disorders, and infectious diseases [7].

The primary difference between biopharmaceuticals and traditional pharmaceuticals is the method by which the drugs are produced: biopharmaceuticals are manufactured in living organisms such as bacteria, yeast, and mammalian cells, whereas pharmaceuticals are manufactured through a series of chemical synthesis.

Biotechnology technology refers to the large and growing array of scientific tools that use living cells and their molecules to make biological products for many different industries. Human and animal health care, agriculture, forestry, environment, and specialty chemicals are among the industries that have benefited most from biotechnology.

The economic promise of biotechnology is extraordinary. At present, it is a $70 billion sector worldwide, and it is estimated to become a market of at least $120 billion annually by 2020. Although biotechnology is a high-growth sector, moving a promising research discovery to market is an exceedingly complex, costly, and challenging undertaking.

Biotech opportunities largely mirror those in the pharmaceutical industry. The key difference is that biotech firms are much more focused on research because they are still developing their initial products. Biotech firms tend to expand their marketing and sales forces when and if a viable product nears US Food and Drug Administration (FDA) approval. Biotech companies tend to be concentrated in geographical clusters, often near prominent research universities and leading hospitals.

The challenges of starting a biotechnology company in the United States include raising capital, building strategic partnerships, recruiting, and motivating and retaining top scientific talent and compliance with regulatory bodies. Commercializing a biotechnology product entails challenges in manufacturing, sales and marketing, reimbursement, and several other unique managerial challenges.

16.4 Pharma Launch Excellence

Launching products into the lucrative pharmaceutical market has never been more crucial and challenging for life science companies seeking to achieve high performance. A product launch nowadays has to be "faster"—enhanced uptake of top line sales, "better"—accelerated growth and higher peak sales, and "cheaper"—executed with fewer resources.

Research shows that many players in the life science industry are facing several market trends that increase the importance of delivering maximum value to customers and to the company with each new product or indication launch. The following trends and implications can be observed:

- Blockbuster patent expiry and weak pipeline enhancing the need to optimize replacement sales from pipeline products and the importance of successful new product launches
- Significant price erosion after patent expiry caused by intense generic competition requiring maximization of product value during patent protection period
- Increased focus on in-licensing requiring capabilities and flexibility to quickly ramp up resources to launch in-licensed products
- Changes in sales model increasing the need to sufficiently align and coordinate resources for launches
- Poor public perception enhancing the need to increase positive perception toward new products and pharmaceutical organizations
- Payer and authority pressures requesting the demonstration of superior product value and benefits
- Intensified and unpredictable health politics environment requesting to ensure an early launch uptake. In order to respond to these dynamics, life science companies need to establish an effective

product launch capability that ensures launch readiness and allows them to accelerate launch uptake to offset sales gaps from patent expiry and maximize sales throughout the patent protected product life cycle.

Despite the importance of an effective product launch process, many companies will experience launch shortcomings that, if not addressed, can threaten the company's future success. Addressing and overcoming these launch weaknesses are a key factor for success for life science companies to become high-performance businesses in the future.

16.4.1 Drivers of Launch Excellence

Understanding the drivers of pharma launch excellence can help companies close the gap between expectations and results. Ahlawat et al. [8] propose that consistent success with drug launches is a function of four interrelated elements: (1) winning launch mind-set, (2) establishing a launch academy, (3) excelling in one of five great decisions, and (4) ensuring a roadmap for fundamentals, as seen in Figure 16.2.

Additionally, management must "think backwards," that is, start from the end and work backward. The end is the optimal price that the new drug can command in the market. We can call this strategic launch excellence, as depicted in Figure 16.3.

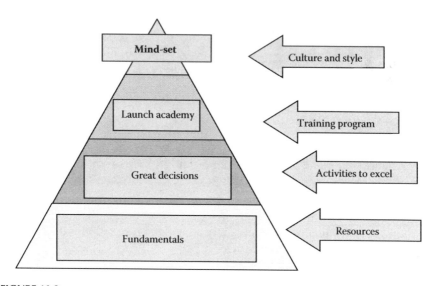

FIGURE 16.2

Pharma launch excellence. Strongly influenced by management. (Modified after DiMasi et al., *J. Health Econ.*, 22, 151–185, 2003.)

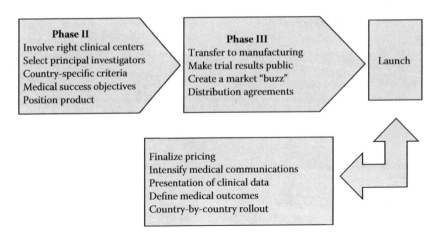

FIGURE 16.3
Key steps in drug launch process. Strategic launch excellence.

16.4.2 Launch Archetypes

Only 25% of pharma launches can be classified as "market disrupters" or "go for the gold" launches. These involve drugs that are strongly differentiated from competing products and treat diseases with a high perceived burden. Examples include Zytiga, Johnson & Johnson's prostate cancer treatment, and Januvia, Merck & Co.'s drug to lower blood sugar levels in people with type 2 diabetes.

At the lower extreme of differentiation, more than half of upcoming launches are "trend setter" products in well-established disease areas, and their priority will be to find a way to "stand out from the crowd."

These launches must find or create an edge that will allow the drug to be positioned effectively for particular patient segments and create clear differentiation from existing competitors.

Roughly 15% of launches are called "breakthrough therapies" by the FDA [9] and are the subject of a specific guidance document [10]. A breakthrough therapy is a drug

- Intended alone or in combination with one or more other drugs to treat a serious or life-threatening disease or condition
- That may demonstrate substantial improvement over existing therapies on one or more clinically significant end points (based on preliminary clinical evidence), such as substantial treatment effects observed early in clinical development

If a drug is designated as breakthrough therapy, FDA will expedite the development and review of such drug. All requests for breakthrough

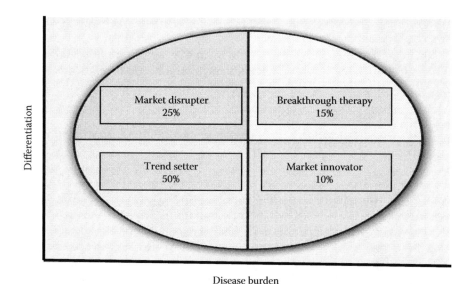

FIGURE 16.4
Launch archetypes. (Modified after DiMasi et al., *J. Health Econ.*, 22, 151–185, 2003.)

therapy designation are reviewed within 60 days of receipt, and FDA will either grant or deny the request.

The priority is to establish unmet needs effectively to ensure access for a targeted population to a well-differentiated treatment. Ahlawat et al. call these launches "category creators," for example, Gardasil, with its development and launch into the unestablished human papillomavirus market.

Finally, the remaining 10% of launches face the substantial challenge of launching an undifferentiated product in an unestablished disease area. Once the decision to market such a product has occurred, the priority for these "market innovator" launches will depend on securing access for the product and effectively establishing unmet needs.

Although no two launches are the same, even for drugs with similar profiles, knowing the four archetypes a product launch falls into can help companies identify the strategic choices they need to make to meet or exceed launch expectations. These four launch archetypes are presented in Figure 16.4.

16.4.3 Speed to Market

Speed to market is a key component to achieving success for any company launching a new product. It provides the distinctive opportunity to establish loyal customers and set the benchmark for consumer expectations. Timing is everything, and getting there first means capturing market share, revenue, profits, and customer mindshare.

Nowhere is timing more crucial than in the pharmaceutical industry. When drug patents expire, generic drug manufacturers play a waiting game with approvals from the FDA. Once approvals come through—often on unpredictable days such as Fridays or holidays—it's a sprint to the pharmacy shelf or the distributor's warehouse. The supply chain network must be ready to deliver when authorization comes, without wasting time or resources.

As the old adage says: Time is Money. The speedier the time to market, the lower the drug development costs. Critically, the failure rate for drugs in Phase III is too high—around 40%, according to a team of researchers at Sagient Research Systems and Biotechnology Industry Organization. From a value-creation perspective, this is perhaps the most inefficient outcome possible. Since the cost of research and development (R&D) increases sharply from one phase of clinical development to the next, failing in Phase III is a very inefficient use of capital that could have been better deployed on other assets.

This is diagrammatically seen in Figure 16.5, where time to marketing is illustrated. What is not easily seen is that as the product proceeds through the different phases, costs escalate exponentially.

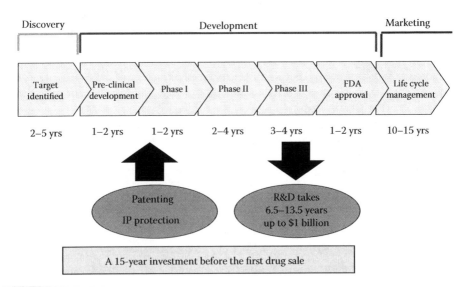

FIGURE 16.5
Time to marketing means lots of money.

16.4.4 Managing Launch Uncertainties

Over the next 3 years, pharmaceutical companies are expected to launch some 400 products and indications yearly, up 146% from 2005. By 2015, sales from products launched in the past 5 years should account for more than US $80 billion worldwide. In an era of patent cliffs and shrinking pipelines, capturing full value from every product launch is critical, but with only about a third of launches meeting or exceeding analysts' expectations, the challenge is considerable and unlikely to get any easier [11].

The importance of getting drug launch correctly the first time and the difficulty of recovering from a slow start suggest that there is an overwhelming need for a consistent and reproducible approach to ensure launch success.

In many ways, launch is like rocket science. Hundreds of activities all need to happen at exquisitely predefined moments to a certain standard. The three main sources of launch uncertainty are as follows:

1. *Regulatory and market access.* Launch preparation starts long before final decisions are taken on a drug's label or pricing and reimbursement. A product is commercialized almost immediately after its approval by the European Medicines Agency or FDA, leaving little room for a company to correct its course if payers make unexpected decisions.

   Changes in payers' priorities and policies, unpredictable label changes, and budget cuts can all have major consequences for a product's launch strategy, tactics, and eventual success.

2. *Clinical data analysis.* In principle, a pharma company enters the launch phase as soon as the clinical data from its Phase III registration trial is published. However, data analysis often continues, with subgroup analysis and statistical elaboration of efficacy and safety data.

   Findings from these analyses, as well as challenging interpretations of results by "antagonist" investigators, can have a considerable impact on a product's launch plan.

3. *Market reaction.* Competitors' clinical results, shifts in medical practice, disruptive innovations, and competitors' negative counter-messaging can radically alter a new product's market situation before launch and impair its eventual outcome.

16.4.5 New Drug Pricing and Reimbursement

In most markets, new drug pricing and reimbursement conditions are the single most important value drivers at the time of your launch. Although many country and regional payers are becoming increasingly sophisticated in their health economic assessments, market access conditions are in practice often influenced by a range of other factors including political agendas, informal social networks within institutions, and emotional drivers such as family members with a specific medical condition.

Pharmaceutical companies, on the other hand, tend to focus on pharmacoeconomic models and technical issues, failing to address the political and personal factors that play a part in payers' decision-making and thereby limiting the effectiveness of their value proposition.

By generating deep insights into your stakeholders' (regulatory, payers, hospitals, physicians, patients, societal values) attitudes and their approach to pricing and reimbursement decisions, companies can gain a better understanding of their priorities and concerns, shed light on how the process for updating formularies and protocols really works, weigh up the relative influence of different stakeholders in the final decision, and assess which arguments for articulating a product's value will resonate most with payers.

16.4.6 Tools into Payer's Priorities and Needs

Different tools exist for gaining insights into payers' priorities and needs: Your "persuading" armamentarium consists of the following:

- *In-depth interviews* are permissible in most countries. Interviews should be thoroughly prepared and carefully structured, with easy-to-use analytical and visual support materials that are detailed enough to enable interviewers to explore how payers actually reach their decisions. One effective approach is to show payers a range of different modules that might be used to launch the new brand and ask them to classify each module as strong or weak. By repeating this exercise with multiple payers, companies can identify which topics and arguments are most compelling and then use them in the value story they develop about their brand.

- *Focus groups* are allowed in some markets, although they can be harder to execute than interviews. Companies can use similar research techniques for payers as for physicians or patients. The advantage of focus groups over interviews is the opportunity to hear a range of views and opposing perspectives within the group.

- *Mock protocol committees*, often involving former members of payer bodies, are the most suitable forum for developing insights into budget impact analyses or the structure of pharmacoeconomic models, but less useful for deriving emotional insights.

- *Advance notification*, whether formal or informal, is becoming common practice in a number of countries throughout the world. Companies can use interactive modeling tools to help them understand a payer's financial constraints, approach to product evaluation, and decision-making priorities. These tools allow users to vary parameters such as price/volume trade-offs and population restrictions so as to test the payer's likely response to different scenarios [12].

16.5 Glocalization of Health Care

The global health care industry is going through a period of "glocalization," a term that combines the words "globalization" and "localization" to describe the adaptation of global products or services to accommodate the needs of people in a specific locale. The term first appeared in a late 1980s publication of the *Harvard Business Review*. At a 1997 conference on "Globalization and Indigenous Culture," sociologist Roland Robertson stated that glocalization means the simultaneity—i.e., the co-presence—of both universalizing and particularizing tendencies [13].

Typically associated with efforts by large consumer companies to boost sales by tailoring their products and menus to appeal to local tastes, glocalization also applies to health care: Industry issues are global, even if care is usually delivered locally. While the effects of these issues are influenced by local factors, many challenges are shared around the world to varying degrees, as are the opportunities to innovate.

Total global health spending was expected to rise by 2.6% in 2013 before accelerating to an average of 5.3% a year over the next 4 years (2014–2017). This growth will place enormous pressure on governments, health care delivery systems, insurers, and consumers in both developed and emerging markets to deal with issues such as an aging population, the rising prevalence of numerous chronic diseases, soaring costs, uneven quality, imbalanced access to care owing to workforce shortages, infrastructure limitations and patient locations, and disruptive technologies.

Across the globe, there have never been more health care challenges than there are today. However, these challenges can push stakeholders to innovate in new and exciting ways and to generate scientific, medical, and care delivery breakthroughs that can improve the health of people worldwide. This chapter examines the current state of the sector, describes the top issues facing stakeholders, provides a snapshot of activity in a number of geographic markets, and suggests considerations for 2016 and beyond.

16.5.1 Global Health Care Spending Patterns

No industry seems more out of step with prevailing efforts to reduce government costs than the health care sector [14]. Health care expenditures, for both providers and payers in public and private settings, is a very costly segment. The Economist Intelligence Unit estimates that global health care spending as a percentage of gross domestic product (GDP) will average 10.5% in 2014 (unchanged from 2013), with regional percentages of

- 17% in North America
- 11% in Western Europe
- 8% in Latin America
- 7% in Asia/Australasia
- 6% in the Middle East/Africa

Among developed nations, health is the second-largest category of government spending, after social protection programs (i.e., social assistance, health/unemployment insurance).

Most of the countries across the globe are facing a formidable challenge to manage the rapidly increasing cost of health care. Although spending rose by just an estimated 1.9% in 2012, it is expected to pick up again, with total spending rising by 2.6% in nominal terms in 2013 and by an annual average of 5.3% until 2017. Given projected population growth, spending per capita is anticipated to rise by an average of 4.4% a year from 2014 to 2017.

16.5.2 Effect of Income on Health Care Expenditures

Concurrently, the number of high-income households (those earning more than $25,000 a year) is expected to increase by approximately 10%, to more than 500 million, with more than one-half of that growth coming from Asia. Governments in many emerging markets are taking note of this economic growth and planning to roll out public health care services to meet consumers' rising expectations.

A glance at expenditures by country reveals a strong correlation between income levels and health outlays. Advanced economies like the United States, Europe, and Japan spend about twice as much of their income (12% of GDP) on health care as emerging/developing economies (6% of GDP, on average). Overall, about two-thirds of the $8 trillion in global health care spending occurs in advanced economies, with the United States accounting for $3 trillion, or 40% of the total, as seen in Table 16.1.

Health care spending varies disproportionately with income for two reasons. (1) Health care spending is a "superior" good, where demand rises more than proportionately with income [15]. As countries become richer, households are naturally willing to forego more discretionary consumption in favor of medical advances capable of extending life and improving its quality. (2) Advanced economies also tend to be older societies. The share of the population over 64 years of age is equal to approximately 24% of the population between 15 and 64 years in advanced economies.

TABLE 16.1

Health Spending and per Capita Income, Holding Other Factors Constant

Percentile	GDP per Capita ($)	Health Care Spending Share of GDP
25	12,000	7
50	20,000	8
75	35,000	9
95	56,100	10

16.5.3 Life Expectancy and Demand for Health Care

Life expectancy is projected to increase from an estimated 72.6 years in 2012 to 73.7 years by 2017, bringing the number of people over age 65 to approximately 560 million worldwide, or more than 10% of the total global population. In Western Europe, the proportion will hit 20%; in Japan, it will reach 27%. The aging population will create additional demand for health care services in 2017 and beyond.

Every year, health care expenditures rise appreciably owing to the growth and aging of the population. Although policymakers can do practically nothing to affect these factors, it is important to understand and anticipate the fiscal impact of such demographic changes [16].

With aging populations, an increase in the number of those inflicted with chronic ailments requires more health care spending, government initiatives to increase the access to care in both industrialized and emerging markets, and treatment advancements expected to drive sector expansion; thus, pressure to reduce health care costs remains and is escalating. Heavy government debts and constraints on tax revenue, combined with the pressures of aging populations, are forcing health payers to make difficult decisions on benefit levels.

Europe remains under particular pressure, and not just in those countries most affected by the regional economic crisis. After forcing through painful cuts to drug prices, wages, and staffing levels, some governments are now using the crisis as a chance to push through broader reforms to health care funding or provision. The goal is that these reforms may make increased health care expenditures more sustainable in the future.

16.5.4 Global Health Care Sector Top Issues

There are four major issues that governments, health care providers, payers, and consumers face: (1) aging population and chronic diseases, (2) cost and quality, (3) access to care, and (4) technology. As evidence of the trend toward glocalization, many of the challenges and opportunities emanating from each of these issues can be both global and market specific.

1. **Aging population and chronic diseases**

   The shared, long-term trends of an aging population and an increase in people inflicted with chronic diseases are expected to drive demand for health care services in both developed and emerging economies in 2014 and beyond.

   Aging populations and increasing life expectancies are anticipated to place a huge burden on the health care system in markets such as Western Europe, Japan, and—surprisingly—China, where it is expected to combine with a sharp decline in the number of young people. (China's decline may be related to the impact of family size policies.) The global population age 60 or above has tripled over the last 50 years and is expected to more than triple again over the next half-century, to reach nearly 2 billion in 2050.

   Europe currently has the world's highest proportion of older individuals and is projected to retain that distinction for at least the next 50 years: About 37% of the European population is projected to be aged 60 or older in 2050. In contrast, only 10% of Africa's population is projected to be older than 60 years in 2050. The current growth rate of the older population, at 1.9%, is significantly higher than that of the total population at 1.2%, and the spread between the two rates is expected to become even larger as the baby-boom generation starts reaching older ages in several parts of the world. Mexico has a young population—nearly 30% were 14 years old or younger in 2011; however, by 2017, about 7.5% will be 65 or older, placing a greater strain on public health care services and boosting spending on chronic, age-related diseases.

   Another shared demographic trend creating increased health care demand is the spread of chronic diseases—heart disease, stroke, cancer, chronic respiratory diseases, diabetes, and mental illness, among others—which is attributable to the aging population, more sedentary lifestyles, diet changes, and rising obesity levels, as well as improved diagnostics.

2. **Chronic diseases**

   Chronic diseases are, by far, the leading cause of mortality in the world, representing 63% of all deaths. Cancer and heart disease are becoming major killers, even in emerging markets. Africa, the Middle East, Asia, and Latin America are experiencing epidemics in diabetes and cardiovascular illnesses. China, with 92 million diabetics, has overtaken India (80 million) as the world leader in diabetes cases, according to the International Diabetes Federation. The cost of treatment for diabetes and other chronic diseases—which may be out of reach for many consumers, especially in emerging markets—is expected to compel a more intense focus on disease education and prevention by governments and health care practitioners while life sciences companies continue to develop innovative new medicines to address many of these diseases.

The transformational changes taking place in the global health care sector can be disconcerting and challenging, but they can also push participants to innovate in new and exciting ways. Additionally, shared health care challenges may lead to shared solutions if individual countries endeavor to learn from other nations' successful practices and adapt them to local needs.

3. **Aging population and chronic diseases**

Many of the world's countries are working individually and collaboratively to address age-related care and cost challenges, and to control and prevent chronic diseases. The World Health Organization is endeavoring to create global awareness about chronic diseases and intervene against them; the organization has set a goal of achieving an additional annual reduction of 2% in the global mortality rate from chronic diseases in the next 10 years, which is projected to prevent 36 million premature deaths by 2015. Additionally, health plans and providers in the United States and other nations are collaborating to innovate in approaches to wellness and prevention. Lifestyle-related habits and chronic diseases contribute to 75% of health costs and patients often get off track in their treatment regimen.

16.5.5 Global Health Care Costs

In the global struggle to manage the cost of health care, payers, providers, and policymakers are transitioning from a focus on volume to a focus on value—improving outcomes while also maintaining or lowering costs. Concurrently, numerous countries are instituting cost-containment measures, such as new physician incentive models, prescription drug price cuts and controls, comparative effectiveness, and evidence-based medicine. Care continues to move outside costly settings such as hospitals to more affordable retail clinics and mHealth applications. Consumers value the convenience, and costs can be as little as one-third of a traditional health care site.

Most national health care systems have been encouraging greater use of generic drugs; in the United States, for example, the proportion of prescriptions filled by generics has risen from around half to 80% over the last decade. Brazil is making branded generics and proprietary drugs of greater interest to pharmaceutical companies, and in China, recent reforms have put intense pressure on the prices of all drugs, including generic and over-the-counter medicines. In another cost-containment approach, Germany and several other countries have turned to value-based pricing for new drugs, which allows a price differential from existing offerings—including generics—based on a new product's demonstrated superiority. Finally, some countries are increasingly mandating drug set prices: India, Brazil, and China, for example, have national lists of essential drugs with set prices.

16.5.6 Access to Care

Nations around the globe are taking steps to address patient access issues by helping to ease the health care workforce shortage. In the United States, for example, health care industry employment rose from 8.7% of the total US civilian workforce in 1998 to 10.5% in 2008, and is projected to increase to 11.9% (19.8 million) by 2018. Several US initiatives are planned at the federal level to address workforce-related issues: The National Health Care Workforce Commission, a 15-member committee appointed by the General Accountability Office, is required to review health care workforce supply and demand and make recommendations regarding national priorities and policy.

The National Center for Health Workforce Analysis is developing guidelines for a uniform minimum health data set across health professionals in order to improve data collection and comparisons over time. Also, competitive grants are provided to enable state partnerships to conduct comprehensive planning and carry out health care workforce development strategies at state and local levels. In Australia, the government has launched the Australian General Practice Training program to increase the number of trainee general practitioners. In 2011, the country's health minister reported that the administration was halfway to achieving its goal of adding another 600 to the program by 2014. China's Ministry of Civil Affairs has set an ambitious target to train 6 million caregivers by the end of 2020. The South African National Department of Health's 2012/2013–2016/strategic plan includes programs around equitable staffing, health workforce development, recruitment, and retention. Other tactics used by various countries' health systems include recruiting quality nurses from low-income and middle-income countries to meet staffing needs and identifying incentives to attract new providers to a specific hospital or to join the profession.

From an infrastructure perspective, hospitals in India are expected to add more than 1.8 million beds to achieve a target of two beds per 1000 people by 2025. The Saudi Arabian government has identified investment in health care infrastructure as a priority; the 2013 budget includes funding for 19 new hospitals, on top of the 102 currently under construction. The Chinese government has consistently increased its health care expenditure budget to expand its primary care infrastructure and insurance reimbursement coverage.

16.5.7 Health Information Technology

Health information technology and innovation are becoming important contributors to improve the quality of care, reduce the cost of care, and, most importantly, improve patient outcomes. Advancements such as electronic health records, mHealth applications, e-prescribing, and predictive analytics are being used to better understand diseases and potential treatments and to identify similarities across patients to improve the quality of care. Industry leaders are applying advanced analytics to improve disease management, to drive more focused sales and marketing efforts, and to build new analytics platforms that combine internal and external data to create new business models for coordinating care across the health care ecosystem. Looking a few years out, the power of technology could enable countries to experiment with virtual health care delivery systems.

16.6 The Typical Biotech Entrepreneur

The typical biotech entrepreneur who starts a company usually comes from one of four background types, although individuals from any background can start a biotechnology company—as long as they have the ideas, skills, and motivation. The four most common backgrounds of life science entrepreneurs include the following [17]:

1. The **Scientist/Physician/Bioengineer** who comes from an academic institution (University, Research Foundation, Nonprofit Research Institute)
2. The **Scientist/Physician/Bioengineer** who comes from within the life science industry such as another biotechnology company
3. A **Businessperson**, such as a former executive in the life science, pharmaceutical, or venture capital industry, who is not a Scientist/Physician/Bioengineer
4. A **Core Group of Individuals** that emanated from another life science organization within the industry group.

The biotech entrepreneur is usually an accomplished scientist, bioengineer, physician, or businessperson. Most often, but not always, they have a PhD, MD, MBA, or a combination of these educational backgrounds. These individuals usually have well-paying and secure positions, and are already experiencing some degree of success in their current position. Frequently, a biotech entrepreneur voluntarily leaves their comfortable world and steps into an industry that carries uncertainties and risks unique to any other business.

Successful Biotech Entrepreneurs Share the following Characteristics:

- Have a strong desire to take control and be independent
- Are not afraid to work hard and put in long hours to achieve personal and business goals

- Are highly optimistic about what the future holds for their businesses and for themselves personally
- Are very self-confident in their abilities
- Set goals and develop an action plan to reach their goals and then reward themselves when they have reached and exceeded those goals (big and small)
- Prepared to handle stress and welcome challenges
- Are not procrastinators, but proactive in their approach to completing jobs and tasks in full, correctly, and on time
- Have a competitive and winning spirit
- Are accountable, accepting personal responsibility for their decisions and actions
- Take the initiative, lead others, and are willing to delegate
- Are independent thinkers and workers
- Take calculated risks and understand that in the absence of risk, success is seldom if ever achieved
- Communicate exceptionally well and respect everyone's right to an opinion even when others disagree
- Are proficient time managers and use time-saving systems
- Are persistent and not easily discouraged
- Are highly organized
- Think and react logically and not emotionally
- Are knowledge hungry and never stop looking for ways to become better in all areas of business
- Have realistic business expectations
- Are great planners
- Are proficient problem solvers and decisive decision-makers
- Keep an open mind, are flexible, and are adaptable to change when change is beneficial
- Are good listeners

16.7 Struggle over Social Media

In 1 year alone—from 2012 to 2013—the number of social network users around the world rose from 1.47 billion to 1.73 billion (about 25% of the world's population), which is an 18% increase [18]. By 2017, the global social network audience is expected to total 2.55 billion [19]. More than 72% of all

Internet users regularly access social networking sites [20]. In the United States, people spend 16 min every hour using social media.

At issue here is the fact that start-up risk management policies and procedures are not designed for, quite literally, minute-by-minute monitoring of social media chatter to identify brand, strategy, compliance, legal, and market risks.

Among corporations, establishing a social media presence is now more than accepted—it is expected. Among Fortune 500 firms, 77% have active Twitter accounts, 70% have Facebook pages, and 69% have YouTube accounts. As a start-up attempting to commercialize a product, social media is a tempting target because of its reach and low cost. The impact of social media is discussed in the subsequent paragraph.

16.7.1 Interactive Social Media

The Internet and interactive social media provide an efficient, low-cost way to send fast messages to millions of people and to targeted patient populations, but pharma companies have been slow to take advantage of these methods, largely because of FDA rules that control what manufacturers can state about their products. FDA has been rolling out new guidelines for using interactive media in recent months [21].

The irony of the social media marketing debate is that patients increasingly turn to the Internet to search for health information, identify possible treatments, and confirm diagnoses. The FDA itself is a heavy user of social media.

In June 2014, the FDA issued its widely anticipated "Guidance for Industry Internet/Social Media Platforms with Character Space Limitations— Presenting Risk and Benefit Information for Prescription Drugs and Medical Devices." The draft guidance intended to describe FDA's current thinking about how manufacturers, packers, and distributors (firms) of prescription human and animal drugs (drugs) and medical devices for human use (devices) that choose to present benefit information should present both benefit and risk information within advertising and promotional labeling (sometimes collectively referred to in this guidance document as "promotion") of their FDA-regulated medical products on electronic/digital platforms that are associated with character space limitations—specifically on the Internet and through social media or other technological venues (Internet/social media).

Examples of Internet/social media platforms with character space limitations include online microblog messaging (e.g., messages on Twitter or "tweets," which are currently limited to 140 character spaces per tweet) and online paid search (e.g., "sponsored links" on search engines such as Google and Yahoo, which have limited character spaces as well as other platform-imposed considerations).

16.7.2 Social Media Increases Its Benefits

A recent survey of physicians [22] found that more than 50% of practices responding used Facebook as a platform, and 87% of those physicians under the age of 55 used some form of social media. With the Centers for Medicare and Medicaid Services requiring increased use of digitalized data under the Meaningful Use guidelines, the government is actively encouraging certain actors in the health care system to increase their use of technology to enhance patient engagement [23].

The draft guidance gives marketers some leeway to correct misinformation on drugs and medical devices posted on the Internet by independent third parties. Corrections of "user-generated content" have to be "truthful and not misleading," apply only to messages outside company control, and should not be used as "a springboard to engage in promotional messaging." Marketers should address only the specific misinformation cited, but are not expected to continually monitor the site and track further comments.

A final guidance is slated to address the FDA's concerns about using links to other Internet sites that discuss drug risks and benefits. FDA has warned against connecting to off-label information, and that a "one-click" process for linking to full risk and benefit information does not satisfy its requirements for fair balance and full disclosure.

Even with the new advisories, pharma companies may continue to lag far behind other industries in utilizing the Internet to communicate important information to the public. Drug makers have been using social media primarily for corporate operations—announcing financial reports, hiring employees, recruiting clinical trial investigators and participants, and disease awareness. Nonetheless, there is continuing disagreement over how effective the Internet is for detecting adverse drug events.

16.8 Pharma Launch Business Plan

The potential for value creation is a central driver of the high-risk, high-reward pharm business model. The odds are daunting, but historically, the companies that succeed in bringing breakthrough products to market—and the investors who back them—have reaped handsome returns. In doing so, these pharm transition from creating value to *capturing* it—generating revenues and earning profits.

Your strategy behind [24] producing a pharm business plan provides you with an excellent opportunity to consider all the facets of a business or a new venture, challenging feasibility and providing greater confidence in decision-making. The process will also help you identify and clarify future financing needs and is a necessary step in raising external finance.

Your business plan should define your strategy planning process and your new venture's competitive advantage and opportunities. Your business plan should detail the broad action points derived from strategy planning, establishing corporate goals, setting objectives, and how you propose to measure successful achievement of milestones.

For a biotech company, there can be three different strategy models. For example, in biopharmaceuticals:

1. Virtual company (few employees, mostly outsourced)
2. Fully integrated pharmaceutical company
3. Strategically partnered, royalty-based pharmaceutical company

16.8.1 What Is Different about Pharma Launches?

The engine driving pharma value capture is, of course, R&D—the years-long process of identifying and testing via sequential clinical trials. As a product journeys from the laboratory to the marketplace, there are discrete events—for instance, completed phases of clinical trials and strategic alliances—at which key stakeholders step up or step down its valuation or the valuation of its developer. These inflection points are critical for both companies and their backers, since value can only be captured if it is recognized and rewarded by others.

Writing a business plan is never easy. Writing one for a biotech company has additional complications (inflection points) owing to the particular characteristics of the industry, some of which we set out below:

- Technology—capturing and conveying the market potential of new technology is critical. Major technological leaps forward, protected by excellent patents, may be valueless without a clear route to market. Multiple applications from the same technology make it a "platform" from which to build even greater value. An understanding of the potential value of the sales from your technology is critical. It is essential to ensure that ownership of any intellectual property is well protected.

- Team—your team should be skilled in technology, proof-of-principle techniques, milestone management, and commercial goals. In short, the skills and experience of your team need to fit the strategy imperatives of the business.

- Timescales—unlike most development stage businesses, biotech companies can take years to get from concept, through proof of principle, to approvals, and finally product sales. It is not unusual for this to take 15 years for biopharmaceutical companies and 10 years for agricultural biotechnology companies.

- Strategy—the costs of developing a new drug are high and significant funding is required to develop a marketable product. Companies must have a dear strategy defining when and if they plan to enter into collaborative agreements in order to gain access to other technology or skills, to help with funding, and in time to provide assistance with marketing and distribution requirements. In the future, the company may need to seek access to public equity markets to raise the significant sums required to develop a marketable product. The timing of entry to such markets should be considered at an early stage.

- Transitions—a biotech company will develop through several stages, as the resource needs for progressing potential products increase. The costs of research trials geometrically escalate through the development phases. Expect management, cultural and cash requirement changes occur.

- Milestones—a journey of several years' duration can be difficult to plot. Funders want to know how you will reach your destination. Large investments in pharma are only made if there is clarity about intended usage and milestones, against which progress can be measured. Future funding will only happen if milestones are achieved.

- Value building—in technology terms, in IPR terms, in commercial terms, and in overall business terms, you are "building value." Financial investors, strategic partners, regulators, and payers all play a role in measuring a biotech product's value. However, the ways in which these groups award value are notoriously inefficient—in other words, there is a disconnect between the creation of value by a biotech company and the timing and extent to which this value is acknowledged by other parties.

- Clinical trials uncertainties—the slow and opaque process of clinical trials—in which results are revealed only at a few discrete points— means a development company's stakeholders have few mechanisms of measuring and recognizing the value that is being created along the way [25].

- Funding—often the most difficult cash is that which gets a company from concept, through proof of principle, and toward the stage when the next plan would have more solid commercial foundations. There are no easy answers to funding this money, but it has to be found by the start-up team if the funds of the later rounds are to follow.

- Deals—it is an inevitable fact that biotech companies will enter into "deals." They do them to acquire technology, to fund developments, share rights/risks, sail distribution rights, and speed up the building of a business. Deals are an important source of funds and an end point in the value chain to market. They are not easy, and doing deals correctly is a core skill for the team.

- Sales—no matter how hard you try to explain, there will always be a majority of people who don't understand how you can build a biotech business if you are not yet selling anything. The financial community that deals with biotech companies understands why sales are not present in most biotech financial projections; however, that does not mean that they don't think about sales. Indeed, assessing product sales potential is a key skill requiring careful market analysis, scientific advisory networks, and business evaluation models.

- Credibility/advice—venture capitalists and other funders take big risks with large sums of money in biotech. They will look very carefully at businesses that appear to have the potential to really create value. In the final analysis though, the team and its scientific and other advisers will need to have very high credentials and be recognized, probably internationally, as experts in their fields. If a team or plan lacks sufficient credibility, then it is unlikely to attract funding.

References

1. http://www.forbes.com/sites/matthewherper/2015/07/29/the-top-drug-launches-of-all-time/
2. http://www.evercore.com/investment-banking/institutional-equities
3. http://www.ipi.org/docLib/20150414_HighCostofInventingNewDrugs.pdf
4. DiMasi, J.A., Hansen, R.W., and Grabowski, H.G. The price of innovation: New estimates of drug development costs. *J. Health Econ.*, 22, 151–185, 2003.
5. Lawlor, M. Difference between Pharmaceutical and Biotechnology, 2013, http://www.morganmckinley.ie/article/difference-between-pharmaceutical-and-biotechnology.
6. https://en.wikipedia.org/wiki/Pharmaceutical_industry
7. Deloitte's 2014 Global Life Sciences Outlook: Resilience and Reinvention in a Changing Marketplace.
8. Ahlawat, H., Chierchia, G., and van Arkel, P. Beyond the storm, launch excellence in the new normal, http://www.mckinsey.com/~/media/McKinsey/dot com/client_service/Pharma%20and%20Medical%20Products/PMP%20NEW /PDFs/PMP_.
9. http://www.fda.gov/RegulatoryInformation/Legislation/SignificantAmend mentstotheFDCAct/FDASIA/ucm329491.htm
10. http://www.fda.gov/downloads/Drugs/GuidanceComplianceRegulatory Information/Guidances/UCM358301.pdf
11. Beyond the storm. Pharmaceutical and Medical Products Practice 2013, McKinsey & Co., http://www.mckinsey.com/~/media/McKinsey/dotcom/cli ent_service/Pharma%20and%20Medical%20Products/PMP%20NEW/PDFs /PMP_Beyond_the_storm_Launch_excellence_in_the_new_normal.ashx.

12. For a broader perspective on using deep customer insights in pharma marketing, see *The Eye of the Storm*, McKinsey & Company, 2008.
13. https://en.wikipedia.org/wiki/Glocalization
14. https://www.carlyle.com/about-carlyle/market-commentary/2016-global-health-care-outlook
15. Hall, R. and Jones, C. The value of life and the rise in health spending, *The Quarterly Journal of Economics*, 2007.
16. Mendelson, D.N. and Schwartz, W.B. Health care costs. The effects of aging and population growth on health care costs. *Health Affairs*, 12(1), 119–125, 1993. doi: 10.1377/hlthaff.12.1.119, http://content.healthaffairs.org/.
17. What makes a biotech entrepreneur? http://www.springer.com/cda/content/document/cda_downloaddocument/9781441900630-c2.pdf?SGWID=0-0-45-855351-p173887155.
18. Culp, S. A Comprehensive Approach to Managing Social Media Risk and Compliance, http://www.accenture.com/sitecollectiondocuments/financial-services/accenture-comprehensive-approach-managing-social-media-risk-compliance.pdf.
19. Social Networking Reaches Nearly One in Four Around the World, eMarketer Inc., June 18, 2013, http://www.emarketer.com/Article/Social-Networking-Reaches-Nearly-One-Four-Around-World/1009976.
20. The Growth of Social Media in 2014: 40+ Surprising Stats [Infographic], *Socially Stacked*, January 23, 2014, http://www.sociallystacked.com/2014/01/ the-growth-of-social-media-in-2014-40-surprising-stats-infographic/#sthash.t4GoW1Bc.KxNuUnDR.dpbs.
21. Wechsler, J. Stuggle over social media continues. *Pharmaceutical Executive*, August 2014, http://www.pharmexec.com/social-media-struggles-continue.
22. Which social media tools are physician practices in love with? *Med City News*, http://medcitynews.com/2013/10/social-media-tools-physician-practices-love/.
23. http://www.forbes.com/sites/johnosborn/2014/05/13/fda-draft-guidance-takes-the-social-out-of-social-media/
24. Biobusiness Plan, http://www.masterclassbiobusiness.nl/downloads/BP.pdf.
25. http://www.ey.com/Publication/vwLUAssets/EY-beyond-borders-unlocking-value/$FILE/EY-beyond-borders-unlocking-value.pdf

17

Launching Medical Device Products

17.1 Introduction

The United States remains the largest medical device market in the world with a market size of around $110 billion in 2012, and is expected to reach $133 billion by 2016. The US market value represented approximately 38% of the global medical device market in 2012. US exports of medical devices in key product categories identified by the Department of Commerce exceeded $44 billion in 2012, or more than a 7% increase from the previous year [1].

There are more than 6500 medical device companies in the United States, mostly small and medium-sized enterprises (SMEs). More than 80% of medical device companies have fewer than 50 employees, and many (notably innovative start-up companies) have little or no sales revenue. Medical device companies are located throughout the country, but are mainly concentrated in regions known for other high-technology industries, such as microelectronics and biotechnology. The states with the highest number of medical device companies include California, Florida, New York, Pennsylvania, Michigan, Massachusetts, Illinois, Minnesota, and Georgia. Other states with significant sector employment include Washington, Wisconsin, and Texas.

US medical device companies are highly regarded globally for their innovations and high-technology products. Investment in medical device research and development (R&D) more than doubled during the 1990s, and R&D investment in the domestic sector remains more than twice the average for all US manufacturers.

The United States also holds a competitive advantage in several industries that the medical device industry relies on, including microelectronics, telecommunications, instrumentation, biotechnology, and software development. Collaborations have led to recent advances including neurostimulators, stent technologies, biomarkers, robotic assistance, and implantable electronic devices. Since the industry is fueled by innovation and the ongoing quest for better ways of treating or diagnosing medical problems, the future growth of this sector remains positive.

17.2 Medical Devices Economic Activity

In measuring economic activity, such as the nation's production or national health expenditures, it is necessary to clearly define the boundary of the activity being measured. To develop a clear "device boundary," we adopted a working definition based on a standard dictionary definition of "device," something "made, particularly for a working purpose; an invention or contrivance, especially a mechanical or electrical one, and without pharmacological activity." The device boundary would have eliminated in vitro diagnostic substances (NAICS 325413). These commodities are "substances" rather than devices. Also included in the US Food and Drug Administration (FDA) definitions are in vitro diagnostic substances and equipment.

To further determine the "medical boundary," we use manufacturing categories in NAICS (the North American Industry Classification System) because the data from which the estimates were developed are from the federal government statistical system, and that system is currently based on NAICS for industry data. The medical boundary narrows the economic activity universe to the nine categories shown below with their NAICS codes.

334510—Electromedical and electrotherapeutic apparatus

334517—Irradiation apparatus

339111—Laboratory apparatus and furniture

339112—Surgical and medical instruments

339113—Surgical apparatus and supplies

339114—Dental equipment and supplies

339115—Ophthalmic goods

339116—Dental laboratories

We exclude dental equipment and supplies (NAICS 339114) and dental laboratories (NAICS 339116), either because complete corresponding data were unavailable for all elements of the analysis (in the case of dental laboratories) or because dental care and related expenses are typically financed through different health care insurance mechanisms than the other products considered in our analysis.

17.2.1 Innovating Medical Devices

Medical devices differ from drugs in that they do not achieve their intended use through chemical reaction and are not metabolized in the body. Medical devices range in nature and complexity from simple tongue depressors and bandages to complex programmable pacemakers, implantable artificial hearts, coronary stents, and sophisticated imaging systems.

According to Davidov [2], surgeons are often on the front line of medical device innovation because of their clinical background and hands-on use of devices. This experience also allows surgeons to clearly see the shortcomings of existing technology.

Whether it is a stapler that misfires, an awkward laparoscopic instrument, or a hard-to-implant bioprosthesis, the "end-user" surgeon quickly recognizes suboptimal performance. For this reason, surgeon-innovators have pioneered many successful surgical products, such as central line catheters, pulse oximeters, implantable pacemakers, pacemaker-defibrillators, balloon-tipped catheters, coronary stents, and so on. Because of their technical understanding of surgical needs and design, surgeons account for more than one-third of all medical device patents in the United States.

17.2.2 History and Overview

In the "good old days" (before the Medical Device Regulation act of 1976), bringing a new medical device to market was a lot easier. It was essentially a two-step process: (1) develop a product that met a perceived medical need, and (2) build a working prototype, display it in your booth at a medical show, and, if doctors like it, start selling the product.

Needless to say, that is not the case anymore. Nowadays, obtaining FDA approval is a multiyear process. Reimbursement issues and increased regulatory requirements are now front and center. While the FDA may approve the device as safe and efficacious, the Centers for Medicare and Medicaid Services (CMS) may withhold reimbursement. Thus, medical device developers must make a compelling case that the new device reduces health care costs.

The role of medical technology in health care costs has long been a source of debate and controversy. It has been widely asserted that health care technology can be cost increasing, owing to price and volume effects, both for medical technologies themselves and related services. Other findings have suggested that returns on spending on medical technologies can far exceed their costs, particularly when longer-term benefits are measured in terms of productivity and reduced disability. Yet, surprisingly, very little analysis has been conducted on the direct costs to the health system of medical devices themselves.

According to AdvaMed, an industry advocacy group, changes in medical practice attributed to medical technology encompass a variety of factors. These factors include (1) development of new medical procedures; (2) improvements in existing procedures; (3) increases in the number of procedures performed because of increased safety, effectiveness, or convenience; (4) development of new pharmaceutical products; and (5) development and use of new and improved medical devices and diagnostics.

While medical device spending has grown at about the same rate as national health expenditures overall, prices for medical devices have actually grown far more slowly than the Medical Consumer Price Index (MCPI) or even the overall Consumer Price Index (CPI). Over the 21-year period from 1989 to 2010, medical device prices have increased at an average annual rate of only 1.0%, compared to 4.7% for the MCPI and 2.7% for the CPI. This relatively slow rate of price increase suggests that the industry is highly price competitive.

During much of the 22-year period, 1989–2010, a significant driver of changed medical practice has been the development of new medical devices—from stents to implantable defibrillators, to artificial hips and knees, to new imaging modalities, to new diagnostic tests, to new surgical tools. In view of the conventional wisdom about the role of medical technology in driving up costs, it is surprising that the cost of medical devices has risen little as a share of total national health expenditures. It is also striking that, unlike most other areas of medicine, the prices of medical devices have actually been growing more slowly compared to not only the MCPI but also the CPI as a whole.

17.3 FDA Device Classification

The US FDA classifies medical devices into three classes based on the risk the device poses to the patient or the user and the intended use [3]. Consequently, class I devices are considered non–life-sustaining and class II devices are defined as more sophisticated and pose more risks than class I. Class III devices support or sustain life, and their failure would be life-threatening. They serve to prevent impairment of human health, or may present a potential risk of illness or injury [4]. Part 860 of 21 CFR provides detailed information on "medical device classification procedures," as seen in Figure 17.1.

Classification	Examples	Required submission
Class I (low risk)	Bandages, gloves, surgical instruments	510(k)
Class II (moderate risk)	Infusion pumps, wound dressings, catheters	510(k) IDE possible
Class III (high risk)	Heart valves, stents, vascular grafts	PMA approval IDE probable

FIGURE 17.1
FDA medical device classification.

In practice, to determine the class of a medical device, the applicant can search the device classification database, which was set up by the US FDA. Approximately 1700 different generic types of devices, grouped into 16 medical specialties, have been defined. Each of these generic types of devices is assigned to one of three regulatory classes based on the level of control necessary to assure the safety and effectiveness of the device.

17.4 Regulatory Pathways for Device Registrations

The device classification determines the marketing authorization process, which can be a premarket notification (PMN [510(k)]), a premarket approval (PMA), or an exemption from the aforementioned. These will be outlined in the following paragraphs.

17.4.1 Premarket Notification

A PMN, also known under the term "510(k)," is relevant for devices, for which no exemption is defined in the regulation and which are not subject to a PMA. It is applicable to most of the class II devices. The aim of a PMN submission is to demonstrate that a device, which is planned to be marketed in the United States, is "substantially equivalent" to a so-called predicate device, a device already legally marketed [5].

Determining whether a device is "substantially equivalent" involves an evaluation of the intended use and the technological characteristics. However, it does not necessarily mean that the devices must be identical. Once the FDA has confirmed that the device is substantially equivalent by sending a letter to the applicant, the device is considered as FDA "cleared" and can be distributed on the US market. 21 CFR, Part 807, Subpart E defines requirements, like content and format, for a 510(k) application [6].

17.4.2 Premarket Approval

The PMA process, which applies to all medical devices of class III, involves a scientific and regulatory review evaluating safety and effectiveness of a medical device. The aim of the PMA is to demonstrate that there is sufficient scientific evidence to assure safety and effectiveness of the device. This type of a device marketing application is the strictest one and is covered by 21 CFR, Part 814, Subpart B. A PMA process for a medical device runs through similar steps as the registration process for a medicinal product in the United States: 45 days after submission of the application, the US FDA will notify the applicant on the acceptance for filing. The review starts and after involvement of the advisory committee's recommendation, the process is finalized with an approval.

These two procedures, 510(k) and PMA, imply that all devices, which cannot be considered as substantially equivalent to a marketed device and which are not classified by the regulation, would have to go through a PMA procedure, like a class III device. For this case, the US FDA offers two further options: The so-called de novo process and device exemptions.

17.4.3 De Novo Process

The "de novo process" is applicable to low-risk devices. Devices for which applicants of a 510(k) receive a "not substantially equivalent" letter would be placed into the category of class III. In these cases, the applicant can request a "de novo classification" of the device into class I or II within 30 days from the receipt of the letter. If the US FDA classifies the device into class I or II, the applicant will receive an approval to market the device and the device is then considered a "predicate device" for other firms to submit a 510(k). If the result of the de novo process is that the device remains a class III device, the applicant has to submit a PMA [7].

Table 17.1 shows the review timelines for the three mentioned procedures, 510(k), PMA and the de novo process. However, the US FDA reveals on their website that a PMA review usually takes longer and can take up to 2 years [8].

17.4.4 Device Exemptions

Most devices of class I and some of the class II devices are exempted from the PMN requirements. Nevertheless, these devices are subject to other general control; for example, all medical devices must be manufactured under a quality assurance program, suitable for the intended use and have an "establishment registration" and device listing [9].

In addition to this, there is also a device exemption for "humanitarian use devices." This is similar to the principle of an orphan drug. If a device is intended to treat or diagnose a disease or condition that affects or is manifested in fewer than 4000 patients in the United States per year, the applicant needs to submit a PMA, but is exempted from some of the requirements [10].

TABLE 17.1

FDA Review Timeline Range

Procedure	Review Timelines
510(k)	90–120 days
De novo	60–90 days
PMA	180–360 days

17.5 Increased Regulatory Environment

Device manufacturers may face increased regulation from the FDA as the FDA reviews its 510(k) clearance program, sometimes referred to as the "fast track" approval process for medical devices. Most devices receive FDA approval through one of two review processes, 510(k) or PMA. PMA is the more stringent of the two approval procedures and requires the submission of clinical trial data. PMA approval can take up to 2 years, whereas receiving 510(k) approval can theoretically take as little as 3 months [11].

Device manufacturers decide which regulatory review course to pursue (PMA or 510(k)), but the FDA has 60 days to comment on the appropriate course of action. The majority of devices in the United States reach market through the 510(k) process. In response to numerous recalls of medical equipment approved through the 510(k) process, critics charge that this process is not as vigorous and robust as is necessary. The FDA's guidelines are vague with regard to which approval process should be followed for specific devices and this lack of clarity may have allowed high-risk medical devices to be approved through 510(k) rather than a more robust PMA process.

Critics also assert that the penalties for submitting inaccurate data are not severe enough, there are too few experts reviewing each 510(k) submission, and postapproval monitoring and surveillance is severely lacking. In September 2009, the FDA commissioned the Institute of Medicine to conduct a thorough review of the 510(k) process and recommend changes. The Institute of Medicine's recommended changes making the 510(k) approval process more rigorous, which will lead to higher costs, lengthen the time to market and lower approval rates for medical device manufacturers.

The FDA has already implemented some changes to the PMA advisory panels. From May 1, 2010, the FDA has required separate votes by outside experts on the safety and effectiveness of a medical device up for PMA review. Before, the FDA only required the expert advisory panel to simply vote on the approvability of the PMA application for the device. In addition, panels now vote by ballot, rather than by a show of hands, and the votes will be made public. The new balloting procedure is intended to allow panel members to vote without the immediate influence of other members [12].

In addition to the FDA implementing changes, the Center for Devices and Radiological Health (CDRH), which is responsible for ensuring the safety and effectiveness of medical devices, is in the process of implementing changes to keep the advisory panel members focused on the science as opposed to the regulatory issues. The medical device industry has issues with the panels in their current form as a result of inexperience, lack of expertise, and potential conflicts of interest of members sitting on the panels. However, the CDRH contends that the pool of qualified, experienced candidates that are interested in sitting on these panels is limited.

17.5.1 Global Regulatory Scrutiny

Across the developed world, makers of medical devices face a perfect storm of increased regulatory scrutiny, more stringent reimbursement requirements, and aggressive new procurement practices. In search of new top-line growth, manufacturers are looking to a land some call OUS, for Outside the United States, and others call BRIC, for Brazil, Russia, India, and China.

However, seeking salvation in emerging markets brings its own challenges, not least in talent recruitment, management, and retention, but how did we get here? Not so long ago, medical devices were seen as the less risky alternative to biotech in the race to apply innovative technology to health care. Devices typically faced lower regulatory hurdles, shorter time to market, and fewer outright failures than biopharmaceuticals.

In addition, acquisitions by big players often provided a quick exit strategy for founders and early-stage investors, but that has changed. Technological innovation is still prized, but it only gets a player a seat at the table. A series of high-profile recalls and other self-inflicted wounds have prompted politicians to view medical devices with a sharper eye and, in turn, urge the FDA to raise the bar on clinical trial outcomes.

Health care reform in the United States and diminished government revenues across the European market have netted tougher reimbursement protocols. At the same time, providers have become savvier bargainers, shifting major purchase decisions from surgeons to supply chain specialists schooled in the tough procurement protocols of heavy industry.

Factor the stagnation since the 2008 financial crisis, and it is no surprise that makers of medical devices face an unfriendly environment with no respite in sight. In this tough climate, the robust economic growth in Asia and parts of South America is like a bright light in the darkness, and device companies have focused on those markets, but making headway in what used to be called the Third World is not easy, and results have been variable.

17.5.2 Headwinds Hitting the Industry

When major newspapers like *The New York Times* or the *Washington Post* run front-page headlines about failing hip implants, faulty heart defibrillators, and overused arterial stents, politicians react, and despite the popular rhetoric about reducing regulations to benefit business, congress's inevitable reaction to these news stories is to publically criticize the FDA and to demand tougher legislation with device makers. FDA officials respond by asking for more detailed data, more relevant end points, and more clinical trials, all of which increases the cost and time required to bring a new device to market [13].

Approval times in the United States have become so protracted that many device makers now launch new products in Europe (or elsewhere) rather than wait for the FDA. In some cases, FDA review has taken so long that companies are already selling second- or third-generation devices abroad while still awaiting initial approval in the United States.

While regulatory delays have a negative impact on device companies' revenues, they also restrict patients' access to advances in health care technology. Industry leaders say that the FDA is well aware of these problems and its negative consequences.

In Europe, the headwind to medical device innovation is reimbursement. A CE Mark—indicating that the product has met the European Union (EU) safety or efficacy requirements—contrary to popular opinion—does not necessarily mean that the product is market-ready. Health care payers want more comprehensive trials to establish clinical efficacy and to demonstrate a compelling health care economic advantage. In other words, the new device must be shown to lower health care costs; otherwise, it will not be approved.

17.5.3 Need for Comprehensive Solutions

In such a market, product features and price alone do not drive the buying process. Sales executives must be able to address cost-of-care and efficiency improvements, value-added services, and comprehensive solutions. They must also understand the needs of varied stakeholders—including clinicians, procurement staff, hospital executives, and local policymakers—and be able to communicate effectively with each type of stakeholder. This requires not only solid relationship-building and negotiating skills but also a firm understanding of health economics and the mechanics of reimbursement.

Often overlooked, quality assurance is an area ripe for transformation. This is a critical function for all device companies, but of greatest significance in implants, where product failures can be tragic for patients, and reports of defects often make front-page news.

17.6 Hospital Spending and Payor Trends

Equipment and device manufacturers are significantly affected by the spending habits of their key customers, namely, hospitals. Hospital spending has declined over the past several years owing to the overall economic decline. S&P estimates that capital expenditures of publicly traded hospital chains will continue to decline [14].

Industry analysts reason that manufacturers of high ticket purchases (e.g., magnetic resonance imaging [MRI] and radiation therapy equipment) have proportionately been affected more by decreased spending than manufacturers of devices that may be implanted as part of a nonelective surgery (e.g., pacemakers, stents, etc.).

Cost containment and comparative effectiveness research (CER) continue to be major focuses of both public and private payors. The American Recovery and Reinvestment Act of 2009 set aside $1.1 billion for CER efforts, which will undoubtedly lead to further margin pressure as device manufacturers will be forced to defend their product's effectiveness and pricing versus that of alternative solutions. Such trends could spur additional industry consolidation as smaller manufacturers may lack the resources to rebut claims of a device's ineffectiveness.

17.6.1 Nonregulatory Policy Areas

There are a number of key nonregulatory areas that significantly affect the viability of the US medical device industry, ranging from financial investments to legislative changes to innovation and product convergence [15].

- *Reimbursement Rates:* Valuation and reimbursement of products by public- and private-sector financial entities are crucial to the success of the medical device industry. The US market is so large that reimbursement decisions made in the United States have the potential to impact the viability of manufacturing the product for other markets. In the United States, there are several unrelated government organizations involved in establishing reimbursement rates.

    The Department of Health and Human Services' Center for Medical and Medicaid Services (HHS/CMS) administers both the Medicaid and Medicare program that covers the reimbursement of medical devices. In addition, the Veterans Administration is the key agency responsible for negotiating an agreement with manufacturers/distributors of medical devices (Federal Supply Schedules) for procurement of medical devices by certain government agencies.

- *Impact of Health Care Reform:* In March 2010, the US House of Representatives passed the Patient Protection and Affordable Care Act (H.R. 3590). The bill had been previously approved by the Senate in December 2009 and was subsequently signed into law by President Obama. Health care reform will have a wide-ranging impact and will impose new mandates on individuals, employers, medical service providers, and health product manufacturers.

- *Comparative Effectiveness and Benefits:* As policymakers contend with rising health care costs, it is likely that some form of comparative effectiveness, a system based on the relative benefits a product delivers, will be implemented or expanded both in the United States and abroad.

    Comparative effectiveness employs research that compares the clinical effectiveness of different drugs, devices, and procedures with an eye toward improving quality of care. However, issues remain as to who should conduct the research or when and how cost-effectiveness should be factored.

- *Attracting Venture Capital:* SMEs with limited earnings in the early stages of development, and the medical device sector is particularly reliant on venture capital funding. Venture capitalists need a predictable system in order to assess risk, and when uncertainties prevent access to venture capital funds, there tends to be a precipitous reduction in innovative activity.

  The downturn in the US economy, which accelerated in late 2008, took a toll on the valuation of medical device start-ups seeking injections of capital. A number of venture capital firms, including some longtime investors, began withdrawing from early-stage investing as the economic slump deepened, choosing instead to hold on to investment capital until higher levels of certainty asset valuations return.

- *Group Purchasing Organizations (GPOs) Negotiations:* GPOs negotiate contracts with health product suppliers on behalf of cooperatives of health care facilities. The role that GPOs play in the health care system has come under scrutiny by Congress in recent years.

  With the economic downturn in recent years, the bond between hospitals and GPOs seems to be strengthening. The recession prompted some hospitals to enact cost-cutting initiatives, including in the area of product procurement. Hospital materials management departments have been empowered by administrators to make money-saving decisions. For the future, products that provide superior clinical value and contain costs will likely attract investors.

- *Industry Consolidation—M&A activity:* In the medical device industry, small firms faced with devoting significant resources to innovations often merge with larger firms with the financial resources necessary to bring products to market. The results were mutually beneficial— larger firms receive the benefit of the new technology and, therefore, maintain market share; small firms can afford to continue to produce and get the benefit of the large firms devoting resources to continued incremental improvements that are crucial in the industry.

  This trend has continued in part owing to economic realities in 2009 that led to further consolidation in the medical device sector, in terms of company mergers, companies combining profit centers, and companies outsourcing for greater efficiencies. There are two prominent examples: In 2009, Abbott Labs and Covidien (now Medtronic) made significant acquisitions adding to their product portfolio while Medtronic took major steps to consolidate its various businesses into two major groups. International joint ventures designed to developing health care technologies and establishing local R&D capabilities have also grown in size and significance. Asia—notably China and Korea— have been the site of a number of collaborations with US firms. Some firms are also gravitating toward a launch in Europe followed by a move to the United States or perhaps a move to China or India. It definitely adds a level of complexity to the development process.

- *Patient Demographics:* Marked increases in the average age of US and foreign populations are already influencing the direction of the medical device industry through the changing health needs of senior citizens and shifts in thinking on how and where they will be treated. As pressures mount to contain costs, expensive and extended stays in health care facilities will be discouraged and health care will be increasingly delivered in alternative settings such as nursing homes, hospices, and, especially, the patient's own home.

  Home health care is one of the fastest-growing segments of the industry and is branching out into new areas. What used to be limited to only the lowest-technology products is now encompassing a proliferation of high-technology medical devices that are intended to be used by unskilled health care workers or patients. In addition, demographics and technological advances will continue to increase demand for advanced medical device products (such as pacemakers and defibrillators) well into the 21st century.

- *Health Information Technologies (HIT):* The 2009 American Recovery and Reinvestment Act (ARRA) appropriated approximately $19 billion toward increased utilization of HIT, including requiring "meaningful use" of electronic health records (EHRs), and new governance boards for setting HIT policy and standards. ARRA also conferred statutory authority upon the HHS Office of the National Coordinator for Health Information Technology (ONC). Development and application of relevant HIT standards (including increasing medical device interoperability) have been an ongoing focus of key stakeholders since 2005.

  At the end of 2009, ONC published draft rules for public comment specifying the conditions where federal programs will reimburse for meaningful use of EHRs. The use of HIT-related medical devices alone, however, will not provide all of the promising synergies and benefits for delivering effective and efficient health care. Reviewing treatment and decision-making processes, while expanding the range of services available to patients, are additional elements that will enable the medical device industry to play an increasingly critical role in the rollout of HIT.

- *Product Convergence:* As medical device and biotechnology products converge, medical devices will act as delivery systems for pharmaceutical treatments and research resulting from genetic engineering and biotechnology research. Many industry experts not only view the impending convergence of medical devices with biotechnology and nanotechnology with cautious optimism but also warn that if the regulatory and reimbursement issues are not addressed, problems will ensue as convergence takes place.

17.7 Industry Characteristics

The US medical devices industry is known for producing high-quality products using advanced technology resulting from significant investment in R&D. The medical device industry is highly entrepreneurial. According to the US Department of Commerce, Bureau of the Census, there were approximately 5300 medical device companies in the United States in 2007, mostly SMEs. In 2007, approximately 73% of medical device companies had fewer than 20 employees, with 15% having as many as 100 employees [16].

Major US medical device companies include Medtronic, GE Healthcare Technologies, Johnson & Johnson, St. Jude, Boston Scientific, Baxter, Becton Dickinson, Beckman Coulter, Abbott Labs, and Stryker Corporation. In addition, the following trade associations closely follow the medical device industry: Advanced Medical Technology Association (AdvaMed), Medical Device Manufacturers Association, Medical Imaging Technology Association, Dental Trade Alliance, and the International Association of Medical Equipment Remarketers & Servicers.

Announcements of progress in medical technology that allow for earlier detection of diseases and more effective treatment options are now almost daily occurrences. Particularly notable technological advances in the industry in recent years included new developments in neurology (e.g., deep-brain-stimulation devices for treating symptoms of Parkinson's), cardiology (e.g., artificial device designed to replace diseased heart valves), and HIT (e.g., "data liquidity" to facilitate information sharing, wireless telemedicine devices, systems designed to track the cardiac activity of patients with implanted medical devices).

Scientists have used nanosensors for the quick detection of cancers through blood tests, with nanomaterial also enabling the release of medicine at targeted organs. Collaborations have led to advances in biomarkers, robotic assistance, implantable electronic devices, liquid bandages/wound dressings, and ingestible diagnostic devices (capsules).

Minimally invasive surgery has also seen major gains—an exciting example of this trend is an endoscopic technique that integrates nanotechnology and diagnostic imaging. Capsule endoscopy, which involves swallowing a tiny wireless camera pill that takes thousands of pictures as it travels through the digestive track, gives physicians more detailed information about hard-to-navigate sections of the digestive tract compared with earlier endoscopic technologies. The ability to navigate and detect conditions in the small intestine is the most promising aspect of this new technology; providing physicians with an unprecedented and real-time view of the small intestine lining.

17.7.1 Major Markets and Determinants Driving Demand

Although the end users of certain medical devices such as pacemakers and insulin pumps are patients, devices are primarily marketed to health care providers. Only hospitals and other large health care provider groups have the purchasing power to buy expensive equipment such as an MRI machine or a computed tomography scanner. Like the pharmaceutical industry, the demand of medical devices is largely based on insurance coverage, age demographics, and the health of the public—the sicker the insured population, the greater the demand for medical devices. Medical specialists also place a high demand on new technologies to better serve their patients. The demand for better devices necessitates the industry to develop new and innovative products [17].

17.7.2 Medical Device Industry SWOT Analysis

The United States is currently the undisputed global leader in medtech innovation, but can it continue to maintain that position? As the medical device industry enters 2015, the United States remains the world leader by market re, with a total revenue of around $110 billion—around one-third of the 0 billion global pie. However, the US medical device industry also faces tifaceted challenges that are hampering growth [18].

recent years, the furious pace of growth the US medtech industry had n accustomed to has slowed. Through 2020, the US medtech market is 'ed to expand by only 5%, down significantly from its 15% growth rate le ago. To improve its prospects, the industry will need to capitalize rengths, overcome its weaknesses, seize opportunities for growth, ess threats that could hamper its progress. The SWOT analysis is zed in Figure 17.2.

ical Device Industry: Strengths

ical device industry boasts many strengths, including market ize, R&D investment, academic institutions, and strong finance

ished Market

ed States continues to command a leadership role in the al device space. As of October 2014, US companies held

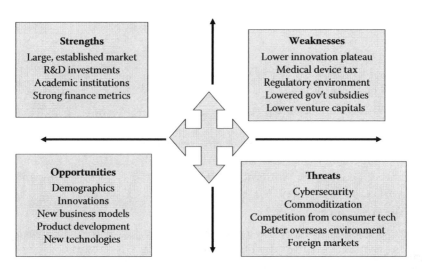

Strengths
Large, established market
R&D investments
Academic institutions
Strong finance metrics

Weaknesses
Lower innovation plateau
Medical device tax
Regulatory environment
Lowered gov't subsidies
Lower venture capitals

Opportunities
Demographics
Innovations
New business models
Product development
New technologies

Threats
Cybersecurity
Commoditization
Competition from consumer tech
Better overseas environment
Foreign markets

FIGURE 17.2
Medical device industry SWOT analysis.

four of the top five rankings for medical device companies with the most revenue and represent 22 of the top 40 spots. Overall, US companies account for almost two-thirds of the total revenue for the top 40 medical device companies, followed by Germany with 14% and Japan with 7%.

An aging population and increased availability of health care as a result of the Affordable Care Act should continue to keep the United States well positioned in the medtech space. US medical device exports grew at a compound annual growth rate of 4.5% from 2008 to 2013 and are expected to increase at similar rates in the future, according to Bloomberg.

Growing economies in Asia and Africa, where gross domestic product is predicted to rise by more than 5.5%, also bode well for US companies, which enjoy good brand recognition and reputations there.

R&D Investment

While the United States is expected to continue to play a leading role in medical device R&D for many years to come, its dominance is eroding. After declining in 2009 for only the second time since the 1950s, according to the National Science Board, R&D spending across all US industries has rebounded—although gains of $2.9 billion in 2010 and $7.3 billion in 2011 were unimpressive.

Larger medical device manufacturers, in particular, have been slow to dedicate more dollars to R&D. From 2013 through 2020, large corporations in the industry with a projected spending of $1 billion or more are expected to grow their R&D budgets by approximately 3%, while the rest of the industry is expected to increase R&D spending by more than 5%, according to Evaluate.

Academic Institutions

The United States is home to 141 accredited medical schools and approximately 400 major teaching hospitals and health systems— many of which consistently rank among the best in the world— according to the Association of American Medical Colleges. Many of these academic institutions partner with medical device companies to collaborate on R&D of new technologies.

Strong Finance Metrics

While growth in the industry has slowed over the past decade, revenues still grew at a faster pace than GDP. Renewed confidence in the medtech sector was evidenced by strong improvement in market capitalizations, which surged 37% in 2013, compared with a 4% growth in 2012. More than 70% of US medtech companies saw their market cap increase, and nearly a quarter saw their share prices grow 100% or more, according to Ernst & Young.

In addition, there has been a strong market for mergers and acquisitions (M&A) in the medtech sector. The total deal value during the first three quarters of 2014 was considerably higher than that in the same period in 2013, while the number of M&A deals rose 20%.

The period from mid-2013 through mid-2014 was also promising for small and midsize companies, with 31 US and European medtech IPOs raising $1.5 billion in funding. This illustrates investors' faith and confidence in the industry's future prospects.

17.7.4 Medical Device Industry: Weaknesses

To maintain its enviable position as the worldwide leader in medtech innovation, the US medical device industry must overcome weaknesses including an innovation plateau, the medical device tax, a tough regulatory environment, inferior government subsidies for R&D, and a lack of venture capital for start-ups. The following are major weaknesses of the industry.

Lower Innovation Plateau

A major reason for slowing growth in the medtech industry has been a gradual shift from risky blue-sky research to more evolutionary research. Large, established corporations, especially, have turned to more predictable research with a more easily measured return on investment. Unfortunately, low-risk or incremental improvements in medical device products do not justify price increases in the eyes of payers.

In contrast, smaller companies outside the United States can accept a larger magnitude of risk owing to their more nimble nature and less burdensome regulatory environment, which could lead to greater innovation.

Medical Device Tax

The medical device sector has been negatively affected by a 2.3% excise tax on sales of medical devices in United States implemented in 2013. According to a February 2014 status report from AdvaMed, as many as 165,000 US jobs have been lost as a result of the tax, and nearly one-third of respondents to a survey by the trade group said that they had reduced R&D investment because of the tax.

The device tax also places US companies at a disadvantage against foreign competitors by raising the US companies' effective tax rate. Furthermore, it often forces US companies to lower the price of their products in order to remain competitive in the global marketplace. Additionally, the higher tax rate reduces companies' resources for capital investments, R&D, clinical trials, manufacturing improvements, and investments in start-ups.

Regulatory Environment

Increased regulatory scrutiny by the FDA has led to increased costs for development of new products. For example, US regulations such as unique device identification, which went into effect in September 2013, add to the growing cost of compliance for companies looking to do business in the United States.

US medical device manufacturers should also be concerned about foreign regulations, particularly in China, which is pursuing policies that favor domestic manufacturers. This may force US medical device manufacturers that want to sell in China to manufacture there. This creates a predicament because companies will need to rely on China's intellectual property laws and enforcement, which have been major concerns to date.

Foreign regulations are also an issue in the EU, where new laws will soon replace the EU's Medical Device Directives. Areas of concern for medtech companies in the proposed legislation include enhanced competence requirements for notified bodies, approaches toward clinical evaluations, and the definition of single-use devices. While there is still ambiguity as to when the final version of the legislation will go into effect and what it will look like, companies will eventually have to comply with the new regulations.

Lowered Government Subsidies for R&D

The R&D tax credit has been vital to sustaining US innovation, but the temporary credit has often been allowed to lapse since its enactment in 1981. Without permanent status, businesses can't fully rely on the R&D tax credit in financial budgeting and forecasting. A permanent credit would give companies the confidence to invest in R&D, knowing that a certain amount of their expenses would be offset come tax time.

The US R&D tax credit is also inferior to others around the globe. The United States currently ranks 22nd in the world for federal R&D tax subsidies, with countries in Europe, Asia, and South America providing greater incentives for businesses to move there.

Venture Capital

Venture capital firms allocated just 7% of their funding to health care in 2013, down from 13% in 2009. Because of long times to market and stringent FDA regulations, early-stage companies have had an especially hard time attracting venture capital. Angel investors have stepped in to provide essential capital to start-up medtech companies, but more funding is needed to keep the industry's innovation pipeline flowing.

17.7.5 Medical Device Industry: Opportunities

To maintain its position as the global leader in medtech innovation, the US medical device industry will need to seize opportunities presented by demographics, service and business model innovations, innovation in product development, and new technologies.

Demographics

From 2000 to 2011, the U.S. population over the age of 65 increased 18%, a rate that is expected to continue for at least 20 years. This trend is significant for medtech because the elderly use more health resources compared with their younger counterparts.

Despite its inclusion of the medical device tax, the Affordable Care Act has provided another tailwind for the medical device industry. The law has been credited with reducing the number of Americans without health insurance by 8 million. In particular, it has extended coverage to people with preexisting conditions and low incomes, groups that tend to need more health treatments that require medical devices.

New Business Models

Because of lower reimbursement rates, many medtech companies are enhancing their products with service offerings that offer additional value for their customers, such as increasing operating room efficiency or reducing hospital visits. By having a suite of offerings designed to address the continuum of care in a given disease area, medical device companies can help provider groups meet important care metrics necessary for reimbursement and simplify the contracting complexity health care buyers face.

Innovation in Product Development

One way medical device companies are combating higher development and commercialization costs is through use of data technologies to increase productivity at each stage of product development. Companies are now mining information from tools in service, clinical trials, genetics, and demographics to perform analyses that provide insights into trials and generate new ideas, while reducing costs by drawing conclusions faster.

With the recent explosion in mobile platforms, interactive graphical user interfaces (GUIs) have become commonplace in medical devices. However, research into recent patient incidents and product recalls has found GUI design most often to be the primary culprit. GUI development is therefore a critical element in most present-day medical device efforts. Considerations of how systems can be designed for integration with medical platforms and end users are essential for the safety, efficacy, and ultimate success of new devices.

Application of New Technologies

Some segments of medical device manufacturing are being transformed by the use of 3-D printing, with medical applications accounting for 16.4% of the $2.2-billion additive manufacturing market in 2012, according to a study published by Deloitte University Press. Relatively small medical devices, such as hearing aids or dental retainer molds, are currently best suited for additive manufacturing, but future medical applications include grafting skin onto burn victims, printing blood vessels and heart tissue, making prostheses that resemble the original missing limb, studying cancer with printed cells, and even creating replacement organs for the human body.

Another technology with niche applications in medical device manufacturing is flexible automation. The robotics incorporated into these systems can provide the capability to process different products through the same system and are reconfigurable for new products, thereby reducing costs, improving production flexibility, and shortening product development life cycles. As a result, robots are being used increasingly in various areas of medical device manufacturing, including assembly, dispensing, quality control, and packaging.

Software development will also continue to play a major role in medtech innovation as the shift to mobile platforms allows personal electronic devices to transmit patient data to doctors, manage documentation and records, and provide identification and traceability of medical devices.

17.7.6 Medical Device Industry: Threats

In its quest to remain the world leader in medtech innovation, the US medical device industry will have to fend off threats such as cybersecurity, product commoditization, competition from consumer tech companies, better business environments abroad, and foreign markets.

Cybersecurity

Cybersecurity threats have become a growing concern, with numerous hacking attempts aimed at medical device companies over the past year. As a result, the US government has taken notice. The US Department of Homeland Security has more than 20 open investigations into cybersecurity flaws in medical devices and hospital equipment, according to an October 2014 report by Reuters. FDA issued its final guidance on cybersecurity in 2014, providing examples of what reviewers expect to see during premarket review.

Product Commoditization

Medtech companies have been pressured by payers to lower prices on widely available devices. A report by AdvaMed found that prices for artificial knees, pacemakers, and drug-eluting stents dropped by 17%, 26%, and 34%, respectively, in real dollars adjusted by the consumer price index for medical care from 2007 to 2011. Many other device categories also faced price declines of significant magnitude [19].

As medical devices become more portable—and thus more prevalent—it will be easier for offshore competitors to bring similar products to market faster and at lower prices. US companies need to ensure that their devices can be differentiated and demand premium pricing based on their capabilities. One way to accomplish this is through software downloads, which can keep device features and functionality updated without the need for hardware replacement.

Companies must also focus on process improvements and Lean manufacturing to become more efficient.

Competition from Consumer Technology

Seeing traditional medtech players slow to adopt mobile, analytics, and cloud solutions, consumer technology firms have sensed an opportunity and are starting to enter the medtech space.

Google is investing in smart contact lenses, and other consumer tech competitors include Apple, AT&T, Canon, Intel, Motorola, Reebok, Qualcomm, Samsung, Sony, and Verizon. Many of these firms are focusing on functionalities such as wireless communication, portability, and seamless integration with other devices to enable more personalized care. Moreover, they have a head start on the medtech industry given their brand recognition and familiarity among consumers.

Better Business Environments Abroad

The United States's 35% corporate tax rate is not competitive with that of many countries in Europe, including Germany, Switzerland, and Ireland. The higher tax rate has caused several large-profile corporations, including giant Medtronic, to switch to offshore domiciles.

The United States is also declining in its relative attractiveness in areas including intellectual property rights, difficulty and length of time of the approval process, and economic freedom.

Foreign Markets

In Japan, the world's second-largest medical device market, the government is making an effort to increase the availability and accessibility of foreign products and technologies through initiatives such as a new Pharmaceutical and Medical Device Law (PMDL), which went into effect last year. Although implementation of the PMDL won't necessarily make Japanese registration easy, it should at least make the process less challenging and more transparent, which should benefit US companies wanting to do business in Japan.

China, the world's third-largest medical device market, is also one of the world's fastest growing. The United States is China's leading supplier of medical devices, and slow growth in US health care spending may encourage US firms to further penetrate the Chinese market. However, barriers including challenging regulatory procedures, inconsistent reimbursement policies, complex tendering for purchasing medical devices, and tariffs on China's most commonly imported devices may continue to hamper expansion in China by US companies.

Israel is also becoming a significant player in medtech innovation, thanks to its technological know-how, infrastructure, tax credits, incentives, grants, culture of innovation, and entrepreneurship. Israel also enjoys a high ranking in ease and speed of regulatory approval. As a result, the acquisition rate of early- to mid-stage Israeli medtech firms has accelerated over the past few years.

17.8 Launching Your Medical Device

In its comprehensive white paper *Launching a Medical Device? Read This First!*, Schwartz MSL Healthcare [20] argues that often launch is defined as the moment when FDA clearance or approval is obtained. However, many companies don't declare "launch" until sufficient inventory is available and enough clinicians have been trained or gained usage experience. We will define "launch" as the moment in time when your product is set to be introduced to the marketplace.

Schwartz classifies medical device launches into three tiers: (1) game changers; (2) challengers, and (3) fundamentals, as seen in Figure 17.3.

17.8.1 Tier 1 Products

Game changers: A new product is worthy of tier 1 if it demonstrates strong potential to fundamentally change or disrupt a market. To determine if your product is tier 1, consider the following questions:

- Does the new product offer first-of-its-kind functionality? Does it have third-party validation (such as peer-reviewed data, presentation of data at a professional meeting, government mandate, advocacy group support, or a favorable professional society position statement)?
- Does the new product require and has it received FDA approval or FDA clearance? By our definition, all products that have gone through the PMA process are automatically classified as tier 1.

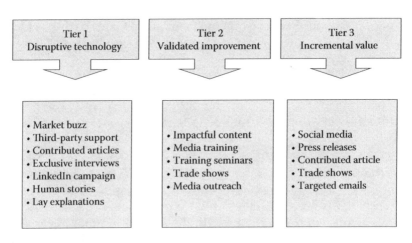

FIGURE 17.3
Product launch spectrum.

- Does the new product demonstrate strong potential to affect clinical or professional practices or a standard of care to the eventual point of change?
- Does the new product affect multiple audiences (such as consumers, physicians and hospitals)?

17.8.2 Tier 2 Products

A tier 2 product offers significant value to an industry, but is unlikely to fundamentally change practices. The product demonstrates many of the following characteristics. To determine if your product is tier 2, consider the following questions:

- Does the new product offer functionality that already exists, but is vastly improved over the status quo?

  Ideally, the improvement should be third-party validated with published data, a position statement from an advocacy group, or public support from a notable industry thought leader. In addition, the advance in form or function should create significant new benefits for clinicians and patients.
- Does the new product require and has it received FDA clearance?

  The FDA clearance may not confer a radically different application of existing technology, but some form of significant improvement should exist and ideally be third-party validated.
- Does the new product deliver a benefit that was previously unavailable?
- While the product is unlikely to change a standard of care, it offers a benefit of significant value that was previously unavailable, and this feature was a significant deterrent to adoption and accessibility. Examples include broad insurance reimbursement, significant availability improvement, or a pediatric indication.

17.8.3 Tier 3 Products

A wide range of products may qualify as tier 3 products, but, typically, a tier 3 product has at least one of the following characteristics. To determine if your product is tier 3, consider the following:

- Does the new product reveal a significant finding that may be only incrementally better than the status quo or "catches-up" to the competition?
- Is the new product important to a narrow or niche audience?
- Does the new product have limited value to my company outside a specific department?

17.9 Medical Device Launch Worksheet

Table 17.2 can be very useful to help you analyze your product launch category and allow you to stand out from the crowd.

TABLE 17.2

Analyzing Your Product Launch Category

Critical Questions	Your (Truthful) Answer
What are the key benefits of your new product? How does it differentiate from your competitors?	
What makes this product unique/first-of-its-kind/or best-of-its-kind?	
What market need does your product address?	
What is the market for this new product? Can you accurately quantify or qualify it?	
Are there competing technologies? If yes, what are they and how are they the same or different?	
Who is the target audience for this new product? Physicians, hospitals, laboratories, patients?	
How does the new product serve to evolve the marketplace or industry? Is the market ready for evolution?	
Why is the new product significant for existing customers, patients, strategic partners, or other stakeholders?	
How will this product help us acquire customers, patients, partners, or investors?	
Is the product FDA-approved/cleared? If so, what was the date of approval/clearance?	
When do we want to publically release the availability of this new product?	
Is there an industry event/tradeshow that makes the timing particularly relevant?	
Who are the third-party validators for this new product? Can we quote them in a press release? Are they open to speaking with media as third-party spokespeople?	
Does the product have peer-reviewed data, presentation of data at a professional meeting, government mandate, advocacy group support or a favorable professional society position statement? If so, provide details.	
Is the sales team trained? What is the sales plan (e.g., full-scale availability on day 1, slow rollout by region, limited number of trial sites, etc.)?	
How will marketing support this launch (e.g., advertising, etc.)? Is there an integrated approach to the launch?	

(Continued)

TABLE 17.2 (CONTINUED)

Analyzing Your Product Launch Category

Critical Questions	Your (Truthful) Answer
Is manufacturing ramped up? Is there sufficient inventory to meet potential demand?	
Are there any data points, metrics, industry stats that support the need for this new product in the marketplace?	
Is there a customer or physician we can quote in a press release? Will they speak to the media?	
Is the website content/landing page ready? Is the web content optimized for search?	

References

1. The Medical Device Industry in the United States, http://selectusa.commerce .gov/industry-snapshots/medical-device-industry-united-states.
2. Davidov, T. How to Commercialize Your Novel Medical or Surgical Device Association for Academic Surgery, October 2013.
3. US FDA (United States Food and Drug Administration). Classify Your Medical Device, http://www.fda.gov/MedicalDevices/DeviceRegulationandGuidance /Overview/ClassifyYourDevice/default.htm.
4. US FDA (United States Food and Drug Administration). Premarket Approval (PMA),http://www.fda.gov/MedicalDevices/DeviceRegulationandGuidance /HowtoMarketYourDevice/PremarketSubmissions/PremarketApprovalPMA /ucm2007514.htm.
5. US FDA (United States Food and Drug Administration). Premarket Notification (510k), http://www.fda.gov/MedicalDevices/DeviceRegulationandGuidance /HowtoMarketYourDevice/PremarketSubmissions/PremarketNotification 510k/default.htm.
6. US FDA (United States Food and Drug Administration). Code of Federal Regulations, Title 21, Volume 8, April 1, 2013.
7. US FDA (United States Food and Drug Administration). Special Considerations, http://www.fda.gov/MedicalDevices/DeviceRegulationandGuidance/How toMarketYourDevice/PremarketSubmissions/PremarketNotification510k /ucm134578.htm.
8. Masterson, F. and Cormican, K. Overview of the regulation of medical devices and drugs in the European Union and the United States. *Therapeutic Innovation & Regulatory Science*, September 6, 2013.
9. US FDA (United States Food and Drug Administration). Class I/II Exemptions, http://www.fda.gov/MedicalDevices/DeviceRegulationandGuidance/Overview /ClassifyYourDevice/ucm051549.htm.

10. US FDA (United States Food and Drug Administration). Humanitarian Device Exemption, http://www.fda.gov/MedicalDevices/DeviceRegulationand Guidance/HowtoMarketYourDevice/PremarketSubmissions/Humanitarian DeviceExemption/default.htm.

11. Andrews R.J., Hauptman, R.A., Hickey, C.T. SRR. Medical device and equipment overview, http://www.srr.com/assets/pdf/medical-device-and-equipment -industry-overview.pdf.

12. Weixel, N. *Medical Devices Law and Industry Report*, The Bureau of National Affairs, June 2010.

13. Araùjo, R., Arons, R., Bucher, J., Hagle, U., Li, L., and Ruh, R. Medical device industry: The changing business and talent landscape. Korn Ferry Institute, September 2011, www.kornferryinstitute.com.

14. Industry Surveys Healthcare: Products & Supplies, Standard & Poor, February 2010.

15. Medical Devices Industry Assessment, http://ita.doc.gov/td/health/medical %20device%20industry%20assessment%20final%20ii%203-24-10.pdf.

16. Manufacturing: Industry Series: Detailed Statistics by Industry for the United States; U.S. Department of Commerce, Bureau of the Census.

17. Zhong, H. Primer: The Medical Device Industry, June 2012. American Action Forum, http://americanactionforum.org/sites/default/files/OHC_MedDevInd Primer.pdf.

18. Hartford, J. Medical Device Industry: Strengths, Weaknesses, Opportunities, and Threats. *Medical Device Business*, January 12, 2015, http://www.mddionline .com/article/us-medical-device-industry-swot-analysis-01-12-2015.

19. http://advamed2016.com/download/files/Press%20Releases/Press_Release -Study_Shows_Declining_Prices.PDF

20. http://files.schwartzmsl.com/files/whitepapers/SchwartzMSL_Medical _Device_Product_Launch_Guidebook_aug13.pdf?utm_source=hs_automation &utm_medium=email&utm_content=12526513&_hsenc=p2ANqtz--McScO3v LZ27TZbp4ZFQrKVOgsWo6gb5N5P8LVQRof8djO4wwFmXIakOBgSgX3WzH DC3fJ-xPqCH31wdOlYtK_zeo-2A&_hsmi=12526513

18

Launching High-Tech Products

18.1 Introduction

Technology (from the Greek *techne* meaning "art, skill, dexterity, proficiency, etc.") is the practical application of knowledge or science for industrial or commercial purposes. Technology can be found embedded into computers, devices, machines, and factories that can be operated by individuals with minimal training of the inner workings of the instrument.

High technology, or high tech, in its current definition, includes any technical or highly specialized technological equipment, instrument, or application [1]. It is mostly used to describe advanced computer electronics, but may include other "technologies" that are dated, everyday, widespread, or commoditized.

Examples of current high-tech products include the following:

- Wireless communications
- Aerospace
- Biotech
- Telecommunications
- Advanced electronic devices
- Medical telemetry
- Internet
- Industrial robotics
- Miniaturized devices
- Semiconductors

The Organisation for Economic Co-Operation and Development (OECD) [2] has indicated that using research intensity as an industry classification indicator is also possible. The OECD takes not only the manufacturing rate but also the usage rate of technology into account. Furthermore, OECD's product-based classification supports the technology intensity approach. It can be concluded that companies in a high-technology industry do not necessary produce high-technology products and vice versa.

TABLE 18.1

OECD High-Tech Product Classification and Intensity Approach

Industry Name	Total R&D-Intensity (1999, in %)	OECD ISIC Rev. 3
Biotechnology and pharmaceuticals	10.46	2423
Aircraft and spacecraft	10.29	353
Medical, precision, and optical instruments	9.69	33
Radio, television, and communication equipment	7.48	32
Office, accounting, and computing machinery	7.21	30
Electrical machinery and apparatus	3.60	31
Motor vehicles, trailers, and semitrailers	3.51	34
Railroad and transport equipment	3.11	352 + 359
Chemical and chemical products	2.85	24 (excl. 2423)
Machinery and equipment	2.20	29

The OECD's classification is shown in Table 18.1 (stable since 1973).

Furthermore, OECD's product-based classification supports the technology intensity approach. It can be concluded that companies in a high-technology industry do not necessary produce high-technology products and vice versa.

18.2 Are You at the Launch Stage?

Your high-tech start-up has developed a working prototype of your innovative product. This is great news because you are now at the product launch stage, and product launch is the lifeblood of high-tech companies.

Most high-tech companies fail in their attempt to launch their new product. According to research published in August 2007 by the Boston Consulting Group, 50% of the 2500 senior executives surveyed were satisfied with the financial performance of their product launch, and only 38% of companies ranked their launches as highly successful [3].

To ensure launch success, make absolutely sure that you

- Put your entire focus on your customer, not your product
- Get opinion leaders and influencers to back your product and its benefits
- Brief industry analysts about the benefits of your product
- Turn your launch into a media spectacle
- Only release a product that early adopters will brag about and show off
- Expect "big bang" press interest only if your product is revolutionary

18.3 Marketing High-Tech Products

In 1991, Geoffrey A. Moore published his influential book *Crossing the Chasm: Marketing and Selling High-Tech Products to Mainstream Customers*, now considered the bible for entrepreneurial marketing. The book focuses on the specifics of marketing high-tech products during the early start-up period. Moore's exploration and expansion of the diffusions of innovations model have had a significant and lasting impact on high-tech entrepreneurship [4].

Everett Rogers, a professor of communication studies, popularized a theory on the spread of innovations in his book *Diffusion of Innovations* [5]. The book, which was first published in 1962 and now in its fifth edition, is considered a classic. Rogers argued that diffusion is the process by which an innovation is communicated through certain channels over time among the participants in a social system. He divided the participants into five categories: (1) innovators, (2) early adopters, (3) early majority, (4) late majority, and (5) laggards [6], as seen in Figure 18.1.

Figure 18.1 is the classical adoption cycle that accompanies any innovation into the market. The entrepreneur's marketing challenge is to quickly move from the innovator/early adopter cycle to the majority of customers. As the figure shows, the early market consists of the **"innovators or techies"** who are eager to be at the forefront of any technology and make a name for themselves if it is proven successful. For the **early adopters**, the technology represents a

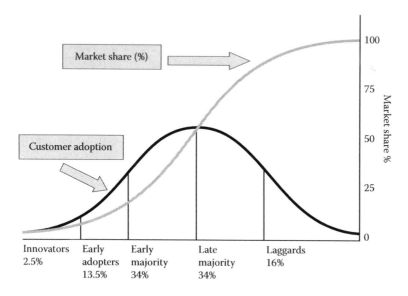

FIGURE 18.1
Rogers' diffusion of innovations.

TABLE 18.2

Characteristics of Diffusion Participants

Market Buyer Types	Characteristics and Idiosyncrasies
Innovators (technology enthusiasts) (techies)	Derive value from pure technology advances Willing to spend hours to make product work Demand immediate access to technical service Being first is part of their reward
Early adopters (visionaries)	Match technology to a strategic advantage Willing to accept risk Willing to be internal product champions Looking for substantial ROI
Early majority (pragmatists)	Regarded as "technology leaders" Communicate with others (word of mouth) Will only buy when you are "established" Price savvy Demand quality and service
Late majority (conservatives)	Wait until product has become the "standard" Like pre-assembled, easy-to-use products Demand competitive prices Afraid of discontinuous innovations
Laggards (ultra conservatives) (risk allergic)	Show no opinion leadership Last to adopt any innovation Focused on "tradition" Avoid change at all costs Oldest of all adopters

change agent, and they are the champions of change, and set the standards. For the **early majority**, improving technology is their priority—they want "evolution not revolution." The **late majority** wait until a platform or application becomes the de facto industry standard and are price-sensitive and very demanding. The **laggards** (risk allergic) wait for turn-key applications with guaranteed results and no surprises. This is summarized in Table 18.2.

Thus, introducing a high-tech product that is new to both the firm and the market requires the greatest expenditure of both effort and resources, thus representing the greatest uncertainty and risk. The marketing challenge for the entrepreneur is twofold: (1) communicating the product/service availability and (2) persuading the early adopters.

18.4 Crossing the Dreaded Chasm

For any start-up, crossing the chasm, that is, becoming the industry standard and becoming profitable, is its most pressing strategic goal. To accomplish that goal, the firm must persuade the pragmatists to adopt their product/service.

Pragmatists demand a total solution to their problem ("pain"); they want the whole product. The whole product is defined as the minimum set of market requirements to compel a radical change and achieve market superiority.

Crossing the chasm is the whole enchilada. The dreaded "chasm" concept [7] is visually presented in Figure 18.2.

The chasm is created because the early majority does not hear the early adopters' findings. The early majority wants, first and foremost, large productivity improvements that lead to cost reductions, and they want bug-free products, ready to use right out of the package. The concept introduces entrepreneurs to five thought-provoking concepts:

1. Technology is adopted in predictable stages by distinct groups.
2. The first two groups (influencers) compose the early market and will predict the success or failure of your product.
3. The bell shape of the curve forecasts that sales will grow exponentially if you can overcome the "chasm" or "Valley of Death."
4. Chasms are caused by the different product needs and buying habits of each group.
5. Completely different marketing and sales strategies are necessary to win each successive group of customers.

A classical example of successful customer focus comes from one of Apple's products: Step 1: charge the battery. Step 2: there is no step 2. You are now ready to go.

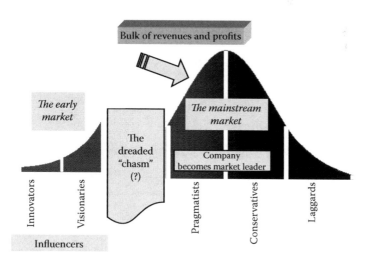

FIGURE 18.2
The chasm. Going from loss to profitability.

18.5 Your Pioneer Strategy

Pioneers are the ones with the tomahawks on their backs.

Question: How can a start-up aspire to become a market leader in the face of gigantic competition? Answer: by the marketing concept of a pioneer strategy.

Marketing gurus have long debated the conundrum "Is it better to be a pioneer or a follower?" Potential sources of competitive advantage available to pioneers are as follows:

- First-mover advantage
- First choice of market segmentation
- Defining the rules of standardization
- Early distribution advantage
- Setting prices (optimizing margins and revenues)
- Creating high barriers to entry

Despite these early entry advantages, many pioneers fail to capitalize on their potential by abandoning the product, going out of business, or getting acquired before their product matures. Followers have the ability to

- Exploit any pioneer mistakes (product, marketing, technical)
- Use more advanced technologies
- Exploit the pioneer's limited financial resources
- Skimming the market (cherry picking)
- Competing on lower price, greater availability, and superior technical support

18.6 Your Product Launch Strategies

Pragmatic marketing [8] recommends the matrix shown in Table 18.3 to ensure a successful product launch and avoid an impending launch disaster.

18.7 Secrets to a Successful Launch

Michael Shoppel and Philip Davis, in their BetaSphere white paper [9], state that, each year, millions of dollars are wasted when products enter the market

TABLE 18.3

Recommended Actions

Tactics	Recommended Actions
Goals for product launch	Establish launch goals with your executive team as early as possible and communicate them in meaningful ways throughout your organization.
Launch "checklist"	Once launch goals are established, formulate the launch strategy and then define the deliverables.
Time frames and expectations	Evaluate launch goals against the ability of the organization to execute. Then develop a plan of action to fill the readiness gaps.
Sales enablers	Become an expert on how and why your buyers buy.
Sales tools and collateral readings	Focus on gaining a deep understanding of your buyers, then build collateral and sales tools to influence them throughout the buying process.
Name "launch owner"	Assign the responsibility for achieving the launch goals to a launch owner and provide them with the flexibility and resources to make it happen.
Depend on market evidence	Make launch planning decisions based on market evidence not guesses, or hunches.
Do not mimic your competitor	An intimate knowledge of buyers and the buying process provides the best guidance for the most effective launch tactics.
Current customers migration plan	Ensure that the migration to a new version of your product is smooth and straightforward for current customers (if you have existing customers).
Create a cross-functional team	Make participation in a cross-functional launch team a priority and reward their contribution.

ill-prepared to meet customer expectations and requirements. Insufficient customer feedback and lack of customer involvement during the development process are the key reasons for unsuccessful launches. Conversely, feedback from customers in your target market is the number one factor leading to successful product and website introductions.

Customer-oriented development organizations have long championed the principle of active collaboration with target users during the development process, but even the most ardent promoters of bringing customers and partners into the product development process confront challenges when attempting to migrate the concept into practice.

Early access programs, alpha and beta programs, pilot programs, and field trials are examples of customer feedback programs. These programs have both quantitative (e.g., find and fix bugs, assess interoperability, evaluate performance, etc.) and qualitative goals (e.g., market readiness, user acceptance, feature set completeness). These programs are logistically complex and require a high degree of interaction with customers and your development team. While product teams are in many cases well prepared to manage the complexity of developing products, they are typically untrained, unequipped, and unprepared for simultaneously managing customer feedback. Successfully validating your product with feedback from your target market will maximize market acceptance and minimize post-launch costs. In this white paper, we will explore the five key factors leading to successful customer feedback programs. These are the five secrets of a successful launch.

18.7.1 Value of Customer Feedback during Development

Shoppel and Davis further recommend that return on investment (ROI) in customer feedback programs can be measured by the following formula:

quantity + quality + timeliness of customer feedback divided by program-specific costs + opportunity costs.

While maximizing ROI for a customer feedback program is a primary objective, minimizing the opportunity costs associated with underexecuted programs is of equal or greater importance.

Opportunity costs include unscheduled or costly follow-up releases to "fix" the product, higher-than-expected support costs, weaker-than-expected market acceptance, lost customer feedback to validate and endorse the product, and lost marketing feedback to understand importance/satisfaction indicators that drive the development of the next release.

1. **Traditional ROI criteria:** For most organizations, baseline reasons for inviting current and prospective customers to evaluate new or next generation products and services include the following:
   - Evaluating and tuning performance across multiple customer configurations and environments
   - Obtaining suggestions and requests for enhancements
   - Gathering usability feedback and statistics
   - Finding and fixing bugs
   - Avoiding incompatibilities with complementary products
2. **Newer ROI criteria:** Competition, product complexity, and the number of stakeholders in new product introductions are all increasing, while development cycle time is decreasing. These factors have raised the bar by which customer feedback programs are measured, including the following:
   - Gathering feedback for use in marketing and public relations
   - Preparing the entire organization for the "real" launch
   - Creating word-of-mouth "buzz" among highly valued, early adopter customers who act as references in the marketplace
   - Preparing third-party developers

- Preparing the channel (sales force, distributors, retailers, and product and service trainers)
- Forging stronger working relationships with key customers

In summary, the execution of a successful product launch begins months before the actual launch, and it starts with successful incorporation of feedback from your target market.

18.7.2 Adequate Resources for Program Execution

The weeks immediately preceding a product launch are typically the most hectic for any product development team. There are literally hundreds of critical activities that must be accomplished. Examples include the following:

- Finalize the product.
- Press and analyst briefings.
- Create and print marketing collateral.
- Notify/train the sales force and channels.
- Complete the documentation.

It is a fact of product development that customer feedback programs occur at a time in the development process when product teams are at their busiest. Customers need the maximum amount of attention and support when product teams have the least time to spare. At this most hectic time, additional resources are also required to ensure the success of the customer feedback programs. These tasks encompass the following:

- Program planning and process management
- Target customer profiling, recruiting, and qualification
- Product fulfillment
- Proactive customer engagement, follow-up, and feedback management
- Rapid resolution of customer problems, "preventive" technical support
- Feedback analysis and metric reporting to the product team and management
- Measurement of ROI

Your organization makes an impression with each point of contact, from recruiting, to regular interaction and follow-up, through program wrap up. Customers state that the most unsatisfactory aspect of participating in customer feedback programs is lack of communication from the product or service provider. In the words of one customer: "Give me some assurance that

I'm not wasting my time. If my feedback goes unanswered, then I'm not sure if you didn't get it, it's unimportant, or it's being ignored. Raise my confidence level in your company."

Product teams find it difficult to estimate the time, resources, and intracompany (and in some cases intercompany) collaboration required to successfully prepare and execute customer feedback programs. In addition, resources must be available to evaluate program results and prioritize actions. In the vast majority of cases, resource requirements are significantly underestimated and those resources are then siphoned from these critical tasks to accomplish other activities. As a result, the effectiveness of the launch is put at risk.

- Do you know what your target customers really think about your product?
- Are you certain it is easy to use?
- Does it interoperate in the different customer environments?

The only way to know for certain is to ask your target customers—and that requires resources.

18.7.3 Defining Objectives Clearly

The ultimate success of the product launch can almost always be traced to understanding the requirements of your target market. The amount of time initially invested in defining and prioritizing your feedback objectives directly affects the quantity and quality of information learned. This typically falls into two major categories:

1. Customer feedback objectives
2. Product team/management objectives

Customer feedback objectives typically include bugs and showstoppers; ease of installation and ease of use; testimonials; and customer assessment of features, functionality, quality, performance, and overall value. Product team/management objectives typically include achieving high customer participation, identifying and fixing bugs of a certain severity and priority as quickly as possible, verifying system and software compatibility on real-world customer configurations, and testing internal processes (e.g., technical/customer support). It is critical that Marketing, Engineering, Quality Assurance, and Customer Service/Technical Support staff schedule sufficient time to prepare a plan and establish complementary goals. With continually decreasing product development cycles, there is no time for rework. Without a set of objectives, the process for obtaining and incorporating customer feedback becomes ad hoc and unpredictable.

18.7.4 Defining the Right Process

A process that is scalable, unobtrusive to the product team, and highly responsive to customers provides product teams with the greatest leverage and flexibility. An ideal program minimizes product team overhead and interruptions while maximizing customer participation, feedback, satisfaction with the process, and ultimately the quality of information received.

The scope of your program (number of participants, their geographic distribution, anticipated technical support requirements, product fulfillment logistics, frequency of upgrades and revisions, product complexity, and feedback management processes) establishes your requirements for management and support resources. Even the simplest programs typically require a substantial time investment by a minimum of three to four team members to be effective. Defining a process for generating the greatest quantity and quality of feedback from customers is arguably the most difficult task, as it requires the greatest ongoing commitment of time to execute successfully. Methods for managing feedback and problem resolution typically include the following:

- Proactive, outbound telephone support
- E-mail/newsgroup communication
- Web-based surveys, bug tracking, and feedback management
- On-site interviews

Most organizations have traditionally employed a combination of the first two methods.

Web-based communication offers a host of new benefits to both product teams and customers, and the case for making the Web an integral part of customer feedback programs has become extremely compelling. On-site feedback collection, because of its cost, is typically reserved for the most technically sophisticated, high-end products with few customers.

18.7.5 Recruiting Motivated Evaluators

Selecting the appropriate quantity of target customers with the right characteristics is a crucial step in setting up and carrying out a successful program. Recruiting a sample of customers whose system configurations and usage patterns reflect the target market for the product or service should be the goal of any customer feedback program—it is the only way to capture real-world, premarket product feedback and customer experiences that cannot be duplicated internally by any Quality Assurance team.

The first step in developing the appropriate testing group is to define a matrix of target requirements, which includes qualifying criteria such as

- Knowledge, experience, and usage level
- System configuration and usage environment

- Availability/desire to test and provide feedback
- Testimonial potential

The number of target customers to include in your program is a function of the type of product or service, the aggregate amount of product/service usage you need for meaningful results, and the selection criteria defined above. There is no magic formula.

The objective is to create a sample no larger than you can adequately manage, and no smaller than will meet your matrix coverage requirements. In general, you will want to include the largest number of target customers that can be effectively managed and supported.

Incentives: While incentives can support program objectives and serve as a form of appreciation, their success varies depending on the type of feedback being elicited, the type of product or service being evaluated, and the incentive being offered. More important than offering incentives is recruiting target customers who are motivated to use the product or service, and to provide high-quality feedback at the frequency desired. No form of incentive will make an enthusiast out of someone either marginally interested or pressured into participating in a customer feedback program.

Your best incentive plan is a commitment to offer easy-to-use feedback mechanisms, personal recognition, appreciation, and time for quality feedback. Feedback *to* customers equals feedback *from* customers. Current or prospective customers need to feel that their efforts are being well spent, which means they need acknowledgment and support.

Because customers are generally *not* being financially compensated for their feedback, they reasonably expect greater interaction and technical support for their contribution to making your product or service better.

18.7.6 Managing Customer Feedback

The acquisition, analysis, and distribution of customer feedback are three of the most challenging areas of customer feedback management for product teams. Success depends on process, people, and technology.

Most technology companies have not yet made investments to establish an infrastructure for effectively communicating with customers during product development. This is reflected by industry average participation rates of less than 15% during customer feedback programs. For most programs, particularly those that are open to everyone (such as public betas), the overwhelming majority of users who obtain or use the product or service provide no feedback at all.

By contrast, programs that employ advanced feedback management systems and provide the support staff necessary for proactively communicating with customers can consistently achieve participation rates in the 70%–100% range, producing substantially greater feedback than industry norms. The good news is that product teams *can* measurably improve participation and productivity, independent of the product or service under evaluation, by focusing on communication and innovative feedback management.

18.7.7 Feedback Acquisition, Analysis, and Distribution

A central goal of effective customer feedback programs is the collection, analysis, and distribution of meaningful data in real time. For collection, this means actively soliciting feedback from customers, as well as providing mechanisms that make it convenient for customers to give feedback.

By analysis, we mean quantifying and qualifying feedback to inform product team and management decision-making during development, and for distribution, this means presenting structured, organized, actionable feedback as it arrives to feedback stakeholders.

The most important element of being able to process feedback quickly is having predefined metrics and categories (e.g., bugs by severity and priority, suggestions by importance, and measurements of customer progress ranging from installation to achieving specific usage levels). The customer graphical presentation of feedback during development can provide a wealth of information to the product team and management, and can objectively represent product performance and customer sentiment at a given point in time.

18.8 Why Do High-Tech Launches Fail So Often?

According to Fortune [10], depending on the study, up to 80% of new product launches fail. The deadliest reasons are as follows [11]:

- *Insignificant target market*—must be large enough to be profitable.
- *Poor product quality/performance*—product has to work adequately, meet customer needs.
  - *Problem of trade-offs*—company may mismanage a trade-off in benefits.
- *Inconsequential product differentiation*—product is not a great improvement on competitive offerings.
- *Poor positioning*—diet beer versus light beer.
- *Inadequate budget*—biggest reason small companies fail is inadequate capital.
- *Inadequate competitive analysis*—reaction of current incumbents, products from new entrants.
- *Blinders (= "Vision"?)*—company may have preconception that is never questioned (especially for high tech).

- *No protocol*—clear statement of target market, its needs, what product would do; difficult for smaller companies in competitive industries.
- *Bad timing*—"Better never than late" relative to competitors. First-movers may have the advantage. Relative to customer trends, may not want to be early; too much education required.
- *Poor execution of marketing mix*—wrong price, wrong distribution, wrong advertising campaign. "Bad advertising can kill a good product."

18.8.1 Famous High-Tech Launch Disasters

The phenomenon occurs over and over again in every product category, whether high tech, low tech, consumer products, or business-to-business products, and it goes for major international companies, as well as start-ups. The following are product launch disasters that have become legends [12]:

Kodak's Photo CD. *Take it now, and show it later.* Kodak offered film camera customers the ability to put their pictures on a compact disc and view them on their TVs. It was 10 years ahead of its time and marketed to customers who were not ready for it. Viable early adopter market in corporate marketing departments ignored.

Apple's Newton. *Or the Apple that fell from the tree.* They were right about the Personal Digital Assistant market but 5 years too soon. Yet they spent like they were in an existing and growing market.

Webvan. *Groceries on demand: the killer app of the Internet.* The company spent money like a drunken sailor. Even in the Internet Bubble, costs and infrastructure grew faster than the customer base.

Sony's MiniDisc players. *Size doesn't matter.* A smaller version of the CD wildly popular in Japan. The United States isn't Japan, and the product flopped in the US market.

Motorola's Iridium satellite-based phone system. *Call from anywhere.* An engineering triumph and built to support a customer base of millions. No one asked the customer if they wanted it, or needed it. Costs ran into the billions.

18.9 The Special Case of Launching Software Products

Before product launch, any new software is generally subjected an alpha and a beta testing program, meaning the product is subjected to practical use under expected operating conditions. Under this scenario, the process should proceed as follows:

- Alpha testing: done in-house.
- Beta testing: done at the customer site (is the product free of bugs?).
- Enable a feedback loop, and learn from the experience.
- Talk to your customers, and then *listen* carefully.
- Make it easy for customers to report bugs or use problems.
- Your beta customers will be the core of your influencer base.

The term *beta test* is believed to originate from an IBM hardware product test convention, dating back to punched card tabulating and sorting machines. Hardware first went through an alpha test for preliminary functionality and small-scale manufacturing feasibility. Then came a beta test, by people or groups other than the developers, to verify that the hardware correctly performed the functions it was supposed to and that it could be manufactured at scales necessary for the market.

And finally, a c test to verify final safety. With the advent of programmable computers and the first shareable software programs, IBM used the same terminology for testing software. As other companies began developing software for their own use, and for distribution to others, the terminology stuck—and is now part of our common vocabulary.

Figure 18.3 shows a classical like/dislike format used to evaluate your customer's initial reaction to the software product mockup being tested.

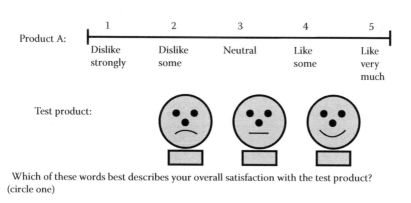

FIGURE 18.3
Like/dislike matrix.

18.9.1 Software Testing

According to Wikipedia, software testing is an investigation conducted to provide stakeholders with information about the quality of the product or service under test [13]. Software testing can also provide an objective, independent view of the software to allow the business to appreciate and understand the risks of software implementation. Test techniques include the process of executing a program or application with the intent of finding software bugs (errors or other defects).

It involves the execution of a software component or system component to evaluate one or more properties of interest. In general, these properties indicate the extent to which the component or system under test

- Meets the requirements that guided its design and development
- Responds correctly to all kinds of inputs
- Performs its functions within an acceptable time
- Is sufficiently usable
- Can be installed and run in its intended environments
- Achieves the general result its stakeholders desire

As the number of possible tests for even simple software components is practically infinite, all software testing uses some strategy to select tests that are feasible for the available time and resources. As a result, software testing typically (but not exclusively) attempts to execute a program or application with the intent of finding software bugs (errors or other defects). The job of testing is an iterative process as when one bug is fixed, it can illuminate other, deeper bugs, or can even create new ones. Software testing can provide objective, independent information about the quality of software and risk of its failure to users and sponsors.

18.9.2 Defining Software Testing

Some authorities [14] argue that a verification method, testing, is a paradox. Testing a program to assess its quality is, in theory, akin to sticking pins into a doll—very small pins, very large doll. The way out of the paradox is to set realistic expectations from the start.

Meyer further opines that testing a program tells us little about its quality, since 10 or even 10 million test runs are a drop in the ocean of possible cases. There are connections between tests and quality, but they are tenuous: A successful test is only relevant to quality assessment if it previously failed, then it shows the removal of a failure and usually of a fault. Meyer follows the IEEE standard terminology: An unsatisfactory program execution is a "failure," pointing to a "fault" in the program, itself the result of a "mistake" in the programmer's thinking. The informal term "bug" can refer to any of these phenomena.

According to Atwood [15], and based on the software release life cycle, below is how he characterizes each phase of software development:

Pre-Alpha	The software is still under active development and not feature complete or ready for consumption by anyone other than software developers. There may be milestones during the pre-alpha that deliver specific sets of functionality and nightly builds for other developers or users who are comfortable living on the absolute bleeding edge.
Alpha	The software is complete enough for *internal* testing. This is typically done by people other than the software engineers who wrote it, but still within the same organization or community that developed the software.
Beta	The software is complete enough for *external* testing—that is, by groups outside the organization or community that developed the software. Beta software is usually feature complete, but may have known limitations or bugs. Betas are either closed (private) and limited to a specific set of users, or they can be open to the general public.
Release candidate (aka gamma or delta)	The software is almost ready for final release. No feature development or enhancement of the software is undertaken; tightly scoped bug fixes are the only code you're allowed to write in this phase, and even then *only* for the most heinous and debilitating of bugs. One of the most experienced software developers I ever worked with characterized the release candidate development phase thusly: "does this bug kill small children?"
Gold	The software is finished—and by finished, we mean there are no showstopping, little-children-killing bugs in it. *That we know of.* There are probably numerous lower-priority bugs triaged into the next point release or service pack, as well.

18.9.3 Beta Phase of Software Testing

Beta, named after the second letter of the Greek alphabet, is the software development phase following alpha. Software in the beta stage is also known as *betaware* [16]. Beta phase generally begins when the software is feature complete but likely to contain a number of known or unknown bugs [17]. Software in the beta phase will generally have many more bugs in it than completed software, as well as speed/performance issues and may still cause crashes or data loss. The focus of beta testing is reducing impacts to users, often incorporating usability testing [18].

The process of delivering a beta version to the users is called *beta release*, and this is typically the first time that the software is available outside of the organization that developed it. Beta version software is often useful for demonstrations and previews within an organization and to prospective customers. Some developers refer to this stage as a *preview, prototype, technical preview/technology preview,* or *early access.* Some software is kept in perpetual beta, where new features and functionality are continually added to the software without establishing a firm "final" release.

Beta testers are people who actively report issues of beta software. They are usually customers or representatives of prospective customers of the organization that develops the software. Beta testers tend to volunteer their services free of charge but often receive versions of the product they test, discounts on the release version, or other incentives.

18.9.4 Resistance to Beta Testing by Staff

> Since you know version 1 is going to suck, hurry up and ship it so you can start working on version 2 immediately.
>
> **Google Proverb**

Frequently, the entrepreneur is faced with fierce internal resistance to product use outside beta testing by the technical staff, as shown below:

- We already spent a fortune on the product.
- Competitors are working on a similar product. We need to rush.
- It suggests management's lack of faith in the product developed.
- Customers have to learn how to use the product.
- Larger competitors will steal our idea and beat us to the market.
- Market research says our product is a winner as it currently stands.
- If it ain't broke, don't fix it.

18.9.5 Effective Beta Testing

Many well-intentioned companies hold beta tests for the wrong reasons, and waste months of time in the process. Michael Bolton [19] offered some practical ways of optimizing your beta test program, as seen below.

The outside beta test can be a very exciting stage in the software development process. Dedicated, loyal customers who are anxious to see your company and its products succeed eagerly download the software, thereby exposing it to a much broader range of platforms than you can hope to have available in your lab—and all for free. The marketing department is thrilled because your product is being exposed to privileged customers who will spread great word of mouth before your product hits the shelves. For the product team, the release of a beta is usually regarded as the last milestone before the retail version of the product ships.

Beta tests can, however, be laden with unfulfilled promise and wasted cycles. Testers don't always find defects or report them—often you'll get a number of beta test reports that say nothing more than "everything's great!". Many of the defects that are reported are trivial. Some testers—especially the better ones—report a few defects, and then are never heard from again. A large beta test might be a useful publicity stunt, but it's debatable that numbers alone improve the quality of the test. Microsoft proudly announces that tens of thousands have beta tested Office and Windows. Ever seen a defect in any of those products?

A beta test, like life itself, is like a sewer: what you get out of it depends on what you put into it. The beta cycle can be used purely as a marketing ploy, with little useful feedback for engineering. However, if you prepare your product carefully, choose your testers wisely, and provide testers with appropriate incentives, you can get useful information from the beta. There are a few issues for which you should prepare:

- Consider the purpose of your beta test. If your organization's priority is solely to send out a trial balloon for the product, prepare to spend several months debating the merits of the feedback with the marketing department and be ready for lots of recriminations later on. If you want useful feedback, prepare your product and your team carefully before the beta release.

- Each defect that an outside beta tester finds costs plenty of time to your organization. It doesn't take many defects before that time begins to turn into staff-months.

- It's essential to prevent the reporting of defects that are already known inside your organization; the easiest way to do this is simply to eliminate those defects before releasing the beta.

- The best outside beta testers cannot match the defect counts for qualified internal testing groups and quality assurance. Make sure that your quality assurance team has had a chance to find defects and that your product teams has resolved them if you wish to get the greatest possible value from an outside test.

- "Beta fatigue" can set in; it's difficult to get outside beta testers to commit their time, especially over a long program.

- Both your installation and uninstallation routines have to be rock solid. Otherwise, later beta versions will not be installed on clean systems—but the released product will.

- If features are missing in an early beta, they won't get the coverage in later cycles than they might have in the early rounds.

In a well-written function, the best way to assure optimal performance is to reduce extra work and wasted cycles inside loops. If function takes a value, does some work, and returns exactly the same value, most people would remove that function from the code, and yet exactly this kind of suboptimal performance appears when a product with plenty of known defects is released to beta test. Consider two scenarios:

Case 0:

- It takes a developer n minutes to fix a defect that he knows about.

Case 1:

- An outside beta tester takes 5 min to test long enough to find a given problem.

- The beta tester takes 2 min to reproduce the problem.
- The beta tester takes 5 min to write up the report.
- The Beta Test Coordinator (BTC), QA person, or program manager takes 3 min to read the report and to consider whether the defect has been reported before.
- The BTC takes 3 min to enter the defect into the defect tracking system.
- It takes 3 min for a developer to read the report and recognize that he knew about the problem already and otherwise process the report.
- The developer takes n minutes to fix the defect (which he already knew about, remember?).
- Having fixed the defect, the developer takes 2 min to note the problem fixed in the defect tracking system.
- The QA person takes 2 min to read the report, in preparation to verify that the problem is fixed.
- The QA person takes 3 min to set up, retest, and verify that the problem is fixed.
- The QA person takes 2 min to check the report off as fixed in the defect tracking system.
- The BTC takes 2 min to write a note to the original beta tester, asking to verify that the problem is fixed.
- The beta tester takes 5 min to retest the problem and to verify that the problem is fixed.
- The beta tester takes 3 min to prepare a message to the BTC confirming the fix.
- The BTC takes 2 min to mark the report as close in the defect tracking system.

Bolton considers most of these time estimates to be hopelessly optimistic in general, although the estimate for each step might be reasonable in a best-case scenario. I haven't included the time associated with processing the same report from two or more different testers. Moreover, I have not included any wait states in this breakdown; there's going to be considerable lag time between the time the tester submits his report and the time that the BTC enters the report in the defect tracker, for instance. Turnaround times of a day are easy to imagine at several of the steps described above.

But even ignoring all those factors, look at the difference between scenarios! In the first case, the developer fixes the known problem before the beta, which takes n minutes. In the second case, a whole bunch of other people get involved pointlessly, and that costs n plus 42 min, according to my highly optimistic assessment. Multiply that by a thousand defect reports—which would not be uncommon for beta test programs that I have observed—and you've got 42,000 staff minutes. That translates to 700 staff hours or 17 staff weeks of wasted time, or to put it another way, you're wasting four people's time for a month for every thousand reports—all to get to exactly the same place you would have been had the beta shipped without the known, fixable defects, and that's just the *wasted* time—never mind the time that the product team needs to do the rest of their jobs. While developers, QA people, and outside testers are distracting themselves with the known defects, the unknown ones still lurk.

If the process above were rendered as a program function in C, most developers would have no problem in identifying the wasted cycles, and immediately would optimize out the unnecessary steps. Why not do in real life what you'd do in a few minutes in front of a debugger?

The most important optimization by far is to eliminate defects as early as possible in the development process. Most people consider fixing defects to be unpleasant; it's a lot more fun and a lot more exciting to add features. However, it's a much better use of time to address problems while they're fresh in your mind, and before the problems become embedded in the program's source. That means subjecting the requirements, the functional specification, and the source itself to review, with the goal of eliminating defects before they start to waste cycles.

Many people equate defects with programming errors. However, to paraphrase Gerald Weinberg, a program that has a lousy design but no programming errors is still a lousy program. The most important person in the program's design is the person who is going to use it. Make sure that the program follows the user's task, rather making the user follow the programmers' functions and procedures. Forestall the first wave of beta test reports—in most betas, you'll get plenty of suggestions on how to improve the user interface or the feature set of the program—by being highly conscious of the user during the design process, by reviewing functional specifications and prototypes carefully, and by performing usability testing on your product long before the beta ships.

Programmers are sometimes resistant to participating in code review. Usually, the problem relates to ego and insecurity; sometimes, additional resistance comes from bad experience. However, review is used by all other forms of engineering. No one would consider working alone to build a bridge, and no engineering company would permit it. Development managers should make sure that the reviews are conducted by the development team with the goal of finding *defects*, not with finding *fault*. Code review is also a very inexpensive way for developers to teach and to learn. If a developer is absolutely certain that his code is robust and free from defects, he is probably wrong, but in any case, you can leverage his pride to suggest that he teach his defect prevention techniques to other developers.

Automated tools, such as Lint and BoundsChecker, can find subtle problems, improving quality while saving enormous amounts of time. Remember also that testing alone tells you neither about the cause of the problem nor where to find it in the code. Unless you choose to look for it, a defect such as a null pointer or a memory leak can easily lie submerged until the product ships to paying customers.

A product's installation program is often written by a junior programmer with relatively little supervision. However, the installation program is critical to assuring a good beta test. If a program cannot be installed at all, you will lose an entire beta cycle for each tester affected by the problem. If the product seems to install correctly but leaves out something crucial, testers will report problems that don't really exist in the core product, netting you nothing but red herrings and unnecessary work. Finally, if the product doesn't uninstall correctly, later beta cycles may fail to identify problems with missing files or configuration settings—those items will be left on the tester's platform from the previous cycle. For this reason, the installation program should be reviewed by senior developers and checked carefully against the product's specifications—another good way for experienced programmers to bring the junior ones along.

Several studies have shown that outside beta testers are dramatically less effective than internal QA staff. There are several reasons for this: QA staff have experience with the product, and often have access to the developers. Good management and a good test plan mean that QA tests more methodically and thoroughly than any outsider could; an outsider usually cannot hope to have the preparation or the discipline that a well-managed QA team can. Outside beta testers might not provide the kind of clarity or consistency that you expect from your own staff. Finally, there's a motivational issue. Your QA department is being paid to test your software; outside testers are typically volunteers.

There are a few obvious ways to improve on this. The first is to qualify your outside testers and to continue to monitor the quantity and quality of problem reports that you receive. If you find that a tester is costing time by returning inadequate reports, drop him from the program. Because of the high cost of processing a report, the quality of beta testers is generally more important than the quantity. Second, prepare your testers; provide them with instructions and tools to help make their reports detailed, consistent, and efficient. Get detailed data on their test platforms once; assign that system an identifier, and make sure that the tester includes the identifier in defect reports. Give your testers clear instructions on testing goals and the areas of the product that you expect them to inspect. If you are aware of any serious problems, note them carefully and clearly. Don't send a product whose feature set is not complete; first, you'll get remarks on the missing features, and second, after you add the feature, it will receive less testing coverage than the rest of the product. On later rounds of the test, use your problem tracking tool to generate a report that indicates clearly which problems have been fixed.

Provide incentives to your testers for producing plenty of clear reports. A free copy of the released software is fine as a courtesy to all of the testers, but it's not likely to be an inducement toward spending several hours on serious testing and clear reporting, which is what you're looking for. Consider substantial monetary awards for the top three providers of useful reports. You should be able to demonstrate easily a good business case for doing this. Current studies suggest that a single technical support call costs a minimum of $20; finding a single defect that generates five calls is worth $100.

Most importantly, remember that you waste your testers' time and your own by releasing beta products without finding and resolving all of the clear, obvious defects first. Beta testers want to find and report defects; if you make defects too easy to find, they'll simply find and report the easy ones. If your product has defects that can be resolved, don't stick to the beta release date just to say that you made it; you'll cause far more work for your product team almost immediately. Check the business case: it's usually worth delaying your beta release for a few days or even weeks, since each known defect that generates a report has a high probability of taking an hour or more of staff time away from your organization.

> A beta test can give you valuable feedback and the assurance that your product works on a wide variety of platforms. By releasing a product that is truly ready for the test, and by preparing your testers properly, you can make sure that the positive feedback does not cost you unnecessary time and effort and helps to improve the quality of your product.

References

1. https://en.wikipedia.org/wiki/High_tech
2. OECD Science, Technology and Industry Scoreboard, http://www.oecd-ili brary.org/docserver/download/9203041e.pdf?expires=1442516370&id=id&acc name=guest&checksum=325B7D018E7EB4B9B79354F135227FCE.
3. Business-to-Business Launch Survey Executive Summary, Schneider Associates, Center for Business Innovation at Babson College, 2007.
4. https://en.m.wikipedia.org/wiki/Crossing_the_Chasm
5. Rogers, E. *Diffusion of Innovations, 5th Edition*. Simon and Schuster, 2003. ISBN 978-0-7432-5823-4.
6. https://en.m.wikipedia.org/wiki/Diffusions_of_innovations
7. http://www.harpercollins.com/authors/6863
8. Pragmatic Marketing. Is your product doomed? http://mediafiles.pragmatic marketing.com/pdf/product_launch_doomed.pdf.
9. Shoppel, M. and Philip Davis, P. The Five Secrets of a Successful Launch. BetaSphere whitepaper. BetaSphere is the leading provider of web-based software and customer feedback solutions, http://i.nl02.net/beta0006/data/beta_white_sosl.pdf.
10. http://fortune.com/2014/09/25/why-startups-fail-according-to-their-founders/
11. Why new products fail? http://web.cba.neu.edu/~srabino/marketing/Why%20 New%20Products%20Fail%20and%20NDP%20phases.ppt.

12. The Four Steps to the Epiphany, http://web.stanford.edu/group/e145/cgi-bin/winter/drupal/upload/handouts/Four_Steps.pdf.
13. Kaner, C. Exploratory Testing (PDF). Florida Institute of Technology, *Quality Assurance Institute Worldwide Annual Software Testing Conference*, Orlando, FL, November 17, 2006. Retrieved November 22, 2014.
14. Meyer, B. ETH Zürich and Eiffel Software Seven Principles of Software Testing, http://se.ethz.ch/~meyer/publications/testing/principles.pdf.
15. Atwood, J. Alpha, Beta, and Sometimes Gamma, July 2008, http://blog.coding horror.com/alpha-beta-and-sometimes-gamma/.
16. Definition of betaware in the Free Online Encyclopedia, *thefreedictionary.com*.
17. Beta Test Management Glossary (PDF).*Centercode Asset Library.* Centercode, Inc.
18. https://en.m.wikipedia.org/wiki/Software_release_life_cycle
19. Bolton, M. DevelopSense, 61 Ashburnham Road Toronto, ON M6H 2K4. ©2003, http://www.developsense.com/EffectiveBetaTesting.html.

Section IV

Pathways to Profitability

19

Practical Methodology for Commercialization

19.1 Introduction

As we have seen in previous chapters, commercialization is the transformation of knowledge into profitable products. Commercialization is thus the final step in the process or cycle of introducing a new product or production method into the market. As such, the launch of a new product is the ultimate stage of new product development and the one where advertising, sales promotion, and other marketing efforts encourage commercial success of the product or method.

Commercialization is broken into phases, from the initial introduction of the product through its mass production and adoption. It takes into account the production, distribution, marketing, sales, and customer support required to achieve commercial success. As a strategy, commercialization requires that a business develop a marketing plan, determine how the product will be supplied to the market, and anticipate barriers to success [1].

The process of commercialization is frequently likened to a funnel. At the widest part of the funnel are the many inventions that a company might have for launching a product. As the funnel narrows, the company weeds out ideas based on logistics, launching costs, consumer trends, the overall economic environment, and technical feasibility. Figure 19.1 shows the commercialization funnel.

19.2 Commercializing Knowledge-Based Products

Knowledge-based products are those products that require intensive knowledge of science, tools, techniques, machines, processes, and so on that solve a market problem, improve a preexisting solution to a problem, and are frequently disruptive technologies.

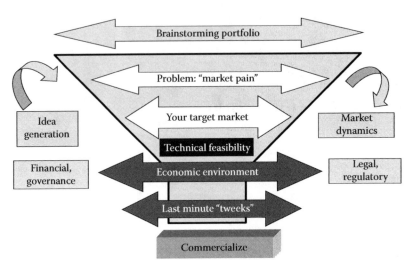

FIGURE 19.1
The commercialization funnel.

Let us make some initial assumptions:

- Your technology actually works under simulated conditions.
- The time for experimentation is over.
- You can manufacture (or outsource) your product at a reasonable cost.
- You can protect and defend your innovation.
- You have financing to support your product launch to the market.

19.2.1 Avoiding Marketing Myopia

Successful start-ups are those firms that can recognize and respond to unmet needs/demands in the market. Unmet needs/demands are plentiful, such as (a) cure for cancer and heart disease, (b) nonpolluting cars, (c) green and sustainable agriculture, (d) desalination of seawater, (e) wireless communications, and so on. However, you can analyze your markets all you want, but there are some parameters that will be noncontrollable, such as

- Demographic trends
- Competitive technologies
- Political/legal environment
- National income

TABLE 19.1

Avoiding Marketing Myopia

Company	Myopic Description	Benefits Description
Apple	We are in the device business	We are in the wireless business
JetBlue Airways	We are in the airline business	We are in the affordable-transportation business
Morgan Stanley	We are in the brokerage business	We are in the financial services business
Revlon	We are in the cosmetics business	We are in the "hope" business

Start-ups need to avoid marketing myopia. Marketing myopia is management's inability to recognize the scope of its business. To avoid marketing myopia, start-ups must broadly define their strategic goals and concentrate on universal customer needs/wants, as depicted in Table 19.1.

19.2.2 Strategic Orientation to Commercialization

You should decide, up front, your marketing orientation. Your marketing orientation will strongly influence your culture and promotional behavior. As Table 19.2 shows, there are four recognized orientations.

Most successful knowledge-based start-ups are customer centric. Customer centric is an approach to doing business that focuses on maximizing customer satisfaction both at the point of sale and after the sale in order to drive profit and gain competitive advantage. The philosophies and operations of customer-centric businesses revolve around their most valuable customers and making sure they are pleased using your product, as summarized in Table 19.3.

TABLE 19.2

Strategic Orientations

1. Market orientation
Based on the customer's perceived values, needs/wants/demands. Focuses on delivering superior customer relationship.

2. Sales orientation
The sales approach will stress those products that the organization can best produce, at the most competitive price.

3. Production orientation
Focuses on the internal manufacturing capability and resources of the firm to manufacture quality products.

4. Societal orientation
A philosophical stance that focuses on preserving or enhancing individual's or societal's long-term interests.

TABLE 19.3

Two Approaches to Knowledge-Based Commercialization as a Start-Up

Technology-Centric Approach *A solution looking for a suitable problem*	**Customer-Centric Approach** *Identifying a commercially relevant problem,* *and then finding a suitable solution*
• Platform technology • Many possible applications • Limited understanding of customer needs • Lack of customer focus • Impossible to prioritize the product features needed • Difficult to assess the commercial viability • High risk	Who are your customers, how many, where • Assess the market potential for your solution • We have a hunch that only we could solve the problem… • How much does the lack of solution cost? • What's the maximum cost to offer attractive ROI to the customers?

19.3 Your Overall Commercialization Plan

Well, you have arrived; you are now ready to commercialize. According to Goyal and Menke of Oracle [2], the following is a comprehensive roadmap to ensure a profitable market launch. Make sure you do not fall into any of the following traps:

Ineffective investments

Too many low-value development initiatives in your company. If your company has too many development initiatives, it is probably trying to develop too many projects that are of low value or outside the company's core strengths. This is an organizational problem in which you fail to prioritize projects because it has no objective way to quantify the value and risks of each project, and because it cannot leverage the company's core strengths. Projects with a high noise level but relatively low value are greenlighted, while other higher-value projects are killed.

Resources overallocated by 200%–300%

Resources are often overallocated by up to 200%–300%, frequently because the company lacks the ability to view the entire development portfolio all at once. This can mean too many projects per person (overloading), or the assignment of people to projects that are outside their actual skill sets, or both. Ineffective allocation of resources in turn leads to various inefficiencies in the productization processes.

Inefficient productization

The key symptoms of inefficient productization include the following:

- Delays of up to 3× over the original schedule, resulting in loss of market opportunity (revenue and market share)
- Budget overruns by 5× caused by constantly changing requirements (moving targets), underestimation of the total cost and time needed to develop the product, and the near impossibility of anticipating product development technical problems and predicting how long it will take to solve them.
- Manufacturing cost overruns caused by the unavailability of parts or by frequent retooling of manufacturing equipment because changes in design.

Products that don't fit the customer

When new product development is inefficient, the final product often does not fit the customer. This means that (1) the product does not solve the customer's core problem, (2) the product is positioned incorrectly so that the wrong customers buy it, or (3) the wrong channel or support is provided for the product.

Low product quality and inadequate customer support

When a high-tech company does not clearly define development modules during the design process, integration testing of the final product is painful. When the company pays too little attention to feedback from its customers, the product gets shipped prematurely. Either way, customers get a poor quality product.

Consequently, the number of customer support calls goes up dramatically, leading to very high support costs, inadequate customer support, and ultimately a loss of business as customers desert the company in droves.

Industry factors unique to high-tech commercialization

Several industry factors contribute to the current lack of profitability in high-tech commercialization, including the following:

Uncertainty

All new high-tech products suffer from uncertainty because of constant changes in the forecasts of their cost, price, margins, and volume. Forecasts of a product's market size and market share also change constantly because of the constantly changing dynamics of competitive forces and new technologies. Finally, there is uncertainty around the technology maturation cycles and customer adoption of new technologies, so it is hard to predict customer receptivity to new products.

Complexity of technology and its many risk factors

By its very complexity, high tech inevitably involves several risks, including the following:

- Technical risks: the technical viability of any initial product idea
- People risks: what are the right skills and the right level of staffing?
- Scheduling risks: delays and project management issues
- Shortages in capital
- Manufacturability issues
- Too many new product choices (too little differentiation) with no effective way to focus on core competencies in order to choose the best options

Platform versus product

It is often necessary to carve a single new product development effort into two projects: a platform project and a specific product project that will use the platform. A platform strategy usually focuses on leveraging a company's key assets to develop sustainable differentiation over an extended period. This platform can manifest itself as a family of products; some products may fail but the overall portfolio based on the platform succeeds. However, when the development effort is not differentiated into platform and product, the company usually loses out on what could have been great future business.

Short product and market life cycles

High-tech companies can no longer keep pace with today's super-short product and market cycles unless they can learn to accelerate their own idea-to-reality cycles.

Industry inflexibility

High-tech companies are often out of touch with changes in the industry, particularly changes in the external technologies on which their own technology depends.

Moreover, they cannot adapt quickly to these changes. For example:

- Customer needs are always changing. It is critical for a company to be able to respond fast to changes in demand.
- Technology gets commoditized quickly, eroding profit margins and revenue when multiple companies offer similar products to the same market. These companies should be

able to change strategy fast, to develop new products and new value propositions quickly.

- New products always depend on the maturation of other infrastructure technologies. For example, a highly advanced CAD application may require a computer with a high-speed microprocessor; if the processor does not exist, the company that makes this CAD application may fail.

Global competition for top-level human capital

Human capital drives new product development in high-tech companies. Unfortunately, there is a global shortage of people with skills in project management (the ability to deliver a project on time, on budget, and on resources) and product management (the ability to decide what products to make, what features these products should have, and, most importantly, what features to leave out).

Increasing role of suppliers as development partners

As companies become highly specialized and recognize their core competencies, they outsource more of the noncore work to other companies. Some of these design partners are suppliers. Thus, companies now need to communicate and coordinate product development with their suppliers. If they cannot manage this communication effectively, inefficient product development is the result.

Increasing role of customers as development partners

Like suppliers, customers are taking on a greater role in product development. This is because customers want increasingly customized products to fit their needs and more options tuned to their particular industry and company. *Leading users are often the best source of breakthrough new product ideas.*

Execution and organizational issues

Your company's leadership or organizational structure often prevents it from executing on new products well. There may be no clear leader to champion potentially viable new products, or the organizational structure may involve too many departments in new product development. In addition, many companies have issues of autonomy versus control.

A development team often needs a great deal of autonomy in order to develop a new product effectively. However, the company headquarters or central planning office, which is usually far removed from the problems this team is trying to solve, sometimes tries to exert too much control over the team. Should this be the case, decentralization may be needed.

19.4 Developing Your Commercialization Strategy

As we have seen, product launch is often the most crucial stage in the life cycle of a start-up. Empirical studies have consistently shown that proficient product launch greatly improves the chances of new product success and even a superior product could fail because of poor launch strategies [3–5].

A product launch involves the largest investment in the entire new product process. The production and marketing expenditures incurred at launch stage often exceed the combined expenditures of all previous development activities [6,7]. This large investment makes successful product launch even more critical for the firm [8].

New product launch is highly risky because new products—either new to the market or to the firm or both—are intrinsically associated with a high level of market uncertainty [9,10]. Forecasts based on prospective market data often cannot accurately capture actual market conditions that are only revealed after initial launch [11,12].

Yet, launch strategies need to be formulated from forecasts and resource commitments made before launch. Firms are exposed to great risk when major discrepancies occur between forecasts and actual market conditions. The sad truth is that commercialization difficulties primarily stem from business issues, not from technology issues, as depicted in Table 19.4.

19.5 "Fat" versus "Narrow" Launch Strategies

Firms can use either (1) a "fat" launch strategy, which involves a large scale of resource commitment and dictates a large target market, large inventory deployment, and large manufacturing capacity; or (2) a "narrow" launch strategy, which involves a small scale of resource commitment and calls for niche marketing featuring small inventory deployment and manufacturing

TABLE 19.4

Business and Technology Issues

Business Issues	Technology Issues
No clear customer sector or segment	Approach already tried elsewhere with no success
Unclear advantages	Small market potential
Benefits and costs unclear	No customers identified
Lack of international experience	Large multinationals as competitors
Inadequate knowledge of markets	References kept as secrets
Inadequate launch budget	Innovation not published in trade journals

capacity. However, because of market uncertainty, the scale of product launch could be either too large or too small compared to actual market demand.

If the forecast is accurate, then the chosen launch strategy matches actual market conditions and the product launch is successful. If the forecast is inaccurate, a fat launch leads to oversupply with excessive inventory and manufacturing capacity, resulting in financial losses; a narrow launch leads to a short supply, resulting in loss of market share and other opportunity costs (see Table 19.5).

Developing your launch strategy depends on the following four key factors:

1. Ensure thorough planning of launch stage.
2. Formal focus by all business functions on the product launch.
3. Demand project sponsorship at an executive level.
4. An evaluation framework and procedure for early market feedback.

Before focusing efforts on developing your product launch strategy, you need to ensure that the product is actually market ready. It is very difficult, time-consuming, and costly to change fundamental elements of the product once the product has been launched. It is well worth having a final internal review of the critical elements before committing to launch. To ensure market readiness, review the four critical elements before launch, as depicted in Figure 19.2.

TABLE 19.5

Forecast-Based Demand at Time of Product Launch

	Actual Demand Lower Than Predicted (Inaccurate)	Actual Demand Accurate
Predicted demand low "Narrow" launch	Success	Small market share Opportunity cost
Predicted demand high	Oversupply with increasing losses	Financial success

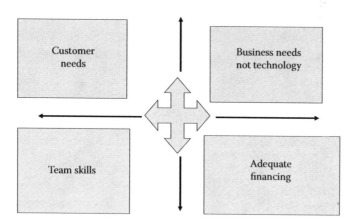

FIGURE 19.2
The four critical elements before launch.

19.6 Marketing Mix: The 4Ps, 4Cs, and the Launch Process

The term *marketing mix* was first coined by Neil Borden, the president of the American Marketing Association in 1953 [13]. The marketing mix is a business tool used in marketing and by marketers. The marketing mix is often crucial when determining a product or brand's launch, and is often associated with the **4Ps**: *price, product, promotion,* and *place* [14].

The **4Cs** are *consumer, cost, communication,* and *convenience.* In contrast to the 4Ps, it focuses on your customer's special needs. The 4Ps and 4Cs can be taken as two sides of the same coin, with one being a buyer's perspective and the other, a seller's. But considering the marketing mix from a 4C perspective is not just an exercise in semantics. Instead, it reflects a change in mind-set to encourage marketers and executives to view their entire process and value chain from the customer's point of view [15]. Figure 19.3 summarizes the launch management process that includes the 4Ps and the 4Cs.

19.6.1 What Are the 4Cs?

According to Entrepreneurial Insights [16], in studying the 4Cs (consumer, cost, communication, and convenience), it makes sense to view them in comparison to the related 4Ps for a more detailed view of both marketing mixes. It may be in the best interest of an entrepreneur to consider both the consumer's point of view and the organization's.

1. **Consumer**

   Here, instead of beginning with a product by itself, the focus is on selling only what the customer specifically wants to buy. This means

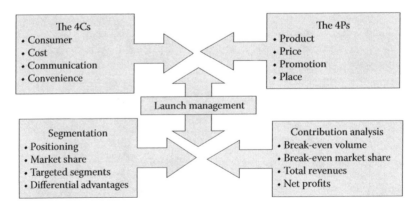

FIGURE 19.3
Launch management at a glance.

that it becomes an absolutely vital activity for the entrepreneur to spend time studying these consumer wants and needs in-depth. Only this detailed understanding will allow a company to sell with accuracy what the customer will buy.

At the core of any marketing effort is the product itself. This, however, is just one piece of the puzzle. The product must be something that the customer finds desirable and there must be something unique about it that sets it apart from the rest of the competition. The most effective way to achieve this is to first find the right untapped market and then develop the product instead of trying to fit a ready-made product into a market. Product testing, therefore, becomes a key element of both the product variable and the customer variable. The understanding should be of what the product can give the customer both in the eyes of the manufacturer and in the eyes of the consumer.

2. Cost

When understood correctly, the cost variable gives more detailed information about the customer than the price variable does. A good way to understand the difference in price and cost is given here. Price is the amount of money that a consumer will be willing to pay to acquire a good or service. On the other hand, cost is the amount that goes into the production of a good or service. This is the sum of the value of all inputs to production such as land, labor, capital, and enterprise.

Within the total cost to satisfy a customer need, price becomes one of the many factors. Other factors may include the cost of time to acquire the product, the cost of conscience when it comes to consuming the product, the total cost of ownership, the cost to change to a new product, and the cost of not selecting an alternative.

There is a common misconception among marketing professionals that the main motivation for a product purchase is the price. Though price-based positioning may provide some initial success, in the long term, this turns out to be a less successful move. If the product is given a price that undercuts cost to gain the market, then the company will be at a disadvantage. If the product is priced at a premium without understanding its value to a customer, it will never be purchased.

Instead, a focus on cost to satisfaction will mean that there is more important information being taken into account than just the purchase price. A focus on this C will help find ways to actually increase the price of the item while decreasing the cost to satisfaction through measures that have a minimal influence on the company's bottom line.

3. Communication

Promotion is a manipulative factor driven only by the seller. Instead, he viewed communication as a more cooperative activity and driven more by the consumer of a product.

A traditional marketing mix uses promotion as a tool to put information about the product in front of the customer. Promotion and its methods continue to evolve with new avenues and means to reach the consumer. Though these methods of promotion remain effective, a niche marketing focus needs a bit more.

Communication will work toward creating a meaningful relationship with the customer with a focus on what they need and what their lifestyle is. The focus is wider and more inclusive of the different forms communication can take. There is more of a give and take between buyer and seller. Looking at advertising as this form of communication can help a marketer understand its market better and increase sales and customer loyalty.

4. **Convenience**

The proliferation of online marketplaces, credit cards, catalogs, and cell phones has made the provision of products to the customer a whole new ballgame. A customer is not bound to actually go to a physical location to meet a need and there is an endless variety of places online to do so. This means that a marketer needs to be aware of how a particular customer group likes to make their purchases in order to make it convenient for them to buy. While place from the 4P model took into account the traditional value chain involved in getting a product into a customer's hand, the convenience variable considers much more.

19.6.2 What Are the 4Ps?

The 4Ps (product, price, promotion, and place) serve as a great place to start planning and evaluating your product launch [17]. A good way to understand the 4Ps is by the questions that you need to ask to define your marketing mix and your launch process.

Product

The product is either a tangible good or an intangible service that is seen to meet a specific customer need or demand. All products follow a logical product life cycle, and it is vital for marketers to understand and plan for the various stages and their unique challenges. It is key to understand those problems that the product is attempting to solve. The benefits offered by the product and all its features need to be understood and the unique selling proposition of the product needs to be studied. In addition, the potential buyers of the product need to be identified and understood.

Price

Getting the right price for a product is extremely important for the success of the company. Unfortunately, sometimes the right price is not easy to determine. Depending on the price elasticity of the product, a 1% increase in price has anywhere from a −20% reduction to a 25% increase in net income.

The most important factor of what ultimately drives price is the customer's perceived "value" of the product. For example, if a company produces software with a unit cost of $10, but the market perceives the product as useful or has the right brand name, the product can then be priced to capture any consumer surplus at $50 or even $80 per unit. However, the product is no longer considered in vogue and thus has little "value"; this time, the product would be priced at only $25.

Price covers the actual amount the end user is expected to pay for a product. How a product is priced will directly affect how it sells. This is linked to what the perceived value of the product is to the customer rather than an objective costing of the product on offer. If a product is priced higher or lower than its perceived value, then it will not sell. This is why it is imperative to understand how a customer sees what you are selling. If there is a positive customer value, then a product may be successfully priced higher than its objective monetary value. Conversely, if a product has little value in the eyes of the consumer, then it may need to be underpriced to sell. Price may also be affected by distribution plans, value chain costs, and markups and how competitors price a rival product.

Another useful tool to help in pricing your product is the "positioning map." This is a helpful framework to analyze where the product's optimal price is positioned against competitors as seen in Figure 19.4.

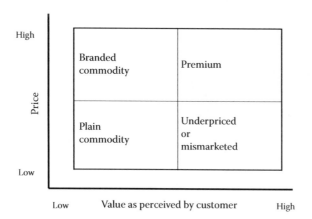

FIGURE 19.4
Price positioning map.

Promotion

The marketing communication strategies and techniques all fall under the promotion heading. These may include advertising, sales promotions, special offers, and public relations. Whatever the channel used, it is necessary for it to be suitable for the product, the price, and the end user it is being marketed to. It is important to differentiate between marketing and promotion. Promotion is just the communication aspect of the entire marketing function.

Place

Place or placement has to do with how the product will be provided to the customer. Distribution is a key element of placement. The placement strategy will help assess what channel is the most suited to a product. How a product is accessed by the end user also needs to complement the rest of the product strategy.

19.7 Your Product "Fit"

In examining the competitiveness of your company's product, whether it is a new product being launched on the market, one needs to examine the product itself. The following are some of the questions that you might find helpful in assessing the competitiveness and "fit" of a product:

- Does the product have the right positioning in the marketplace?
  - Does it serve a particular segment of the market?
  - Is it addressing a mass market or a niche product?
  - Is it differentiated enough to stand out against the competition?
- What kind of brand equity does the product uphold?
  - What are some of the issues/risks associated with the "image" or "perception" of the brand relative to other brands in the market?
  - What are some of the features that can be added to the product that would add to the value or the perception of value to the consumer?
- What are some of the packaging issues that might present an opportunity or impediment to increased sales?
  - Does my packaging reflect the positioning of the product? If mass market, does it have a mass market appeal?
  - What kind of a financial role is the product playing (i.e., cash cow, long-term profit potential, etc.)?

19.8 The Launch Management Process

While R&D is the origin of your knowledge-based innovation and technical differentiation is your competitive advantage, how you launch your product often determines whether it succeeds of fails. In today's competitive global marketplace, a new product generally just gets one opportunity to make an impact, as famously demonstrated by successive Apple new product launches.

A well-planned and executed launch management process will eliminate duplicated efforts and get new products to market faster and cheaper. The first question is: "How do you define launch success?" Without a clear definition of your ultimate goal, it will be nearly impossible to manage the process, reduce risks, or judge the outcome. Table 19.6 summarizes the launch success factors, the 4Ms (*mission, market, message,* and *media*), necessary to define your goals.

The launch managing process will allow you to launch your product to the right market, using the right message through the right media to achieve your launch success, as shown in Figure 19.5.

TABLE 19.6

Defining Launch Success

Revenue Goals	Product Success Goals
Initial market acceptance	Production readiness
Continuing and expanding demand	Timely distribution
Customer satisfaction	Consistent and reproducible product quality

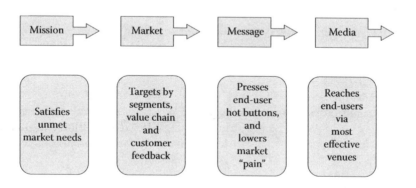

FIGURE 19.5
Managing product launch: The 4Ms.

19.9 Timing Your Product Launch

Time can have a significant bearing on a successful product launch. Your strategy should consider all the relevant internal and external timing factors in order to commit to the ideal time to launch. For example:

Seasonality: If launching into a seasonal market, then the ideal timing may be when the market is in peak phase as this is when most consumers are buying. On the other hand, if you are targeting heavy users of a particular market, then the best time to reach them may be in an off-peak season when they account for most of the buying population.

Internal factors: Like production capacity, they may dictate certain periods for launch as more favorable than others.

Key accounts: Will also dictate timing as they may only have certain times when products can be listed. On average, a lead time of at least 12 weeks should be allowed for a major distributor listing.

Macroeconomics: May also affect timing. For example, if raw ingredients are particularly expensive, then a decision may have to be taken to wait until prices settle or, perhaps, seek an alternative source.

Location: Can significantly affect the success of a launch. There are principally three levels that should be considered within the launch strategy.

Geographical area: What size of area to launch in? This might be a full national launch, a region, or even a cluster of towns. The size of launch area will be driven by the launch objectives. The elected area will depend on what market conditions and consumer profile you need to target. For example, if you are targeting young trendsetters, you may elect certain city-centre areas. The size of your launch market will directly affect the level of investment required and potential sales that can be targeted. It is, therefore, a crucial part of the launch strategy.

Distribution: If your product is not there, your customer cannot buy it. Distribution will be driven by your product positioning and target market. In developing the launch strategy, key distribution channels should be identified. A launch plan should be developed specifically for each account based on factors such as their trading policy, promotional plans, customer profile, and competitive set. This plan should then be presented to each account within their necessary time frames. This presentation is the first stage of securing distribution. Assuming a positive response, further negotiation may take place alongside product sampling. Technical requirements for launch will also need to be supplied, for example, New Product Listing forms, which will provide key technical information such as barcode, case code, sizes, and so on.

Promotion: One of the main marketing tasks at launch is to build awareness and stimulate trial. Not everyone will go on to buy your product a second or third time. Therefore, the key to longer-term success is driving as much first-time trial as possible. Advertising is traditionally the fastest way to build maximum awareness.

19.10 Managing a Successful Launch

There are a lot of elements to manage simultaneously to achieve a successful launch. Moreover, it involves pulling together all the internal functions of the business as well as many external agencies. The task should not be underestimated. At the outset, a project launch team should be established. This should have a team leader who will have the relevant experience and authority within the business to develop the strategy and make it happen. Crucially, the team should also have a team sponsor. This person should be of an executive level and his or her role is to ensure that the business is fully supportive of the launch, the Board is aware of all key elements, and that senior expectations are both met and managed throughout the process.

The launch team should include representatives from all the key internal functions. This will include marketing, sales, production, finance, technical, logistics, and distribution.

At the outset, a critical path should be developed, which includes all the critical operational tasks, dates, and responsibilities. Each function will be responsible for delivering the elements of the critical path with the team leader managing the overall process. Regular status meetings and key task reporting will help ensure every department is working in tandem and the launch is progressing to time.

19.10.1 Beyond Your Launch

Launching the product into the marketplace is not the end; it is the beginning of the next stage. It is critical to plan the management of that next stage before launch. Your launch strategy should include key performance indicators [18,19], which will be monitored to evaluate the product's performance. This may include sales, market share, awareness, and level of market understanding.

Regular reviews will help inform future decisions, for example, if awareness is low, should the advertising or media plan be reviewed? Internal reviews should be regular to ensure that the product is performing at all key levels. Particular attention should be paid to any problems as they arise, for example, production speed or product stability. In addition, reviews of performance versus forecast for sales and profitability will be uppermost in the business' attention throughout the early in-market period. The launch strategy will have set out a time frame for evaluation. Do not be tempted to be too reactive within the early period of launch.

Assess performance carefully and allow time in-market for the performance to build. Ideally, the launch project team should manage the product in-market for at least 6 to 12 months after launch. This team has the greatest knowledge and experience of the product and, given the high level of new information that will have to be evaluated in this period, ensuring that stability at the managerial level makes sense.

19.11 B2B Product Launches

According to Dan Adams, you should think of the expanding power of the Internet, considering the unique behaviors of B2B (business to business) buyers, as shown in Figure 19.6 [20].

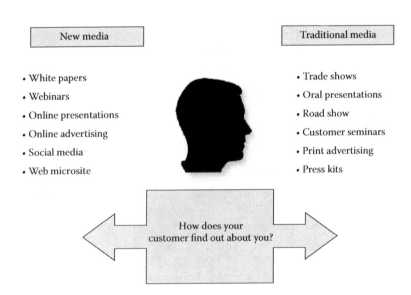

FIGURE 19.6
B2B product launch.

19.11.1 The Five Deadliest B2B Launch Mistakes

The biggest product launch problem encountered by start-ups is lack of preparation: Start-ups are so focused on designing and manufacturing innovative products that they postpone the hard work of getting ready to market their products until too late in the game.

The following are the five deadliest B2B launch mistakes made by start-ups:

1. The product falls short of claims.
2. The product is revolutionary, but no one heard anything about it.
3. The company cannot support fast growth.
4. Product use requires extensive customer education.
5. Failure to develop a post-launch commercialization strategy.

By now, you have your product and it is launch ready. Your business is now poised to introduce the product to market. This post-launch stage, known as commercialization, can be the most testing. This is when your business will need to commit to marketing investment and will rely on key routes to market for their support.

Most importantly, this is the point when you relinquish control to the end user. Now, the end user will decide between product success and failure. Having a clear strategy is crucial to both a successful launch and managing your innovative product in the early stages of its launch life cycle.

19.12 Product Launch and First-Mover Advantage

The product launch involves managing the development and support of a knowledge-intensive product throughout the entire life cycle from product design to product build to post-sale service. It includes the integration of traditional new product introduction (product innovation, design, and collaboration) with sourcing and procurement, supply chain planning and execution, and service—the entire product life cycle [21].

The importance of being first to market is discussed extensively in various sources. Besides the instinctive idea that it is best to be first, other measurable benefits are possible for those that get to the market sooner with innovative products and services:

- Increased sales through longer sales life—The earlier the product reaches the market, relative to the competition, the longer its life cycle.
- Increased margins—The more innovative the product (i.e., the longer it remains on the market with little or no competition), the longer consumers will pay a premium purchase price.

- Increased product loyalty—Getting the first opportunity to attract customers, especially early adopters, offers an advantage in terms of customer loyalty; customers will most likely upgrade, customize, or purchase companion products.

- More resale opportunities—For components, commodities, or products that other companies can private-label, being first to market can often help ensure sales in other channels.

- Greater market responsiveness—The faster companies can bring products to market that satisfy new or changing customer needs, the greater the opportunity to capitalize on those products for margin lift and to increase brand recognition.

- A sustained leadership position—Unlike *best-selling, fastest,* or other superlative market positions, *first* is the market position a competitor cannot take away, and repeated firsts establish companies as innovators and leaders in the market.

19.13 Pharma Launch Parade

Kunst, Natanek, Plantevin, and Eliades from Bain and Company, in their paper entitled "A new pharma launch paradigm: From one size fits all to a tailored product approach," propose that one should move away from a one-size-fits-all approach to a tailored product launch [22].

Many companies have pursued a one-size-fits-all approach to their launches when it comes to positioning, go-to market strategy, and resourcing. That approach may still work for blockbuster assets, but it is less applicable to other pipeline drugs. They claim that the two most meaningful variables were the size of the target population and how payers and providers perceived product differentiation. That insight revealed four distinct product archetypes, each with its own optimal launch approach: (1) Block Buster, (2) Value Buster, (3) Access Buster, and (4) Turnaround Buster.

Plotting product archetypes on two dimensions (perceived value or differentiation and targeted patient population) gives companies a practical approach for planning each launch according to the archetype that best describes its characteristics, as depicted in Figure 19.7.

As Figure 19.7 indicates:

- A traditional **Block Buster** approach will work for products targeting a large patient population and high perceived value and differentiation, but it will continue to require a focus on efficient launch

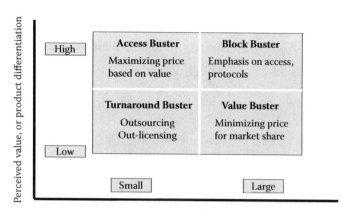

FIGURE 19.7
The four pharma launch archetypes. (Modified after Kunst, M., Natanek, R., Plantevin, L., and Eliades, G. A new pharma launch paradigm: From one size fits all to a tailored product approach. Bain and Company, http://www.bain.com/Images/BAIN_BRIEF_A_new_pharma _launch_paradigm.pdf.)

activities (e.g., Merck's diabetes drug Januvia, which emphasizes digital channels and patient education along with traditional feet-on-the-street and direct to-consumer models).

- For products with a large patient population but perceived *low* differentiation by payers, pursuing a **Value Buster** approach could pay dividends, with a price point 20% to 30% lower to ensure access, and re-sourcing 30% to 50% below the traditional Block Buster (e.g., Sanofi's colorectal product Zaltrap, which was forced to discount price 50% because of perceived similarity in outcomes to those of a competitor).

- For products with a smaller patient population but a *high* perceived differentiation, an **Access Buster** approach will make the most of price based on demonstrated value (e.g., Genentech's highly successful targeted-therapy cancer drug Herceptin, which, while expensive, has retained its price because it demonstrated successful outcomes for HER2-positive types of breast cancer, with a companion diagnostic).

- The most challenging archetype, which we label as **Turnaround Buster**, includes products with a smaller patient population and low perceived differentiation. The best strategy for these products may be to refocus for other indications, delay the launch to capture additional trial outcomes, or simply consider other options, such as outsourcing or out-licensing the technology (e.g., orphan drugs).

19.14 A Recommended Pharmaceutical Product Launch Process

The USC Regulatory Science Program, School of Pharmacy, modified after USC Marshall School of Business, developed a "Technology Readiness Level" for Biomedical Developments [23]. It divides the process into levels as seen below:

Level 1. Basic conceptual development

Basic concept of what the device will do and theoretical principle of how it will work are defined. Design inputs identified and implemented.

Level 2. Proof of concept

Research that validates basic idea and supports feasibility has been done. The design inputs have been defined. Device specifications are defined. A plan for the development of a prototype has been completed. The design process has not yet been initiated.

Level 3. Prototype development

A basic prototype has been designed and built. Development process has been documented.

Level 4. Preclinical research and benchmark testing

Validation tests of device. The device has proven to work under expected conditions in the laboratory. Toxicology and pharmacology studies have been done. Device design has been updated if deemed necessary. Manufacturability and production requirements have been defined.

Level 5. Animal testing

An animal model has been chosen and animal testing has been done to corroborate the safety of the device and to validate design inputs.

Level 6. Clinical trials

A detailed plan for human trials has been developed and executed. The safety and efficacy of the product has been tested. The device design has been validated.

Level 7. Commercialization

The device design has been completed and tested for safety and efficacy. The product is ready for manufacturing and launching.

19.15 A Recommended Medical Device Launch Process

The USC Regulatory Science Program, School of Pharmacy, modified after USC Marshall School of Business, divides the Device Development–Regulatory Readiness process into levels as seen below:

Level 1. Device conception

The development has been identified as a medical device.

Level 2. Regulatory pathway identification

Applicable regulations have been identified. A preliminary regulatory pathway for the device has been identified, along with the resources required to meet product-specific regulations.

Level 3. Regulatory pathway definition

A completed regulatory pathway for the device has been identified. The appropriated notified body (NB) has been chosen. The industry standards that the product will conform to have been identified. Design and quality control systems are in place.

Level 4. Animal testing

Appropriated Institutional Animal Care and Use Committee approval has been obtained. An application for exempt status (Investigation Device Exemption [IDE]) has been submitted. Animal testing has been completed.

Level 5. Preparation for clinical trials

An IDE has been obtained. Clinical studies protocols have been developed. Procedures for inspections by regulatory authority on NB have been established.

Level 6. Clinical trials

Clinical trials have been done after the approval of the Institutional Review Board. Information required in preparation of US Food and Drug Administration (FDA) application/notification to market product has been collected.

Level 7. Regulatory filing

Premarket notification 510(k) or premarket approval has been filed.

Level 8. Postapproval

Clearance for marketing of the device has been obtained. Device has been marketed according to FDA and Federal Trade Commission advertising and labeling rules. Postmarketing device tracking has been performed (class III devices only).

19.16 A Recommended Molecule with Therapeutic Potential Launch Process

Developed with the USC Regulatory Science Program, School of Pharmacy, Drug Development.

Level 1. Molecule identification

A molecule with the potential for therapeutic effect has been identified.

Level 2. Synthesis or extraction of new molecules formulated

Study for the development of new therapeutic agents has begun. Models for pharmacology and toxicology have been designed. Models of manufacturing have been developed. New molecules have been produced. Good Laboratory Practice laboratories have been identified.

Level 3. Preclinical pharmacological/pharmacokinetic testing of compounds

Animals, cell cultures, and tissues, as well as computer models, have been used to explore the pharmacological activity and therapeutic potential of compounds. The potential beneficial activity of compounds has been determined. Drug metabolism has been assessed.

Level 4. Preclinical dosage formulation and stability testing of compounds

The active compounds have the form and strength suitable for human use. Dosage forms and strength have been determined. Design of optimum drug delivery system has been initiated.

Level 5. Preclinical toxicology and safety testing of formulated compounds

The potential risk for the compounds to man and the environment has been tested. Information about dose–response pattern and the toxic effect of the compounds has been obtained.

Level 6. Phase I clinical trial

The new compound has been tested in healthy human subjects on a small-scale basis. The tolerance level at different doses has been established. The pharmacological effects of the metabolism and excretion in humans have been determined.

Level 7. Phase II clinical trial

Controlled clinical testing of a new compound has been conducted in a relatively small number of patients. The new compound's preliminary efficacy and short-term side effects or risks for particular indication or indications in patients with the disease have been evaluated.

Level 8. Phase III clinical trial

Controlled and uncontrolled clinical testing of the new product has been conducted in large patient populations. Additional information about effectiveness and safety to evaluate the benefit–risk relationship of the new drug has been obtained.

Level 9. Commercialization

Clinical trials have been completed. The new drug has been approved and is available for physicians to prescribe.

19.17 A Recommended Drug Development–Regulatory Readiness Process

Developed with the USC Regulatory Science Program, School of Pharmacy.

Level 1. Drug conception

A new potential drug has been identified.

Level 2. Regulatory pathway identified

Applicable regulations have been identified. A preliminary regulatory pathway for the drug has been identified, along with the resources required to meet the drug-specific regulations.

Level 3. Regulatory pathway definition

A completed regulatory pathway for the drug has been identified. Design and quality control systems are in place.

Level 4. Preparation for IND application

Toxicology and pharmacological data have been gathered and a General Investigation Plan has been defined, in preparation for the Investigational New Drug (IND) application.

Level 5. Regulatory Review I

An IND application has been filed and has been approved by the US FDA.

Level 6. Preparation for NDA application

Scientific information about the drug, gathered during the drug discovery and development process, has been documented in preparation for a New Drug Application (NDA).

Level 7. Regulatory review II

An NDA has been filed and has been approved by the US FDA.

Level 8. Monitoring

Periodic reports to FDA have been submitted, including any cases of adverse reactions and appropriated quality-control records.

References

1. Investopedia, http://www.investopedia.com/terms/c/commercialization.asp.
2. Goyal, J. and Menke, J. Commercializing New Technology Profitably and Quickly, Oracle Corporation, 2006, http://www.oracle.com/es/industries/high-tech/022564.pdf.
3. Cooper, R.G. The dimensions of industrial new product success and failure. *Journal of Marketing*, 43(3), 93–103, 1979.
4. Langerak, F., Hultink, E.J., and Robben, H.S.J. The impact of market orientation, product advantage, and launch proficiency on new product performance and organizational performance. *Journal of Product Innovation Management*, 21(2), 79–94, 2004.
5. Montoya-Weiss, M. and Calantone, R. Determinants of new product performance: A review and meta-analysis. *Journal of Product Innovation Management*, 11(5), 397–417, 1994.
6. Beard, C. and Easingwood, C. New product launch—Marketing action and launch tactics for high-technology products. *Industrial Marketing Management*, 25(2), 87–103, 1996.
7. Urban, G. and Hauser, J. *Design and Marketing of New Products*, 2nd ed. Prentice-Hall, Englewood Cliffs, NJ, 1993.
8. Cui, A.S., Zhao, M. and Ravichandran, T. Market Uncertainty and Dynamic New Product Launch Strategies: An Systems Dynamics Model, https://indigo.uic.edu/bitstream/handle/10027/8576/NEW%20PRODUCT%20LAUNCH%20STRATEGIES%20-%20IEEE%20final%20pub.pdf?sequence=1.
9. Bstieler, L. The moderating effect of environmental uncertainty on new product development and time efficiency. *Journal of Product Innovation Management*, 22(3), 266–284, 2005.
10. Chen, J., Reilly, R.R., and Lynn, G.S. The impacts of speed-to-market on new product success: The moderating effects of uncertainty, *IEEE Transactions on Engineering Management*, 52(2), 199–212, 2005.
11. Hitsch, G.J. An empirical model of optimal dynamic product launch and exit under demand uncertainty. *Marketing Science*, 25(1), 25–40, 2006.

12. Luan, Y.J. and Sudhir, K. Forecasting marketing-mix responsiveness for new products, *Journal of Marketing Research*, 47(3), 444–457, 2010.
13. https://en.wikipedia.org/wiki/Marketing_mix
14. McCarthy, J.E. *Basic Marketing. A Managerial Approach*. Irwin, Homewood, IL, 1964.
15. http://www.entrepreneurial-insights.com/understanding-4cs-marketing-mix/
16. Entrepreneurial Insights, http://www.entrepreneurial-insights.com/understanding-4cs-marketing-mix/.
17. http://www.entrepreneurial-insights.com/understanding-marketing-mix-concept-4ps/
18. Warren, J. Integrating KPIs into your company's strategy, http://www.atinternet.com/wp-content/uploads/2012/02/AT_WP_KPI_EN.pdf
19. Peterson, E. The Big Book of Key Performance Indicators, http://www.webanalyticsdemystified.com/downloads/The_Big_Book_of_Key_Performance_Indicators_by_Eric_Peterson.pdf
20. Adams, D. 12 New Rules of B2B Product Launch, http://b2bproductlaunch.com/wp-content/themes/aim-ls/assets/12-New-Rules-of-B2B-Product-Launch.pdf
21. The perfect product launch. IBM. Global Business Services, 2006, http://www-935.ibm.com/services/us/gbs/bus/pdf/ibv-perfect-product-ge510-6281-00.pdf.
22. Kunst, M., Natanek, R., Plantevin, L., and Eliades, G. A new pharma launch paradigm: From one size fits all to a tailored product approach. Bain and Company, http://www.bain.com/Images/BAIN_BRIEF_A_new_pharma_launch_paradigm.pdf.
23. USC Marshall Center for Technology Commercialization University of Southern California, http://www.usc.edu/org/techalliance/pdf/CTC_TRI_Definitions-2007.pdf.

Appendix: Business and Legal Glossary

A

"A" round: Typically the first institutional financing, generally derived from the "A" in Series A Preferred Stock. The venture capitalists invest in a company that was previously financed by founders or angels.

Ab initio: From the start or beginning of something.

Abandonment: Voluntarily giving up a legal right. To surrender, forsake, or cede.

Abatement:

a. Agreeing to reduce payments in some agreed proportion, if there is not enough money to pay them in full.

b. Reducing the bequests in a will, in some proportion, if there are insufficient funds.

c. Cancelling a court order or action.

Abduction: Taking something or someone away by force or muscle power.

Abovementioned: Describing something that has been previously referred or described in the document.

Abscond: When a person fails to appear before the court when required, such as when they have been released on bail and not returned to court.

Absolute: Total, complete, and unconditional.

Absolute discharge: A person who has been convicted of an offense being released without any penalty. (May still be liable to pay compensation.)

Absolute liability: Responsibility without admitting fault or negligence.

Absolute owner: The only legal owner of property such as patents, copyrights, equipment, buildings, land, or vehicles.

Abstract: A summary description and overview of a patent's subject matter.

Abstract of title: Document, drawn up by the seller, summarizing the title deeds to property (such as a house).

Abuse: Contrary to established norms, standards or practice.

Abuse of process: When criminal proceedings are brought against a person without there being any good reason and with malice or malicious intent.

Accelerated depreciation: Provisions yielding larger deductions in the early years of the life of an asset.

Accelerated premium: Guaranteed or enhanced rate of pay for increased production.

Acceleration clause: Provision requiring a party to make payment upon the occurrence of some event or circumstance described in the contract.

Acceleration order: An order by the SEC declaring a registration statement effective (and thereby making sales of securities permissible).

Acceleration request: A letter to the SEC from both the issuer and the managing underwriters requesting that the SEC declare a registration statement effective.

Acceptance: In contract law, when an offer is accepted unconditionally, without duress, thus creating a legally binding agreement.

Acceptor: Person who accepts a draft.

Access: Freedom to approach or to communicate.

Accessory: Someone who encourages or helps another person to commit a crime.

Accessory contract: Contract made to assure the performance of a prior contract.

Accord: Agreement between two parties to settle a dispute.

Accordingly: Word used in legal documents that means therefore or thereby.

Accountable: Liable or responsible to make payment.

Accountant's opinion: A report signed by an independent accounting firm, which describes the scope of the accountant's review or audit and generally expresses their opinion on whether the financial statements are presented in conformity with GAAP.

Accredited investor: A wealthy investor who meets certain SEC requirements for net worth and income as they relate to some restricted offerings. Accredited investors include institutional investors, company directors and executive officers, high net worth individuals, and certain other entities. Some limited partnerships and angel investor networks accept only accredited investors.

Accrual accounting: The most commonly used accounting method, which reports income when earned and expenses when incurred, as opposed to cash basis accounting, which reports income when received and expenses when paid.

Acknowledge: To admit, own, recognize, or accept responsibility.

Acquisition: The act of becoming the owner of property. The process through which one company takes over the controlling interest of another company usually by owning at least 51% of shares.

Action: Using the law to make a claim.

Actionable: Legal grounds for cause of action.

Actionable negligence: Breach or nonperformance of a duty, through negligence or carelessness causing injury.

Actionable tort: A tort for which a legal cause of action exists.

Act of bankruptcy: An act that, if carried out by a person with debts, could have led to bankruptcy proceedings against that person.

Act of God: An unexpected naturally occurring event (such as an earthquake, fire, avalanche or flood) that could not have been anticipated.

Addendum: Something to be added.

Adequate consideration: Reasonable, proportionate, or equal to the value of property.

Adhesion contract: "Take or leave it" a forced contract, without opportunity to bargain.

Ad hoc: Established for a particular and specific purpose. For example, a committee set up to deal with a particular situation is an ad hoc committee.

Adjudge/adjudicate: An official judgment about something.

Administrative agency: Governmental body charged with implementing specific legislation.

Administrative rule making: Power of an administrative agency to make and enforce rules and regulations.

Administrator: Person who has been appointed to manage the affairs of a bankrupt business.

Admissibility of evidence: Evidence can be presented in court. Cannot be hearsay or other evidence of little value to the case.

Admission: One side in a case agreeing that something the other side has alleged is true.

Ad valorem: In proportion to the agreed value.

Adverse witness: A witness who gives evidence that damages the case of the side that asked the witness to testify on their behalf.

Advertise: To announce, make public, inform, publish, or call public attention to any matter.

Advisory board: A group of external advisors to a private equity group or portfolio company. Advice provided varies from overall strategy to portfolio valuation. Less formal than a Board of Directors and without any of the Board of Directors' legal authority.

Affidavit: A written statement that is sworn to be true by the person signing it. Generally, sworn in the presence of a witness.

Affiliate: In close connection, allied, associated; part of the business. A person that controls, is controlled by, or is under common control with (directly or indirectly) the entity specified. The SEC takes the position that a corporate officer, director, or 10% stockholder is presumed to be an affiliate of the corporation. An individual officer's, director's, or 10% stockholder's spouse and children living at home are normally considered affiliates as well.

Affiliate company: Company effectively controlled by another company, branch, division, or subsidiary.

Affinity groups: People who already possess some connection to the developing company, such as customers or suppliers.

Affirmation: Solemnly promising to tell the truth when giving evidence. It is an alternative to swearing an oath during a court proceeding.

Affirm to:

- Solemnly promising to tell the truth in a legal proceeding
- Solemnly promising to tell the truth in an affidavit
- Allowing a contract to continue although it could have been cancelled because it had been fundamentally breached

Aforementioned: Describing something referred to or previously incorporated within the document.

Aforesaid: Describing something which has been said or referred to or previously incorporated within the document.

Aftermarket: Products and accessories sold after the original equipment was sold.

Agency: The legal relationship between a principal and an agent. Fiduciary relation may be employer and proprietor, and principal and independent contractor.

Agent: Someone appointed to act for a principal. Person authorized to act on behalf of the principal.

Aging of accounts: Chronological order of accounts receivable.

Agreed value: Worth or value of property following negotiation or bargaining.

Agreement: A negotiated and legally enforceable understanding between parties.

All hands meeting: A meeting during the public offering process attended by representatives of the issuer, underwriters, their respective lawyers, and issuer's accountants. A public offering will typically involve several all hands meetings to conduct due diligence and to draft the registration statement and prospectus.

Allocation: The number of securities assigned to an investor, broker, or underwriter in an offering.

Allotment: Distribution of shares in a public undertaking or corporation.

Allowance: Deduction, payment, portion assigned, or approved.

Amalgamation: Two or more companies combining.

Ambiguity: Uncertainty of meaning in a written document; doubtfulness. Doubt of meaning between reasonable people.

Amortization: Allocation of the cost of an intangible item over its expected life.

Analyst: A research analyst, usually employed by an investment bank, who "follows" a company and issues reports regarding the condition and prospects of the company and its securities. The quality and reputation of an investment bank's analyst will often be a key component in selecting an underwriter, since analyst coverage of the company after the public offering helps to generate interest in the company's securities.

Ancillary: Auxiliary, collateral, or subordinate.

Angel financing: Capital raised for a private company from independently wealthy investors. This capital is generally used as seed financing.

Angel groups: Organizations, funds, and networks formed for the specific purpose of facilitating angel investments in start-up companies.

Angel investor: A high worth individual who provides capital to one or more start-up companies. Unlike a partner, the person is rarely involved in management.

Angel network: A typically informal network of Angels that invest together as a group.

Annex: To add or join to something of larger importance.

Annual accounts: The summary of an organization's financial transactions during the year covered by their accounts, and a "snapshot" of the assets and liabilities at the end of the fiscal year.

Annual meeting: Yearly meeting of stockholders. Required of public corporations.

Annual report: Yearly report including balance sheet, income statement, and other financial statements. See Form 10-K.

Annuity: A yearly amount paid out to a party.

Antidilution, full ratchet: Antidilution provisions that apply the lowest sale price for any shares of common stock (or equivalents) sold by the company after the issuing of a security with antidilution protection. As an example, if a prior round of financing raised capital at $2.00 per share with investors receiving full ratchet antidilution protection, and a subsequent round of financing was completed at $1.00 per share, the prior round investors would have the right to convert their shares at the $1.00 price, thereby doubling the number of shares they would receive.

Antidilution provision: Provision in convertible securities guaranteeing that conversion privileges are not affected by share reclassifications, splits, dividends, or similar transactions.

Anti-takeover provisions: Provisions in a company's organizational documents that are designed to discourage undesired takeover bids.

Appraisal: Independent value estimate of property.

Apprenticeship: Person who agrees to work for a specified time to learn a trade.

Arbitrage:

- Borrowing money at a low rate of interest to lend out again at a higher rate.
- Buying and selling in different markets to make profits from any price differences.

Arbitration: Act of settling a dispute by using a referee or independent party, thus avoiding costly court expenses.

Arbitration clause: Provision inserted in a contract providing for compulsory arbitration in case of dispute.

Arbitrator: An independent referee who settles a dispute without the need to use the courts, and authorized to render a decision.

Arm's length transaction: Transaction negotiated by unrelated parties, with each action in their own best interests.

Articles: Separate and distinct clauses in a document. Connected series of propositions. One of several items presented as connected or forming a whole.

Assent: Declaration of willingness to perform in compliance with a request.

Asset (asset-based) approach: A general way of determining a value indication of a business, business ownership interest, or security using one or more methods based on the value of the assets net of liabilities.

Assets: Property in general, tangible or intangible.

Assign: To formally transfer something. Appoint, select, or designate.

Assignment: The formal transfer of the rights to a party.

Association: Collection of persons who willingly joined together.

Assumption of risk: Doctrine stating that a plaintiff may not recover for an injury when he voluntarily exposed himself to a known and foreseeable danger.

Attest: The act of signing to witness a signature on a document.

Auction: A process in which an investment bank invites several private equity houses to look at a particular company that is for sale and to offer a bid to buy it.

Audit: Systematic and professional inspection of accounting records.

Audit committee: A committee of the board of directors responsible for selecting and overseeing the work of outside auditors and the conduct of various audit activities, normally composed of independent directors. Public issuers traded on major US markets are now required to appoint an audit committee of not less than three financially knowledgeable independent directors, one of whom must have a background in finance.

Auditor: Person who checks the accuracy, fairness, and acceptability of accounting records.

Auditor's report: A report and opinion, by an independent person or firm, of an organization's financial records, according to applicable standards.

Authorize: To formally empower, to approve an action.

Authorized capital: See Authorized stock issue.

Authorized stock issue: Total number of shares permitted under the articles of organization.

B

"B" round: Typically a second-round financing event whereby professional investors such as venture capitalists provide additional funds after the "A" round of financing. If more than two rounds are consummated, generally the subsequent rounds follow the alphabet (e.g., "C," "D," and so on).

Backdoor listing: A technique used by a private company to become a public company without going through the customary initial public offering process. Such transactions typically involve the private company being merged into a public shell company.

Bailment: Delivery of property from one person (bailor) to another (bailee) who holds the property for a certain period. The ownership of the property is not transferred; that is, there is a change in possession but not title.

Balance sheet: Statement of an entity's financial position, listing assets, liabilities, and owner's equity.

Bank limit: Credit line commitment up to a maximum amount; interest is charged only on the amount actually borrowed.

Bankrupt: Insolvent. Indebted beyond any capability of payment.

Bankruptcy: Procedure by which a person or organization is relieved of debts by a supervised reorganization or liquidation for the benefit of creditors.

Bankruptcy order: Order that takes ownership of the debtor's property away from the debtor and allows the property to be sold. The money raised is divided proportionately between the creditors following strict rules.

Bankruptcy trustee: Person appointed by a court to administer the debtor's property during a bankruptcy proceeding.

Barrier to entry: Economic or technical factor that prevents a competing business to enter a market.

Barter: A way of paying for things by exchanging goods instead of using currency.

Battle of the forms: Conflict between contractual terms during bargaining negotiations.

Benchmarks: Performance goals against which a company's success is measured by investors to help determine whether a company should receive additional funding or whether management should receive bonus stock.

Beneficial interest: Belonging to a person even though someone else is the legal owner. If something really belongs to someone, even if that person does not legally own it, they still derive a beneficial interest.

Beneficial owner: The owner of a property. Beneficial owners have the right

- To the income their property generates
- To use the property for their own purposes

  It can also be a person who owns something even though it is held in someone else's name.

Beneficiary: Person who is designated to benefit from property, an appointment, disposition, or assignment.

Best case: Business scenario based on the assumption that the majority of events affecting the targeted result will be positive.

Best efforts underwriting: An offering in which the investment banker agrees to distribute as much of the offering as possible, and return any unsold shares to the issuer.

Beta: A measure of systematic risk of a stock; the tendency of a stock's price to correlate with changes in a specific index.

Bill of lading: Document recording and enumerating the goods being shipped and the terms under which the goods are being carried.

Bill of sale: Document transferring ownership of goods from one person to another.

Bind: To impose one or more legal duties to a person or organization.

Binding arbitration: See Arbitration.

Binding effect: Requiring obedience and conformity.

Blue sky law: State statute establishing standards for offering and selling securities.

Blue sky laws: A common term that refers to laws passed by various states to protect the public against securities fraud. The term originated when a judge ruled that a stock had as much value as a patch of blue sky.

Board of Directors: Group of individuals elected by the shareholders of a company to promote and safeguard the shareholders' interests, to oversee the general direction of the company and appoint its officers.

Board minutes: Minutes of the meetings of the Board of Directors that record actions taken, typically written after a board meeting and approved at the subsequent meeting.

Bona fide: Latin for genuine, sincere, or in good faith.

Bond: Written promise to repay a debt at an agreed time and at an agreed rate of interest on the debt.

Bonus: A premium paid above and beyond what is expected.

Bonus shares: Additional free shares that a company offers to its shareholders, in proportion to their existing shareholdings.

Book value: The value at which an asset, such as a building or machinery, is carried on a balance sheet.

Brand: A distinguishing name and/or symbol intended to identify goods or services and to differentiate those products from competitors. A product is something that is manufactured; a brand is something bought by a customer.

Breach: Violation or infraction of an obligation or law.

Breach of contract: Failure or violation to carry out a duty under a contract.

Breach of duty: Failure to carry out a duty that is required by contract or law, or doing something the law forbids.

Break clause: A clause in a contract that allows it to be ended before its anticipated date.

Break-even point: A point reached when a company's revenue equals its expenses. In the context of a start-up: point in time when positive cash flow is achieved; generally: point in time when the profit threshold is crossed and a profit is realized.

Break-up fee: A sum agreed between the buyer and seller to be paid by the seller to the buyer if acquisition fails.

Bridge loans: Bridge loan is a short-term loan that is used until a person or company can arrange a more comprehensive longer-term financing. The need for a bridge loan arises when a company runs out of cash before it can obtain more capital investment through long-term debt or equity.

Broker: An agent who acts as an intermediary between bargaining parties.

Broker-dealer: An individual or, more commonly, a group of individuals who have met certain standards and are licensed to buy and sell securities for others (broker) for their own accounts (dealer).

Bulletin board stock (BBS): An over-the-counter (OTC) stock for which bid and ask prices can be obtained from the OTC Bulletin Board operated by the NASD.

Burn rate: The burn rate for a company is the speed per month at which your start-up capital (cash) is being used up before you are able to have positive cash flow. The *burn rate* includes everything that you will outlay money for (wages, marketing, utilities, supplies, licensing, professional fees, computers, etc.).

Business accelerator: A business accelerator is very similar to an incubator but differs in that they usually have a greater focus on companies entering or growing in a national or global market. Business accelerators are more likely to be financed by venture capitalist looking for an opportunity to finance growth potential through defined action plans. Business accelerators will generally offer all of the services offered by a business incubator. The key difference is the level of hands-on involvement.

Business incubator: The definition of a business incubator can be described as a set of programs set up by a government, business alliance, or academic group though a variety of services/training. The intent is to help small companies in the incubator have a better chance of survival through the start-up phase.

Business enterprise: A commercial, industrial, service, or investment entity (or a combination thereof) pursuing an economic activity.

Business incubator: Provides workspace, coaching, and support services to entrepreneurs and early-stage businesses.

Business model: The underlying model of a company's business operation.

Business plan: A business plan is defined for entrepreneurs and micro-enterprises as a method for thinking through your idea. A business plan will answer and identify the Who, What, Why, How, When, and Where, enabling you to create a roadmap for your success.

Business risk: The degree of uncertainty of realizing expected future returns of the business resulting from factors other than financial leverage.

Business valuation: The act or process of determining the value of a business enterprise or ownership interest therein.

Buyback: A corporation's repurchase of stock or bonds it has issued. Also the purchase of a long position to offset a short position.

Buyout: A transaction in which a business, business unit, or company is acquired from the current shareholders (the vendor). Purchase of a company or a controlling interest of a corporation's shares or product line or some business.

Buyout fund: Funds whose strategy is to acquire other businesses and may also include mezzanine debt funds that provide (generally subordinated) debt to facilitate financing buyouts, frequently alongside a right to some of the equity upside.

Buy–sell agreement: An arrangement between owners of a business agreeing to purchase interests of a withdrawing or deceased owner.

By-laws: Rules or administrative provisions adopted for governance purposes.

C

C corporation: A corporation that is subject to taxation as a separate entity. Compare with "S Corporation" and "Limited Liability Company."

Call: A request, demand, or instruction for share redemption before its maturity date.

Call option: A contract that gives the holder the right to purchase securities at a specified price during a specified period of time.

Called-up capital: The totally of shares called by a company when it issues shares. When calls have been made for the whole of the share price and the shareholders have paid, the shares then become paid-up share capital.

Capital: Money or assets available for use by a business. Total value of corporate stock.

Capital allowances: Tax deductions allowances that can be claimed when buying long-term assets, such as machines, to use in a business. The deductions or "claim" are part of the cost against profits before the tax is worked out for the year.

Capital asset pricing model (CAPM): A model in which the cost of capital for any stock or portfolio of stocks equals a risk-free rate plus a risk premium that is proportionate to the systematic risk of the stock or portfolio.

Capital call: Also known as a draw down—When a venture capital or private equity firm has decided where it would like to invest, it will "call" the capital from its investors in order to "draw down" the money. The money will already have been committed to the fund, but this is the actual act of transferring the money so that it reaches the investment target.

Capital gains: The profit realized when a long-term asset held for more than a year is sold or exchanged.

Capital structure: The composition of the invested capital of a business enterprise, the mix of debt and equity financing.

Capital under management: The total amount of funds available to the venture capital or private equity fund managers for future investments plus the amount of funds already invested (at cost) and not yet divested.

Capitalization: The process of converting something into capital. The total amount of long-term financing including stocks, bonds, retained earnings and all other funds. Generally accepted as referring to the sum of a company's long-term debt, stock, and retained earnings. Also called "Invested capital." The items comprising "capitalization" may vary in different jurisdictions. See also Market capitalization.

Capitalization rate: The discount rate used to determine the present value of a stream of future earnings. Equals normalized earnings after taxes divided by present value, expressed as a percentage.

Capitalization ratios: The percentage of a company's total capitalization that each capital component (debt, preferred stock, common stock, other equity) contributes.

Capitalization table or cap table: A table showing the total amount of the various securities issued by a company. This typically includes the amount of investment obtained from each source and the securities distributed—for example, common and preferred shares, options, warrants, and so on—and respective ownership percentages.

Capitalize: To record an outlay as an asset (as opposed to an expense), which is subject to depreciation or amortization.

Carryover: A tax deduction that cannot be taken in a single year, but may be deducted over a 5-year period.

Case law: Law that is based on the precedent established by previous court cases.

Cash basis: The accounting practice of recording sales and expenses only when cash is actually received or paid out, as opposed to accrual basis. Generally, cash basis accounting is simpler than accrual basis accounting.

Cash flow: The movement of cash during a year as a measure of profitability or liquidity.

Cash flows to equity valuation: A variant of the DCF model, where future cash flows to the equity owners of the company are discounted at the cost of the equity, thus directly calculating the equity.

Cause of action: The legal reason someone is entitled to sue someone else.

Certificate: A document in which a fact is formally attested (and sometimes witnessed).

Certificate of incorporation: A document issued by state authority granting a corporation legal status.

Certify: To authenticate, verify, or attest as being true or meeting predetermined criteria.

Champion: A person in another company who likes your product and is willing to help you gain approval in that company.

Chapter 7: The part of the US Bankruptcy Code that provides for liquidation of a company's assets.

Chapter 11: The part of the US Bankruptcy Code that provides for reorganization of a bankrupt company's assets.

Claim:

- To apply for monetary damages
- To apply for a right
- To demand a remedy
- An application for something such as a right
- Assertion of an existing right

Class or class of securities: Classes of securities are securities that share the same terms and benefits. Classes of capital stock are generally alphabetically designated, for example, "Class C Common Stock" or "Class A Preferred Stock."

Clause: A specific section in a contract.

Claw back option: The right to require repayment of funds set aside for a specific purpose that have been disbursed in a manner inconsistent with or contrary to the rules or agreements governing the disbursement. In the context of an acquisition, a buyer may have "Claw Back Rights" with respect to part of the purchase price if the target company fails to meet agreed upon milestones after the acquisition. In the context of a venture capital fund, investors may have claw back rights if interim distributions result in the fund general partner receiving more than the contemplated carried interest.

Close company: A company controlled by five people or fewer, or by its directors.

Closely held: A corporation in which most of the stock is held by a small number of shareholders.

Closing: Closing is the final event to complete the investment, at which time all the legal documents are signed and the funds are transferred.

Co-investment: The syndication of a private equity or venture capital financing round or an investment by individuals (usually general partners) alongside a private equity or VC fund in a financing round and company management's "friends and family."

Collar agreement: Agreed upon adjustments in the number of shares offered in a stock-for-stock exchange to account for price fluctuations before the completion of the deal.

Collateral: Supplementary but secondary and subordinate. Extra security for a debt.

Comfort letter: A letter delivered by the auditors for an issuer at the time of a registered public offering that typically (a) confirms certain numerical information in the registration statement that can be derived from the issuer's financial records and (b) provides limited negative assurances concerning changes in the issuer's financial condition since the last audit.

Comment letter: A letter prepared by an examiner at the SEC setting forth the SEC's questions and comments with regard to an SEC filing, such as a registration statement.

Commercialization: The ultimate step in the process of monetization of innovative ideas.

Commitment: A partner's obligation to provide a certain amount of capital when the managing partner asks for capital.

Committed capital: The total dollar amount of capital contractually committed to a private equity fund.

Committed fund: A venture capital or private equity investment fund that has its capital committed by investors. Cash may be drawn down by the private equity or VC managers usually on a deal-by-deal basis (up to the maximum of each partner's commitment).

Commodity business: A business for which you must have the lowest cost to survive.

Common seal: The seal companies use to authenticate (validate) important company documents. The company's name is engraved on the seal.

Common stock: A unit of ownership of a corporation. In the case of a public company, the stock is traded between investors on various exchanges. Owners of common stock are typically entitled to vote on the selection of directors and other important events and in some cases receive dividends on their holdings. Investors who purchase common stock hope that the stock price will increase so the value of their investment will appreciate. Common stock offers no performance guarantees. Additionally, in the event that a corporation is liquidated, the claims of secured and unsecured creditors and owners of bonds and preferred stock take precedence over the claims of those who own common stock.

Company: A corporation, partnership, or union that carries on business.

Company buyback: Redemption or repurchase by an issuer of its securities.

Compensation: Financial remuneration and other benefits in exchange for services rendered.

Compensation committee: A committee of the board of directors responsible for reviewing and setting the compensation of certain executive officers of the company. The compensation committee may also be responsible for the allocation of stock options to employees. The committee is typically composed of independent (i.e., nonemployee) directors of the company. The definition of an "independent" director may vary from one market to another.

Competition: A market in which rival sellers are trying to gain extra business at one another's expense and thus are forced both to be as efficient as possible and to hold their prices down as much as possible. Competition is thus a sophisticated yet uncoordinated mechanism that sorts out the actions of millions of buyers and sellers and uses the resulting pattern of supply and demand to determine what shall be produced, in what quantities, and at what price. Efforts or action undertaken by two or more commercial interests to attract business from third parties in the same field.

Competitor analysis: Observation and comparison with rival firms in the same sales market with the aim of understanding their strengths and weaknesses more thoroughly.

Concession: Voluntary yielding to a demand in order to reach a settlement.

Condition precedent: An event that must happen before a contract starts.

Condition subsequent: An event that may happen in the future, and if it does, it will affect a contract.

Conditional agreement: An agreement that depends on a certain event happening in the future. If the event does not happen, the agreement will not start to operate.

Conditional sale agreement: An agreement by which the seller remains the owner of the goods until all the installments have been fully paid and all other conditions have been met.

Confidentiality and proprietary rights agreement: An agreement by which an employee, customer, or vendor agrees not to disclose the company's trade secrets or other confidential information to any third party or to use such trade secrets or confidential information other than in connection with company business. Also referred to as a "Nondisclosure Agreement." If such an agreement is made between a company and its employee, the employee typically also agrees to convey to the company all inventions that the employee develops while employed by the company and represents that the employee is not bound by obligations to a former employer that would restrict the employee's services to the company.

Conflict of interest: Term used when fiduciaries also have a private interest or potential gain in a matter.

Consent: Agreement, approval to something given voluntarily. A contract would not be valid unless all the parties consented to the provisions.

Consideration: The price paid for something.

Consolidate: To unite two or more corporations to create one new corporation.

Consolidated financial statements: Financial statements for a company and all of its subsidiaries as if for a single enterprise rather than for the company on a stand-alone basis.

Contract: An agreement between two or more parties (or groups) to do (or not to do) something, thus creating legally enforceable obligations.

Contract for services: A contract under which materials and services are provided by an independent contractor.

Contract of exchange: A contract to exchange goods without money being involved (barter).

Contract of service: The contract or agreement between an employer and an employee.

Contributed capital: Contributed capital represents the portion of capital that was initially raised (committed by venture capital or private equity investors) that has been drawn down in a private equity or VC fund.

Contributory negligence: A doctrine that bars a plaintiff if the damages were partly the plaintiff's own fault or carelessness.

Control: The power to direct the management and policies of a business enterprise.

Control premium: An amount or a percentage by which the pro rata value of a controlling interest exceeds the pro rata value of a noncontrolling interest in a business enterprise, to reflect the power of control.

Conversion rights: Rights by which preferred stock "converts" into common stock. Usually, one has this right at any time after making an investment. Conversion rights may carry with them antidilution protections.

Convertible security: A bond, debenture, or preferred stock that is exchangeable for another type of security (usually common stock) at a prestated price.

Convertible shares: Corporate securities, usually preferred shares or bonds, that may be exchanged for a set number of another security, usually common shares, at a prestated price.

Copyright: Copyright is a form of protection for published and unpublished literary, scientific and artistic works that have been fixed in a tangible or material form.

Corporate charter: The document prepared when a corporation is formed. The charter sets forth the objectives and goals of the corporation, as well as a complete statement of what the corporation can and cannot do while pursuing these goals.

Corporate venturing: Practice of a large company, taking a minority equity position in a smaller company in a related field as a strategic investment.

Corporation: A body that is granted a charter recognizing it as a separate legal entity having its own rights, privileges, and liabilities distinct from those of its members. The primary advantage of a corporation is that it shields its investors from personal liability for any losses the corporation may experience.

Corporation tax: A tax that companies pay on their profits before any distribution.

Cost approach: A general way of determining a value indication of an individual asset by quantifying the amount of money required to replace the future service capability of that asset.

Cost of capital: The expected rate of return that the market requires in order to attract funds to a particular investment.

Counterpart: An exact copy of a document.

Covenant: A contract or legally binding mutual promises. A protective clause in an agreement. Provisions in a venture capital investment agreement, underwriting agreement, or other financing document whereby the investee company agrees whether or not to do something in the future. Covenants may remain in effect as long as the investors hold a stated amount of securities or may terminate on the occurrence of certain events (i.e., completion of a public offering). Affirmative covenants define acts that the company must perform and may include payment of taxes, maintenance of corporate existence, insurance, property and equipment, environmental and legal compliance, representation of venture capital firm on the board, and so on. Negative covenants define acts that the company may not perform and could include a prohibition on mergers, sale or purchase of assets, amendments to its organizational documents, incurring of indebtedness, issuance of securities, distributions and redemption of securities, and so on.

Creditor: One to whom a debt is owed. A person who gives credit for money or goods.

Cross license: When company A wants to use company B's invention, while company B wants to simultaneously use company A's invention.

Cumulative preferred stock: A form of preferred stock that provides if one or more dividends is omitted, those dividends accumulate and must be paid in full before other dividends may be paid on the company's common stock or junior securities.

D

Damage: Loss or injury to a person or property. Monetary compensation for loss or injury.

Damages: Money claimed or awarded by a court as compensation for loss or injury.

Deal: An arrangement for mutual advantage.

Deal flow: The measure of the number of potential investments that a fund reviews in any given period.

Deal structure: An agreement on transaction terms between the investor and the company defining the rights and obligations of the parties involved.

Death spiral deal: A convertible security where the conversion price is tied to the market price (frequently at a fixed percentage discount) at the date of conversion.

Debenture: A debt secured only by the debtor's earning power, not by a lien on any specific asset.

Debt: Money owed; liability on a claim; sum due by agreement.

Debt/equity ratio: A measure of a company's leverage, calculated by dividing funded indebtedness (debt provided by banks and funding sources; not accruals or payables) by common shareholders' equity.

Debt financing: Raising financing for working capital or capital expenditures by selling bonds, bills, or notes to individual and institutional investors.

Debt securities: Debts that can be bought and sold, such as debentures.

Debt service: Cash required in a given period to pay interest and matured principal on outstanding debt.

Debtor: Someone who owes you money due to an obligation.

Declaration: A formal statement, proclamation, or announcement especially in a document.

Deed: Something done or carried as part of an agreement.

Default: Failure to perform a legal or contractual duty. Failure to discharge an obligation when due.

Deficiency letter: A letter sent by the SEC to the issuer of a new issue regarding omissions of material fact in the registration statement.

Defined contribution plan: A retirement plan in which the employer's obligation is to make a definite contribution into the retirement plan and the employee bears the risk of investment performance by the plan. A defined contribution plan is the opposite of a defined benefit plan where the employer's obligation is to make a definite payment to the retired employee and the employer bears the risk of investment performance by the retirement plan.

Delegation: Act of entrusting or empowering another with authority and responsibility.

Delisting: The suspension of the privilege of being listed on an exchange.

Depreciation: The drop in value of an asset due to wear and tear, age, technology, and obsolescence.

Derivative: A financial instrument whose characteristics and value depend on the characteristics and value of another security (typically a commodity, bond, equity, or currency). Examples include futures and options.

Derivative work: Copyrightable creation based on existing products.

Differentiation: Marketing concept denoting the differences between the features, advantages, and benefits of similar product offerings, that is, how competing products and services differ from one another.

Diligence: Attention to detail. See Due diligence.

Dilution: Diminution of monetary value or voting power owing to increase of total number of outstanding shares.

Director: One appointed to manage, guide, and administer a company's business.

Directors and officers insurance: Professional liability coverage for legal expenses and liability to shareholders, creditors, or others caused by actions or omissions by a director or officer of a company.

Disbursement: Payments.

Discount: A reduction from the stated value of something.

Discount for lack of control: An amount or percentage deducted from the pro rata share of value of 100% of an equity interest in a business to reflect the absence of some or all of the powers of control.

Discount for lack of marketability: An amount or percentage deducted from the value of an ownership interest to reflect the relative absence of marketability.

Discount for lack of voting rights: An amount or percentage deducted from the per share value of a minority interest voting share to reflect the absence of voting rights.

Discount rate: A rate of return used to convert a future monetary sum into present value.

Discounted cash flow method: A method within the income approach whereby the present value of future expected net cash flows is calculated using a discount rate. Also known as DCF.

Discounted future earnings method: A method within the income approach whereby the present value of future expected economic benefits is calculated using a discount rate.

Dismissal: Termination without further actions.

Distributor: A wholesaler, jobber, or manufacturer's supplier that sells to retailers.

Distributorship: Person or company that sells to retailers or individual customers.

Dividend: A portion of a company's earning distributed pro rata to shareholders on an annual basis.

Document: The written record supported by references used to support agreements.

Domain name: The unique name that identifies you to all of the other computers on the Internet (your website name).

Down round: A round of equity financing at a valuation lower than a prior round of financing.

Due: Reasonable, proper, expected, just.

Due diligence: Appraisal required by broker-dealers to inform potential shareholders.

E

Early stage: A state of a company that typically has completed its seed stage funding and has assembled a core management team, has demonstrated some proof of its concept, and has minimal revenues and no earnings. VC firms often invest in early-stage companies.

Earnest money: An escrow deposit made by a buyer to show good-faith intentions.

Earnings: Revenue earned from business operations.

Earnings before interest expense and taxes (EBIT): A financial measurement often used in valuing a company.

Earnings before interest expense, taxes, depreciation and amortization (EBITDA): A financial measurement sometimes used in valuing a company.

Earnout: An arrangement in which sellers of a business may receive additional future payments for the business based on economic performance of the sold business or the buyer (including the sold business) after the sale.

Economic benefits: Inflows such as revenues, net income, net cash flows, and so on.

Effective date: The date of the SEC order declaring the registration statement for a public offering to be effective, at which time the sale of shares to the public can commence.

Elevator pitch: An extremely concise presentation of an entrepreneur's idea, business model, company solution, marketing strategy, and competition delivered to potential investors. The pitch should not last more than a few minutes, or the duration of an elevator ride.

Emerging growth company: The definition of *growth company* is a business beyond the start-up phase but not yet mature. The term *emerging growth company* is used to describe a business that is just coming out of a start-up and entering the growth company category. Most candidates for an initial public offering are emerging growth companies.

Emerging growth stock: A popular term to describe shares of companies large enough to have a trading market, but still in the early stages of an expected period of growth.

Employee stock option plan (ESOP): A plan established by a company whereby a certain number of shares are reserved for key employees. Such options to purchase shares usually vest over several years to serve as an incentive for employees to build long-term value for the company.

Employee stock ownership plan: A trust fund established by a company to purchase stock on behalf of employees.

Employment at will: Employment without a contract that may be terminated at any time by either party.

Endorsement: An agreed change to the original terms of a contract.

Entrepreneur: The person who initiates and assumes the financial risks of a new enterprise.

Equity: The owner's interest in property after deduction of all liabilities.

Equity financing: Issuance of shares of common or preferred stock to raise money, especially when share price is high.

Equity kicker: Option for private equity investors to purchase shares at a discount. Typically associated with mezzanine financings where a small number of shares or warrants are added to what is primarily a debt financing.

Equity net cash flows: Those cash flows available to pay out to equity holders (in the form of dividends) after funding operations of the business enterprise, making necessary capital investments, and increasing or decreasing debt financing.

Equity offering: Raising funds by offering part ownership in a corporation through the issuing of shares of a corporation's common or preferred stock.

Equity risk premium: A rate of return added to a risk-free rate to reflect the additional risk of equity instruments over risk-free instruments (a component of the cost of equity capital or equity discount rate).

Escrow: A deed that has been supplied but cannot become effective until a future date, or until a predetermined event happens.

Ex dividend: Without a dividend. If a share is sold ex dividend, the seller will receive the dividend declared just before it was sold.

Ex works: Available directly from the factory.

Excess earnings: That amount of anticipated economic benefits that exceeds an appropriate rate of return on the value of a selected asset base (often net tangible assets) used to generate those anticipated economic benefits.

Excess earnings method: A specific way of determining a value indication of a business, business ownership interest, or security determined as the sum of (a) the value of the assets derived by capitalizing excess earnings and (b) the value of the selected asset base. Also frequently used to value intangible assets. See Excess earnings.

Exchange: The stock exchange on which an issue is listed (NYSE, AMEX, or regional exchanges).

Exchange of contract: Swapping identical contracts.

Exclusive license: A license under which only the licensee holder has any rights.

Execute: To undertake a contract.

Executed: In contract law, describing a document that is made valid (in the eyes of the law) such as by being signed or sealed.

Executive: A corporate officer at the highest levels of management.

Executive director: A person who usually works full time as a director of the company.

Executive resolution: A proposition for consideration by the members of a company at a general meeting of the members.

Exercise price: The price at which shares that are subject to a stock option may be purchased or sold. Also known as the "Strike Price."

Exit: The sale or exchange of a significant amount of company ownership for cash, debt, or equity of another company.
Liquidation of holdings by a private equity fund. Among the various methods of exiting an investment are trade sale, sale by public offering (including IPO), write-offs, repayment of preference shares/ loans, sale to another venture capitalist, and sale to a financial institution.

Exit route: The method by which an investor would realize an investment.

Exit strategy: The way in which a venture capitalist or business owner intends to get out of an investment that he or she has made. Exit strategy is also called liquidity event: The method by which an owner intends to monetize its company. When starting a new company, the founders should plan for a strategy of "cashing in" on their company. Some exit strategies are as follows:

- Listing the company's stock on a stock market and selling the shares held by the owners
- Selling the company to another company/individual

Expansion capital: Also called "Growth Capital." Financing provided for the growth and expansion of a company, which may or may not break even or trade profitably. Growth capital may be used to finance increased production capacity, market or product development, or provide additional working capital.

Expense allowance: An amount paid by the issuer of a security to an underwriter (most common in smaller, higher-risk offerings) to reimburse it for expenses incurred in connection with a securities offering.

An expense allowance may be accountable (reimbursement against documented out-of-pocket expenses) or nonaccountable (typically a percentage of the offering amount without documentation of the expense).

Expert: A person who through education or experience has developed great expertise in a particular area.

F

Face amount: The amount payable under an insurance policy.

Factoring: The buying of account receivables at a discount. The factor agent assumes the risk of collection.

Fair market value: The price, expressed in terms of cash equivalents, at which property would change hands between a hypothetical willing and able buyer and a hypothetical willing and able seller, acting at arm's length in an open and unrestricted market, when neither is under compulsion to buy or sell and when both have reasonable knowledge of the relevant facts.

Fairness opinion: An opinion as to whether or not the consideration in a transaction is fair from a financial point of view.

FASB: The Financial Accounting Standards Board. The quasi-public body primarily responsible for developing rules governing US generally accepted accounting practices.

Fiduciary: One who owes the duties of good faith, trust, confidence, and candor. This includes people such as trustees looking after trust assets for the beneficiaries and company directors running a company for the shareholders' benefit.

Fiduciary relationship: Duty to act for the benefit of others on matters within the scope of the relationship.

Field of use: Segregated market or territories as described in an agreement.

Financial risk: The degree of uncertainty of realizing expected future returns of the business resulting from financial leverage.

Financial markets: Financial markets are the places where financial instruments are traded. For example, the stock market is where the equity in publicly traded corporations is traded. More specifically, the New York Stock Exchange is where the largest publicly traded common stocks, such as General Electric and ExxonMobil, in the United States are traded.

Financial planning: Analysis of the financial situation of a company and forecasting/estimating the company's future financial development, for example, capital requirement, depending on the actions taken by the company.

Financing: Obtaining or providing financial resources or capital for a project or business.

Firm commitment underwriting: An underwriting arrangement in which an underwriter agrees to purchase all of the securities being offered for resale to the public, thereby, in theory, assuming the risk of finding buyers. In practice, this risk is very slight by the time an underwriter becomes legally obligated to purchase the securities from the issuer, as the underwriters will already have "built a book" of investors who have indicated an interest in buying the securities.

First refusal rights: A negotiated obligation of the company or existing investors to offer shares to the company or other existing investors at fair market value or a previously negotiated price, prior to selling shares to new investors.

First round financing: The first offering of shares by a start-up.

First stage capital: First stage capital is the money provided to an entrepreneur who has a proven product, to start commercial production and marketing, not covering market expansion, de-risking, acquisition costs.

First stage/round: The first round of financing that involves an institutional venture capital fund.

Fiscal year: An accounting period of any 12 consecutive months.

Fixed fee: An unvarying amount that does not vary according to any factor.

Flipping: The act of buying shares in an IPO and selling them immediately for a profit. Brokerage firms underwriting new stock issues tend to discourage flipping, and will often try to allocate shares to investors who intend to hold on to the shares for some time. However, the temptation to flip a new issue once it has risen in price sharply is too irresistible for many investors who have been allocated shares in a hot issue.

Float: The number of shares not held by corporate insiders that are freely tradable in the public market or markets on which a company's securities are listed.

Follow-on financing: Subsequent offerings made at a later developmental stage in comparison to the first round.

Follow-on investment: An additional investment by existing investors, which may be provided for in documentation relating to the initial investment.

Force majeure: An unforeseen event that cannot be controlled and that stops duties under an agreement from being carried out.

Forced liquidation value: Liquidation value at which the asset or assets are sold as quickly as possible, such as at an auction.

Foreclosure: Repossession of property.

Form 10-K: This is the annual report that most reporting companies file with the Commission. It provides a comprehensive overview of the registrant's business. The report must be filed within 90 days after the end of the company's fiscal year.

Form 10-KSB: This is the annual report filed by reporting "small business issuers." It provides a comprehensive overview of the company's business, although its requirements call for slightly less detailed information than required by Form 10-K. The report must be filed within 90 days after the end of the company's fiscal year.

Form S-1: The form can be used to register securities for which no other form is authorized or prescribed, except securities of foreign governments or political subdivisions thereof.

Form S-2: This is a simplified optional registration form that may be used by companies that have been required to report under the '34 Act for a minimum of 3 years and have timely filed all required reports during the 12 calendar months and any portion of the month immediately preceding the filing of the registration statement. Unlike Form S-1, it permits incorporation by reference from the company's annual report to stockholders (or annual report on Form 10-K) and periodic reports. Delivery of these incorporated documents as well as the prospectus to investors may be required.

Form SB-2: This form may be used by "small business issuers" to register securities to be sold for cash. This form requires less detailed information about the issuer's business than Form S-1.

Founder vesting: A term imposed on founders in which their ownership is subject to a vesting schedule, typically 4 years. The purpose of this term is to protect investors from an early, unplanned exit by the founder and to provide investors with the equity necessary to attract a new management team.

Founder's stock: Stock issued to the founders of a company at its inception.

Free of encumbrances: No one else having any rights over something.

Full ratchet: An investor protection provision that specifies that options and convertible securities may be exercised relative to the lowest price at which securities were issued since the issuance of the option or convertible security. The full ratchet guarantee prevents dilution, since the proportionate ownership would stay the same as when the investment was initially made.

Fundraising: The process by which venture capitalists themselves raise money to create a fund. These funds are raised from private, corporate, or institutional investors, who make commitments to the fund that will be invested by the general partner.

Futures contract: A binding contract to buy or sell something on a specific date in the future at a fixed price.

G

Gain: An increase in an amount, degree, or value of something.

General damages: Damages that a court will award to compensate for a wrong done without needing specific proof that damage has been done to the claimant.

General partner: A partner in a partnership who has unlimited personal liability for the debts and obligations of the partnership and the right to participate in its management.

General partnership: Form of partnership in which all partners are general partners. See Partnership.

An organizational structure in which each general partner shares in the administration, profits and losses of the operation.

Generally accepted accounting principles (GAAP): The common set of accounting principles, standards, and procedures. GAAP is a combination of authoritative standards set by standard-setting bodies as well as accepted ways of doing accounting. The conventions, standards, rules, regulations, and procedures that define approved accounting principles.

Going concern: See Going concern value.

Going concern value: The value of a business enterprise that is expected to continue to operate into the future. The intangible elements of going concern value result from factors such as having a trained work force, an operational plant, and the necessary licenses, systems, and procedures in place.

Going effective: The time at which the SEC declares a registration statement effective under the Securities Act of 1933, so that sales (not just offers) of the securities being registered can be made.

Going private: Process of changing a public corporation into a private corporation.

Going public: Popular expression for the process of selling stock to the public for the first time.

Golden parachute: Provision granting an upper-level executive lucrative severance benefits.

Good faith: Observance and adherence of reasonable business standards.

Good faith bargaining: Negotiating with open minds in an effort to reach a balanced agreement.

Goodwill: That intangible asset arising as a result of name, reputation, customer loyalty, location, products, and similar factors not separately identified.

Goodwill value: The value attributable to goodwill.

Green shoe: Term for an underwriter's overallotment option. This name derives from the fact that the overallotment option technique was first used in a public offering of the securities of the Green Shoe Company.

Greenmail: Acquiring a large block of a public company's securities and threatening a takeover, tender offer, proxy fight, or other action for the purpose of inducing the company to repurchase the securities at an above-market price.

Ground floor: A term used for the first stage of a new venture or investment opportunity.

Growth capital: A resource supplied to a growing company with capital limitations. Companies that receive this type of funding are beyond the typical venture capital stage. The reasons why a business would seek this capital input can vary from geographic expansion to development of a new product line to a restructuring of the balance sheet.

Guarantee: Assurance that a contract will be fulfilled.

Guarantor: A person or organization that promises to pay a debt owed by a second person, even if the second person fails to repay the debt.

Guideline public company method: A method within the market approach whereby market multiples are derived from market prices of stocks of companies that are engaged in the same or similar lines of business, and that are actively traded on a free and open market.

H

Harassment of debtors: The illegal act of attempting to collect a debt by threatening or constantly acting in a way that humiliates or distresses a debtor.

Hard money: Capital that must earn a return, for example, venture capital.

Hard sell: The illegitimate sales practice of aggressive selling, intimidation, and urgent decision making.

Hedge: A hedge is typically accomplished by making offsetting transactions that will largely eliminate one or more types of risk. Hedging investors can use derivatives and covered warrants to hedge investments. For instance, if an investor owns a particular stock, he can neutralize the impact of an impending fall in price by buying a put option, selling futures, or buying a put warrant.

Hedge fund: A private investment fund that invests in a variety of assets, utilizing investments and strategies with various long and short exposures and degrees of leverage.

Hockey stick projections: The general shape and form of a chart showing revenue, customers, cash, or some other financial or operational measure that increases dramatically at some point in the future. Entrepreneurs often develop business plans with hockey stick charts to impress potential investors.

Holder: Person with the legal possession of any negotiable instrument and who is entitled to receive payments.

Holding company: A company that effectively controls another company, usually by owning more than half of its shares.

Holding period: The length of time an investment remains in a portfolio. Can also mean the length of time an investment must be held in order to qualify for capital gains tax or certain securities law exemptions.

Home-based business: A home-based business is a business whose primary office is in the owner's home. The business can be any size or any type as long as the office itself is located in a home.

Hurdle rate: A rate of return on investment after which economics of the investment are adjusted or capped.
Minimum return (internal rate of return) that must be earned so that an investment is attractive (venture capitalists typically expect 30%–40%).

Hypothecation: A person giving a bank authority to sell goods that have been pledged to the bank as security for a loan.

I

Incentive stock options or ISOs: Stock options that are entitled to special tax treatment under the Internal Revenue Code. The employee who exercises the option does not have to pay tax until the employee actually sells the stock. However, the employee may be subject to alternative minimum tax. The company does not get a tax deduction.

Income: The money received periodically from employment, business activities, and so on.

Income (income-based) approach: A general way of determining a value indication of a business, business ownership interest, security, or intangible asset using one or more methods that convert anticipated economic benefits into a present single amount.

Incorporate: The act of forming a legal corporation.

Incorporation by reference: The technique of making a secondary document part of a primary document.

Incubator: An entity designed to nurture business concepts or new technologies to the point that they become attractive to venture capitalists. An incubator typically provides both physical space and some or all of the services—legal, managerial, or technical—needed for a business concept to be developed. Incubators often are backed by venture firms, which use them to generate early-stage investment opportunities.

Facility specifically designed to foster entrepreneurship and help start-up companies, usually technology-related, to grow through the use of shared resources, management expertise, and intellectual capital.

Independent contractor: One who practices an independent trade, business, or profession in which they offer their services to the public. The person contracting for their services must have the right to control or direct only the result of the work and not the means and methods of accomplishing the result.

Independent director: A member of the board of directors who is not an employee of the company or affiliated with a controlling stockholder of a company.

Initial investment: First venture-backed investment made in an investee company.

Initial public offering (IPO): The sale or distribution of a stock of a portfolio company to the public for the first time. IPOs are often an opportunity for the existing investors (often venture capitalists) to receive significant returns on their original investment. During periods of market downturns or corrections, the opposite is true. The first sale of stock by a private company to the public. IPOs are often smaller, younger companies seeking capital to expand their business.

Insiders: Directors, officers, key employees, and any other persons privy to material nonpublic information relating to a company. This may be further defined in different countries or markets.

Insolvency: Being unable to pay debts as they become due.

Institutional investor: An institution (such as an investment company, mutual fund, insurance company, pension fund, or endowment fund) that generally has substantial assets and experience in investments. In many countries, institutional investors are not protected as fully by securities laws because it is assumed that they are more knowledgeable and better able to protect themselves. They account for a majority of overall trading volume in most major securities markets.

Institutional investors refers mainly to insurance companies, pension funds, and investment companies collecting savings and supplying funds to markets as well as other types of institutional wealth such as endowment funds, foundations, and so on.

Intangible assets: Nonphysical assets such as franchises, trademarks, patents, copyrights, goodwill, equities, mineral rights, securities, and contracts (as distinguished from physical assets) that grant rights and privileges and have value for the owner.

Intangible property: The type of property that does not physically exist, such as a right, or a patent.

Intellectual assets: The knowledge, experience, and skills that have been obtained, preserved, cataloged, and made available for sharing.

Intellectual capital: Sum of all knowledge in an enterprise. Intellectual capital is the sum of intellectual assets and intellectual property.

Intellectual property: Intellectual assets that have been legally protected. Intellectual property is often referred to as IP. Types of intellectual property include patents, trade secrets, know-how, trademarks, and copyrights.

Interest: The legal right to use property.

Internal rate of return (IRR): A discount rate at which the present value of the future cash flows of the investment equals the cost of the investment. Compounded rate of return on an investment that an investor receives on an investment at the time of sale or other exit. Often used in capital budgeting; it's the interest rate that makes net present value of all cash flow equal zero. Essentially, IRR is the return that a company would earn if they expanded or invested in themselves, rather than investing that money abroad.

In-the-money option: An option is described as "in-the-money" when the market price of the underlying security or commodity is higher than the strike price of the option.

Intrapreneur: An intrapreneur is one who takes on entrepreneur-like ventures within a large corporate environment.

Intrinsic value: The value that an investor considers, on the basis of an evaluation or available facts, to be the "true" or "real" value that will become the market value when other investors reach the same conclusion. When the term applies to options, it is the difference between the exercise price or strike price of an option and the market value of the underlying security.

Invention: A patentable device or process created through independent and nonobvious efforts.

Invested capital: The sum of equity and debt in a business enterprise. Debt is typically (a) all interest-bearing debt or (b) long-term interest-bearing debt. When the term is used, it should be supplemented by a specific definition in the given valuation context.

Invested capital net cash flows: Those cash flows available to pay out to equity holders (in the form of dividends) and debt investors (in the form of principal and interest) after funding operations of the business enterprise and making necessary capital investments.

Investment: An expenditure to acquire property or assets expected to produce revenues.

Investment banks: Investment bank is a financial intermediary that performs a variety of services that includes underwriting, acting as an intermediary between an issuer of securities and the investing public, facilitating mergers and other corporate reorganizations, and also acting as a broker for institutional clients.

Investment risk: The degree of uncertainty as to the realization of expected returns.

Investment value: The value to a particular investor based on individual investment requirements and expectations.

Issue price: The price per share deemed to have been paid for a series of preferred stock. This number is important because cumulative dividends, the liquidation preference and conversion ratios are all based on issue price. In some cases, it is not the actual price paid. The most common example is where a company does a bridge financing (a common way for investors to provide capital without having to value the company as a whole) and sells debt that is convertible into the next series of preferred stock sold by the company at a discount to the issue price.

Issued and outstanding stock: Issued stock of a corporation that is still outstanding and has not subsequently been repurchased by the corporation.

Issued share capital: Share capital that has been allocated to shareholders who have subscribed (asked and paid) for the shares.

Issuer: The legal entity offering its securities for sale or subscription, whether it be a corporation, partnership, trust, or other appropriate entity.
The person or entity that sells securities, negotiable instruments or letters of credit.

J

Joint and several liability: Two or more people responsible for repaying a debt. They are each responsible individually (severally) to repay all the debt as well as being responsible as a group.

Joint venture: A legal entity created by two or more businesses joining together to conduct a specific business enterprise with both parties sharing profits and losses. It differs from a strategic alliance in that there is a specific legal entity created.

Judicial precedent: Lower courts must follow the decisions rendered by higher courts in similar cases. This is called judicial precedent, binding precedent, or precedent.

Jurisdiction:

- The geographical territory in which a court can operate
- The legal power it has to deal with particular cases
- The power it has to issue orders

Just-in-time: The controlling of inventory so that materials are delivered just in time for assembly or manufacture.

K

Keogh plan: A tax-deferred retirement program developed to benefit the self-employed.

Key man insurance: A life and/or critical illness insurance policy taken out by a company to provide a cash sum if a key executive dies or becomes ill, thus covering some or all of the resulting financial loss to the business.

Knockoff: An unauthorized copy or imitation of another product for sale at a reduced price.

Know-how: The specialized information, expertise, knowledge, technique, or skill that distinguishes an organization.

Knowledge-based products: Knowledge-based products are based on the development, distribution, and commercialization of advanced high-technology products based on science.

L

Labeling: Under FDA rules, any written, printed, or graphic matter that accompanies a product.

Lagging indicator: An economic indicator that varies after the overall economy has changed. Examples include labor costs, business spending, unemployment rate, prime rate, outstanding bank loans, and inventory book value.

Later stage: A VC or private equity fund investment strategy involving financing for the expansion of a company that is producing, shipping, and increasing its sales volume. Later-stage funds often provide the financing to help a company achieve critical mass in order to position its shareholders for an exit event, for example, an IPO on strategic sale of the company.

Lead investor: The lead investor is a company's principal provider of capital, such as the entity that originates and structures a syndicated deal.

Investor who has contributed the majority share in a private equity joint venture or syndicated deal. See Syndication.

Lead manager/lead underwriter: The single underwriter that assumes leadership and financial responsibility for placing the securities offered in a public offering. On the cover of a prospectus, the lead manager/ underwriter is typically listed on the bottom of the page on the left-hand side, with the other underwriters listed to the right of the lead manager/lead underwriter.

Lease: A contract between the owner of a property and a tenant, giving the tenant sole use of the property for an agreed time in return for rent.

Letter of credit: A document one bank sends to a second bank asking them to pay money to a named person.

Letter of intent: A written statement specifying the preliminary understanding between parties before entering into a contract.

Leveraged buyout: Leveraged buyout or LBO is an acquisition of a business using mostly debt and a small amount of equity. The debt is secured by the assets of the business. In LBO, the acquiring company uses its own assets as collateral for the loan in hopes that the future cash flows will cover the loan payments.

Liabilities: Debts that a person or organization owes.

Liability: Financial or monetary obligation.

License: A revocable authority to do something.

Licensee: The beneficiary of a license to do something.

Lien: The right to keep possession of property owned by someone who owes a debt, until the debt has been discharged.

Limited appraisal: The act or process of determining the value of a business, business ownership interest, security, or intangible asset with limitations in analyses, procedures, or scope.

Limited liability company (LLC): A legal entity that is not taxable itself and distributes the profits to its owners, but shields personal assets from business debt like a corporation.

Limited partnership: Limited partnership is a business organization with one or more general partners, who manage the business and assume legal debts and obligations, and one or more limited partners, who are liable only to the extent of their investments. Limited partnership is the legal structure used by most venture and private equity funds. Limited partners also enjoy rights to the partnership's cash flow, but are not liable for company obligations.

Line of credit: Similar to a business loan, except that the borrower only pays interest on the amount actually used. Much like a credit card, the business makes periodic payments against the outstanding balance.

Liquidation: Liquidation is the sale of the assets of a portfolio company to one or more acquirers when venture capital investors receive some of the proceeds of the sale.

Liquidation preference: The right to receive a specific value for the stock if the business is liquidated.

Liquidation value: The net amount that would be realized if the business is terminated and the assets are sold piecemeal. Liquidation can be either "orderly" or "forced."

Liquidity: Being capable of readily converting to cash. The ability to quickly convert property to cash or pay a liability.

Liquidity event: The way in which an investor plans to close out an investment. Liquidity event is also known as exit strategy.

Liquidity ratio: Ability to readily pay current debts as they become due.

Listed security: A security that has been accepted for trading on an exchange. To become a listed security, the issuer must satisfy the listing requirements of the relevant exchange or regulatory authority.

Listing: The quotation of shares on a recognized stock exchange.

Listing requirements: The standards to be satisfied for a security to be admitted to trading on an exchange. Listing requirements vary among exchanges and regulatory authorities but commonly include financial standards and levels of market capitalization.

Loan: To lend money.

Loan capital: Money borrowed by an organization for business purposes.

Lock-up agreement: Agreement between an underwriter and certain stockholders of a company requiring the stockholders to refrain from selling their shares in the public market for a specified period after a public offering. This period is customarily 180 days after an IPO and 90 days after subsequent offerings, but may range from as little as 30 days to as much as 1 year or more.

Lock-up period: Lock-up period is the period an investor must wait before selling or trading company shares subsequent to an exit. In an initial public offering, the lock-up period is usually determined by the underwriters.

M

Majority control: The degree of control provided by a majority position.

Majority interest: An ownership interest greater than 50% of the voting interest in a business enterprise.

Make or buy: Decision whether to produce a product or service in one's own company (make) or to purchase it from others (buy).

Management buyout: Management buyout or MBO is the term used for the funds provided to enable operating management to acquire a product line or business, which may be at any stage of development, from either a public or private company.

Management fee: Compensation for the management of a venture fund's activities, paid from the fund to the general partner or investment advisor. This compensation generally includes an annual management fee.

Managing underwriters: The underwriters whose names appear on the cover page of the prospectus and who assist the company in preparation of the prospectus and road show and organize the syndicate of underwriters to sell the securities.

Market (market-based) approach: A general way of determining a value indication of a business, business ownership interest, security, or intangible asset by using one or more methods that compare the subject to similar businesses, business ownership interests, securities, or intangible assets that have been sold.

Method of estimating property value by comparing to similar properties.

Market capitalization or market cap: The number of shares outstanding multiplied by the market price of the stock. Market capitalization is a common standard for describing the worth of a public company.

Market maker: Brokerage and securities firms that are required by the rules of a stock market or exchange to both buy and sell securities of a quoted company, for which they act as market maker, at bid and offer prices that they quote.

A securities professional who helps establish a fair and orderly market.

Market multiple: The market value of a company's stock or invested capital divided by a company measure (such as economic benefits, number of customers).

Market overhang: The depressive effect on the market price of a publicly traded security when the market knows that there are a substantial number of shares that are freely tradable and there is reason to believe the holders may sell in the foreseeable future.

Market penetration: Percentage of the number of customers in the target market that use your product or service.

Market share: The percentage of the total market that a firm controls.

Market value: The amount someone is willing to pay for something.

Marketability: The ability to quickly convert property to cash at minimal cost.

Marketing: The process of researching, promoting, selling, and distributing a product or service. Marketing covers a broad range of practices, including advertising, publicity, promotion, pricing, and overall packaging of the goods or services.

The discipline of promoting and creating a need for products and services.

Material information: Information that a reasonable investor would consider an important part of the total mix of information required when deciding to buy or sell a security, to vote for or against a director or merger, or when making some other investment decision.

Mediation: Professional from an independent person (a mediator) to solve differences.

Memorandum: An informal note or record summarizing terms of a transaction or contract.

Merger: A joining together of two previously separate corporations. A true merger in the legal sense occurs when both businesses dissolve and move their assets and liabilities into a newly created entity.

Merger and acquisition method: A method within the market approach whereby pricing multiples are derived from transactions of significant interests in companies engaged in the same or similar lines of business.

Mezzanine capital: Capital provided in the form of subordinated debt with an above market coupon (typically between 12% and 14% per annum) with warrants to buy equity.

Mezzanine debt: Mezzanine debts are debts that incorporate equity-based options, such as warrants, with a lower-priority debt. Mezzanine debt is actually closer to equity than debt, in that the debt is usually only of importance in the event of bankruptcy. Mezzanine debt is often used to finance acquisitions and buyouts, where it can be used to prioritize new owners ahead of existing owners in the event that a bankruptcy occurs.

Mezzanine financing: Mezzanine financing is a late-stage venture capital, usually the final round of financing before an IPO. Mezzanine financing is for a company expecting to go public usually within 6 to 12 months, usually so structured to be repaid from proceeds of a public offerings, or to establish floor price for public offer.

Mezzanine level: Mezzanine level is a term used to describe a company that is somewhere between start-up and IPO. Venture capital committed at the mezzanine level usually has less risk but less potential appreciation than at the start-up level, and more risk but more potential appreciation than in an IPO.

Minority discount: A discount for lack of control applicable to a minority interest.

Minority interest: An ownership interest less than 50% of the voting interest in a business enterprise.

Minutes: A complete record of the meetings held by members and directors of companies.

Mortgage: Using property as security (collateral) for a debt.

Mutual assent: Agreement by both parties to an offer and acceptance.

N

National Association of Securities Dealers (NASD): A self-regulating organization composed of broker/dealers that the SEC recognizes as a substitute for government regulation. Testing of individual brokers and operating requirements for broker/dealers are administered by the NASD.

Negligence: Failure to exercise the proper standard of care.

Negotiable instrument: A document that

- Is signed
- Is an instruction to pay an amount of money
- Can have its ownership changed by changing the name of payee
- Can have its ownership changed simply by delivery to its next owner

Negotiation: The bargaining process to reach agreement.

Net book value: With respect to a business enterprise, the difference between total assets (net of accumulated depreciation, depletion, and amortization) and total liabilities as they appear on the balance sheet (synonymous with Shareholder's equity). With respect to a specific asset, the capitalized cost less accumulated amortization or depreciation as it appears on the books of account of the business enterprise.

Net income: The net earnings of a corporation after deducting all costs of selling, depreciation, interest expense, and taxes.

Net present value: The value, as of a specified date, of future cash inflows less all cash outflows (including the cost of investment) calculated using an appropriate discount rate.

Networking: Developing business contacts to form business relationships, increase your knowledge, expand your business base, or serve the community.

No shop, no solicitation clauses: A no shop, no solicitation, or exclusivity, clause requires the company to negotiate exclusively with the investor, and not solicit an investment proposal from anyone else for a set period after the term sheet is signed. The key provision is the length of time set for the exclusivity period.

Noncompete clause: A clause in an agreement whereby a party agrees not to work for competitor companies or form a new competitive company within a certain period after termination of employment. Permissible scope of such clause is very dependent on local law.

Nondisclosure: The failure by one party to a contract to voluntarily disclose a fact to the other side that would influence their decision to go ahead with the contract.

Nondisclosure agreement (NDA): An agreement between parties to protect the privacy of their ideas when disclosing those ideas to each other.

Nonexclusive license: An agreement giving someone the right to use something but which does not prevent competitors being given similar agreements.

Nonqualified stock options: Stock options that do not qualify for special tax treatment. Accordingly, there are no limitations on the exercise price, person to whom granted, and so on. In the United States, the option holder has no tax at the time of grant, but will have ordinary taxable income at the time of exercise equal to the difference between the exercise price on the date of option exercise and fair market value on that date. The company generally may take a deduction at the same point in an equal amount if the option were issued as compensation. The taxation regime in other countries is often different from this, but nonqualified options are increasingly being used as part of executive remuneration packages.

Novation: Replacing an existing agreement with a new one with different terms, or replaces an original party with a new one.

O

Obligation: A legal or moral duty to do or not to do something.

Obviousness: In patent law, the quality or state of being apparent to someone with similar skills.

Offer: In contract law, a promise to do something, or not to do something. If the promise is accepted, it becomes legally binding.

Offer document: In the context of an acquisition, the document by which the offer or makes the formal legal offer to target shareholders.

Offer period: In the context of an acquisition, the period from announcement of an offer or potential offer until the closing date for the offer or the date when the offer becomes or is declared unconditional as to acceptances (i.e., the acceptance condition that requires a certain percentage of shareholders to accept has been satisfied) or the offer lapses.

Offeree: In contract law, the person who receives a legally binding offer.

Offeror: In contract law, the person who makes the legally binding offer.

Omission: A failure to do or say something.

Opening price: The price at which a security trades at the beginning of a day or, in the case of an initial offering, at the commencement of its first day of trading.

Option: A type of contract under which money is paid for a right to buy or sell goods at a fixed price by a specified date in the future.

Organizational chart: A graphic representation of how authority and responsibility are distributed within a company or other organizations.

Organizational meeting: In the public offering process, the first meeting after the underwriter or underwriters have been selected, attended by representatives of the issuer, underwriters, their respective lawyers, and the issuer's accountants. The initial portion of the meeting is typically spent reviewing the timetable for the proposed public offering, with the remainder being used to familiarize the underwriters and their lawyers with the company's business.

Over-the-counter (OTC): A market for securities made up of dealers who may or may not be members of a formal securities exchange. The over-the-counter market is conducted over the telephone and is a negotiated market rather than an auction market such as the NYSE.

Outsourcing: Purchasing standard operational services from another business. Outsourced services typically including accounting, payroll, IT, advertising, and more.

Outstanding stock: The shares of a corporation's stock that have been issued and are in the hands of the public.

Overallotment option: The option granted to an underwriter in a public offering giving it the option, for a period of anywhere from 15 to 45 days (usually 30 days) after the effective date, to purchase additional securities from the issuer (usually up to 15% of the shares being sold) at the initial price to the public, for the purpose of covering oversubscriptions for the securities. See Green shoe.

Overhang: A large number of securities that may be released into the market, putting downward pressure on the trading price of the shares.

Oversubscription: Occurs when demand for shares exceeds the supply or number of shares offered for sale. As a result, the underwriters or investment bankers must allocate the shares among investors. In private placements, this occurs when a deal is in great demand because of the company's growth prospects.

Owner-employee: Owner-employee is a sole proprietor or any individual who has ownership of at least one-fifth of the capital or profits associated with a given venture.

P

Par: The nominal amount assigned to a security by the issuer. For an equity security in the United States, par is usually a very small amount that no longer bears any relationship to its market price, except for preferred stock, in which case par may be used to calculate dividend payments. For a debt security, par is the amount repaid to the investor when the bond matures (usually, corporate bonds have a par value of $1000; municipal bonds, $5000; and federal bonds, $10,000), which is also called "face value" or "par value."

Partnership: Voluntary association of two or more persons for mutual benefit.

Partnership agreement: A contract clearly specifying the rights and duties between partners.

Party: Someone who has participated in a contract or agreement.

Patent: Official monopoly for a specified time to prevent others from using an invention.

Patent pending: A statement or notice typically found on an article of manufacture or related documentation indicating that a patent has been applied for, but not yet granted.

Payback period: Time elapsed from an investment is made until all negative cash flows relating to an investment are compensated for by positive cash flows.

Payment in kind (PIK): A feature of a security permitting the issuer to pay dividends or interest in the form of additional securities of the same class.

P/E ratio: Price/earnings ratio.

Penetration strategy: Strategy aimed at achieving a defined market share referred to as the "target penetration" level, for example, by introducing a new product at a low price (contrast with "skimming" strategy).

Penny stock: A stock that trades for less than $1.00 per share. Because they are assumed to be especially volatile, penny stocks are subject to heightened regulation. In the United Kingdom, the term *penny share* refers generally to shares trading with a wide spread and is not limited to shares with low trading values.

Performance: Doing what is required under a contract.

Piggyback registration rights: Contractual rights granted to security holders, giving them the right to have their holdings included in a registration statement if and when the issuer files a registration statement.

Pink Sheets LLC: A privately owned company based in New York that provides broker/dealers, issuers, and investors with electronic and print products and information (including quotes) relating to the over-the-counter securities that are not listed on the OTC or Nasdaq Bulletin Board. The name is derived from the fact that historically the information was printed on pink paper.

Pipeline: Pipeline is the flow of upcoming underwriting deals.

Pitch: The set of activities intended to persuade someone to buy a product or take a specific course of action.

Planning: A detailed method, formulated beforehand, for managing a business.

Poison pill: The most famous anti-takeover device. It normally takes the form of granting existing stockholders (other than stockholders who acquire more than a certain percentage of the company) the option (which can only be exercised upon certain events) to buy more stock on very favorable terms as a way of diluting the position of the person trying to take control.

Portfolio company: A portfolio company is a company or entity in which a venture capital firm or buyout firm invests. All of the companies currently backed by a private equity firm can be spoken of as the firm's portfolio.

Positioning: Concept from marketing; refers to where and how a product or a company is or should be placed from the customer's perspective, for example, with respect to various customer segments or in comparison with competitors.

Post-money valuation: The valuation of a company immediately after the most recent round of financing. For example, a venture capitalist may invest $3.5 million in a company valued at $2 million "pre-money" (before the investment was made). As a result, the start-up will have a post-money valuation of $5.5 million.

Preemption: The right to buy property before others are given the chance to buy.

Preemptive right: The right of an investor to participate in a financing to the extent necessary to ensure that, if exercised, its percentage of ownership of the company's securities will remain the same after the financing as it was before.

Preferred dividend: A dividend ordinarily accruing on preferred shares payable where declared and superior in right of payment to common dividends.

Preferred shares: Shares entitled to a fixed dividend. Holders of preferred shares are treated more favorably than ordinary shareholders.

Preliminary prospectus: The form of prospectus used to solicit indications of interest in an issuer's securities before the effectiveness of a registration statement. In the United States, it contains a legend printed in red ink (hence, it is sometimes called a "Red Herring"), indicating its preliminary nature and that it does not contain final pricing information.

Pre-money valuation: The valuation of a company immediately before investors put new funding into the company. Used as the basis for calculating the investors' price per share and percentage of the equity for the new investment.

Present value: The value, as of a specified date, of future economic benefits and/or proceeds from sale, calculated using an appropriate discount rate.

Price/earnings multiple: The price of a share of stock divided by its earnings per share.

Priority date: The date assigned by the Patent Office when you first file a patent application.

Private equity: Private equities are equity securities of unlisted companies. Private equities are generally illiquid and thought of as a long-term investment. Private equity investments are not subject to the same high level of government regulation as stock offerings to the general public. Private equity is also far less liquid than publicly traded stock.

Private investment in public equities (PIPEs): Investments by a hedge fund or private equity fund in unregistered (restricted) securities of a publicly traded company, usually at a discount to the then-prevailing price of the company's registered common stock.

Private limited partnership: A partnership in which all partners have limited liabilities. It thus exhibits elements of partnerships and corporations.

Private placement: Private placement is a term used specifically to denote a private investment in a company that is publicly held. Private equity firms that invest in publicly traded companies sometimes use the acronym PIPEs to describe the activity. Private placements do not have to be registered with organizations such as the SEC because no public offering is involved.

Private placement memorandum: Also known as an offering memorandum or "PPM." A document that outlines the terms of securities to be offered in a private placement. Resembles a business plan in content and structure. A formal description of an investment opportunity written to comply with various federal securities regulations. A properly prepared PPM is designed to provide specific information to the buyers in order to protect sellers from liabilities related to selling unregistered securities. Typically, PPMs contain a complete description of the security offered for sale, the terms of the sales, and fees; capital structure and historical financial statements; a description of the business; summary biographies of the management team; and the numerous risk factors associated with the investment. In practice, the PPM is not generally used in angel or venture capital deals, since most sophisticated investors perform thorough due diligence on their own and do not rely on the summary information provided by a typical PPM.

Pro forma financial statements: Pro forma financial statements are specific financial statements involved in budgeting and planning.

Proceeds: The net amount of monies received by a company from a public offering; "use of proceeds" describes how a company intends to use the money.

Product liability: The liability of manufacturers and sellers to compensate people for goods that have caused injury to people or property.

Profitability: Profitability is the measure of how much money a venture makes after collecting all the revenues and covering all the expenses. If a bookstore has €10,000 in revenue and €3000 in expenses, then the profitability of the bookstore is €7000 per year.

Promisee: A person who has been promised something.

Promisor: A person who has promised to do something.

Promissory note: A written promise to pay an amount of money at a given time.

Prospectus: A formal written offer to sell securities that provides an investor with the necessary information to make an informed decision.

A prospectus explains a proposed or existing business enterprise and must disclose any material risks and information according to the securities laws. A prospectus must be filed with the SEC and be given to all potential investors. Companies offering securities, mutual funds, and offerings of other investment companies including business development companies are required to issue prospectuses describing their history, investment philosophy or objectives, risk factors, and financial statements. Investors should carefully read them before investing.

A stylized formal document giving details of a company's past performance and of its plans for the future. If a public company wants to sell shares publically, it prepares a prospectus.

Provisional patent: A patent filed in the United States Patent and Trademark Office (USPTO) that establishes an early filing date but does not mature into an issued patent unless the applicant files a regular non-provisional patent application within 1 year.

Proviso: In contract law, a clause in a legal document that qualifies another section of the agreement.

Proxy: A person authorized by a shareholder to go to a meeting of shareholders. The proxy can vote at the meeting for the shareholder.

Proxy form: A written form for shareholders by which, if it is delivered to a company at least 48 hours before the shareholders' meeting, the person who is the proxy will be able to vote at that meeting.

Public offering: An offering of stock to the general investing public. The definition of a public offering varies from country to country, but typically implies that the offering is being made to more than a very restricted number of private investors, that road shows promoting the offering will be open to more than a restricted audience, or that the offering is being publicized. For a public offering, registration of prospectus material with a national competent authority is generally compulsory.

Public relations (PR): The deliberate promotion of a specific image for a business. Often confused with publicity, which is simply the materials used in a specific part of a public relations effort. See more information on Public relations from your About.com Advertising Guide.

Put option: A contract that gives the holder the right to sell specified securities at a specified price during a specified period of time.

Q

Qualification: The attributes to make a person eligible for a high position.

Quick asset ratio: The ratio between current assets and its current liabilities.

Quiet period: The period starting at the time the underwriters and the issuer reach a preliminary understanding and continuing until 25 days after the effective date of the registration statement for IPOs and the effective date for subsequent offerings. During this period, there are various restrictions imposed by the SEC on company publicity.

Quorum: The minimum number of qualifying people needed for a meeting to be able to make a decision.

Quotation: A statement that is reproduced, attributed, cited, and dated.

R

Raising capital: Raising capital refers to obtaining capital from investors or venture capital sources.

Ratchet: Ratchets reduce the price at which venture capitalists can convert their debt into preferred stock, which effectively increases their percentage of equity. Often referred to as an "antidilution adjustment."

Recapitalization: Recapitalization is a financing technique used by companies to defend against hostile takeovers. By recapitalization, a company restructures its debt and equity mixture without affecting the total amount of balance sheet equity.

Redemption: Paying off all the money borrowed under an agreement.

Redemption rights: Rights to force the company to purchase shares (a "put") and more infrequently the company's right to force investors to sell their shares (a "call"). A put allows one to liquidate an investment in the event an IPO or public merger becomes unlikely. One may also negotiate a put effective when the company defaults or fails to make payments upon a key employee's death, and so on.

Reduced to practice: Making a working prototype with all the desired features.

Redundancy: Being dismissed from a job because it no longer exists, or is no longer necessary.

Registered secondary offering: An offering of securities by a stockholder (often an affiliate) of a company that requires an effective registration statement to be on file with the SEC before distribution may be effected.

Registered securities: Securities issued in a form allowing the owner's name to be imprinted on the certificate and allowing the issuer to maintain records as to the identity of the owners. Also commonly used in the United States in reference to securities that are registered under the Securities Act of 1933.

Registration: The SEC's review process of all securities intended to be sold to the public. The SEC requires that a registration statement be filed in conjunction with any public securities offering. This document includes operational and financial information about the company, the management, and the purpose of the offering. The registration statement and the prospectus are often referred to interchangeably. Technically, the SEC does not "approve" the disclosures in prospectuses.

Registration rights: Provisions in the investment agreement that allow investors to sell stock via the public market. Means by which one can transfer shares in compliance with the securities laws subject to Lock-Up and Market Stand-off Agreements.

Registration statement: The document required by the Securities Act of 1933 to be filed with the SEC by the issuer of securities before a public offering can be made. The most frequently used registration statement forms include the following: Forms F-1, 2, and 3 for foreign companies, which correspond to Forms S-1, 2, and 3 described below: Form S-1: The most complete version, required for initial public offerings. Form S-2: Intermediate version, used for public companies already registered under the Securities Exchange Act of 1934 that are up to date with their filings and with payments to security holders. Form S-3: Short version, used for public companies already registered under the Securities Exchange Act of 1934 that meet certain additional conditions. Form SB-2: Similar to Form S-1, but somewhat abbreviated for small business issuers. Form U-7 A: form of registration at the state level for offerings by small businesses that are exempt at the federal level because they are below $1 million. Requires somewhat less disclosure. Form 2O-F: This is an integrated form used both as a registration statement to register securities of qualified foreign private issues under Section 12 and as an annual report under Section 13(a) or 15(d) of the Securities Exchange Act of 1934.

Regulation A (or Reg A): A regulation under the Securities Act of 1933 providing for a simplified form of filing with the SEC, used for certain public offerings of not more than $5,000,000 and exempting such offerings from full registration.

Regulation D (or Reg D): A regulation under the Securities Act of 1933 that exempts limited offers and sales of securities from registration if the offering satisfies certain requirements as to the number and nature of investors and the value of the offering. Advertising and resale are restricted. In general, Rule 504 of Reg D is used for offerings of $1 million or less; Rule 505 of Reg D is used for offerings of $5 million or less, with no more than 35 purchasers who are not accredited investors; Rule 506 of Reg D is used for offerings that are more than $5 million, with no more than 35 purchasers who are not accredited investors, but who must be either sophisticated or represented by a purchaser representative. See Accredited investor.

Regulation S (or Reg S): A regulation under the Securities Act of 1933 that exempts from registration certain offers and sales of securities made outside of the United States by US or foreign issuers.

Regulation S-K: An SEC regulation that sets forth in detail the information to be disclosed in registration statements and periodic reports of public companies.

Regulation S-X: An SEC regulation that sets forth in detail the requirements as to the form and content of financial statements used in registration statements and periodic reports of public companies.

Reporting company: An issuer subject to the periodic reporting requirements of the Securities Exchange Act of 1934, such as the requirements to file Form 10-Ks and Form 10-Qs. A prerequisite to listing on the major exchanges in the United States is that the issuer must be a reporting company.

Reporting company forms (periodic reports): The most common forms under the Securities Exchange Act of 1934 include the following: Forms 3, 4, and 5: Reports to the SEC required to be made under Section 16 of the Securities Act of 1934 by directors, executive officers, and certain other insiders of a public company, reporting their trades in securities of that company or its subsidiaries; Form 6-K: The form filed with the SEC by foreign companies subject to the US public company reporting rules for the filing of information that (a) the company is required to make public under the laws of its jurisdiction of incorporation, (b) it files with the securities exchange on which its securities are traded and which was made public by that exchange, or (c) it distributes to its stockholders; Form 8-A: The form filed with the SEC to register a company's class of securities under the Securities Exchange Act of 1934 concurrently with a company's registration of securities under the Securities Act of 1933. Form 8-K: A form required to be filed with the SEC by any US public company upon the occurrence of certain events such as a change in control of the company, significant acquisitions or dispositions of assets, bankruptcy or receivership of the company, changes in the company's independent accountants, and certain other matters. Form 10: A form required to be filed with the SEC to register a company's class of securities under the Securities Exchange Act of 1934 where no other form is prescribed. Generally used when an issuer has more than 500 shareholders in the United States. Form 10-K: A form required to be filed annually with the SEC by any public company with a class of securities registered under the Securities Exchange Act of 1934 that includes a narrative description of the business, audited financial statements, and other information. Form 10-Q: A form required to be filed quarterly with the SEC by any public company with a class of securities registered under the Securities Exchange Act of 1934 that includes unaudited quarterly financial information and certain other information.

Representation:

- Acting on behalf of someone else
- A statement or promise in a contract

Representations and warranties: Provisions in a venture capital investment agreement, underwriting agreement, or other financing document in which the company provides assurances as to the status of its business and other matters, such as the company's capitalization, key personnel, financial information, brokerage, ownership of properties and assets, litigation, and compliance with legal and environmental requirements.

Required rate of return: The minimum rate of return acceptable by investors before they will commit money to an investment at a given level of risk.

Rescission: The cancellation of a contract.

Resolution: An official decision taken by the members of a company during a meeting.

Restricted shares: Shares acquired in a private placement are considered restricted shares and may not be sold in a public offering absent registration, or after an appropriate holding period has expired. Nonaffiliates must wait 1 year after purchasing the shares, after which time they may sell less than 1% of their outstanding shares each quarter. For affiliates, there is a 2-year holding period.

Return: Return is a concept related to earning power. Return seeks to quantify how much a particular venture pays back those willing to take on the risk of failure. Thus, if the venture will pay a return of 200% if successful, then investors could double their money if the venture succeeds.

Return on equity: The amount, expressed as a percentage, earned on a company's common equity for a given period.

Return on invested capital: The amount, expressed as a percentage, earned on a company's total capital for a given period.

Return on investment: Return on investment or ROI is the profit or loss resulting from an investment transaction, usually expressed as an annual percentage return. ROI is a return ratio that compares the net benefits of a project versus its total costs.

Revenues: Revenues are the funds collected by the company in the process of being in business. For example, if a bookstore sells €10,000 in books over the course of a year, that money is the yearly revenue for book sales to the company.

Right of first refusal: A contractual right, frequently granted to venture capitalists, to purchase shares held by other shareholders before such shares may be sold to a third party.

Rights issue: An issue of extra shares by a company. Existing shareholders can buy extra new shares in proportion to the shares they already hold. The shares are usually on sale at a lower price than the stock market price to encourage shareholders to buy. The shareholders can sell the rights if they do not wish to use the privilege.

Rights offering: Issuance of "rights" to current shareholders allowing them to purchase additional shares, usually at a discount to market price. Shareholders who do not exercise these rights are usually diluted by the offering. Rights are often transferable, allowing the holder to sell them on the open market to others who may wish to exercise them. Rights offerings are particularly common to closed-end funds, which cannot otherwise issue additional ordinary shares.

Risk: The probability of loss or damage. In a start-up organization, risk is the chance of losing invested capital. In a new venture, the probability that the business will fail. Risk seeks to quantify how likely a particular event is to happen. For example, if a particular company is very risky, then the probability of that company failing might be as high as 50%. Compare that to another company that has little or no chance of failing and the first company is significantly more risky.

Risk capital: Risk capital are funds earmarked for start-up firms and small businesses with exceptional growth potential.

Risk premium: A rate of return added to a risk-free rate to reflect risk.

Road show: The process during a public offering in which the management of an issuing company and the underwriters meet with groups of prospective investors to stimulate interest in an issuer. Road shows are conducted during the "waiting period" shortly before the registration statement becomes effective. Road shows may take place in multiple cities and countries.

Round of funding: Round of funding is the stage of financing a start-up company is in. The usual progression is from start-up to first round to mezzanine to pre-IPO.

Rounds: Stages of financing of a company. A first round of financing is the initial raising of outside capital. Successive rounds may attract different types of investors as companies mature.

Rule 144: Rule 144 provides for the sale of restricted stock and control stock. Filing with the SEC is required before selling restricted and control stock, and the number of shares that may be sold is limited.

Rule 144A: A safe harbor exemption from the registration requirements of Section 5 of the 1933 Act for resales of certain restricted securities to qualified institutional buyers, which are commonly referred to as "QIBs." In particular, Rule 144A affords safe harbor treatment for reoffers or resales to QIBs—by persons other than issuers—of securities of domestic and foreign issuers that are not listed on a US securities exchange or quoted on a US automated interdealer quotation system. Rule 144A provides that reoffers and resales in compliance with the rule are not "distributions" and that the reseller is therefore not an "underwriter" within the meaning of Section 2(a)(11) of the 1933 Act. If the reseller is not the issuer or a dealer, it can rely on the exemption provided by Section 4(1) of the 1933 Act. If the reseller is a dealer, it can rely on the exemption provided by Section 4(3) of the 1933 Act.

S

S corporation: A corporation that limits its ownership structure to 100 shareholders and disallows certain types of shareholders (e.g., partnerships cannot hold shares in an S corporation). An S corporation does not pay taxes; rather, similar to a partnership, its owners pay taxes on their proportion of the corporation's profits at their individual tax rates.

Sales: The exchange of a product or service for money. Also refers to the profession of that activity or a department within a company that performs that activity.

Sales velocity: The rapidity at which a product penetrates the market, particularly when compared to other related products.

Sales volume: A quantitative measure of sales, either in terms of dollar amount or in terms of the number of units sold.

Satisfaction:

- Paying a debt in its entirety
- Settling an obligation by an act
- Settling an obligation by substituting something satisfactory for what was or is required in the original agreement

Scope: A measure of the market in terms of its breadth, territory, or sales potential.

SEC: The US Securities and Exchange Commission, which is charged with the administration and enforcement of federal securities laws.

SEC 10-K: An annual report to the SEC providing a comprehensive summary of a company's financial performance.

SEC 10-Q: A quarterly unaudited report to the SEC providing a summary of a company's financial performance.

Second stage capital: Second stage capital is the capital provided to expand marketing and meet the growing working capital need of an enterprise that has commenced production but does not have positive cash flows sufficient to take care of its growing needs.

Secondary market: A market or exchange in which securities are bought and sold following their initial sale. Investors in the primary market, by contrast, purchase shares directly from the issuer.

Secondary public offering: Secondary public offering refers to a public offering subsequent to an initial public offering. A secondary public offering can be either an issuer offering or an offering by a group that has purchased the issuer's securities in the public markets.

Securities: Financial instruments such as stocks, shares, debentures, and so on where there is a right to receive interest or dividends from the investment.

Securities Act of 1934: The federal law that established the Securities and Exchange Commission. The act outlaws misrepresentation, manipulation, and other abusive practices in the issuance of securities.

Seed capital: Seed capital is the money used to purchase equity-based interest in a new or existing company. This seed capital is usually quite small because the venture is still in the idea or conceptual stage. Capital invested at the earliest stages of a business start-up.

Seed money: The first round of capital for a start-up business. Seed money usually takes the structure of a loan or an investment in preferred stock or convertible bonds, although sometimes it is common stock. Seed money provides start-up companies with the capital required for their initial development and growth. Angel investors and early-stage venture capital funds often provide seed money.

Seed stage financing: An initial state of a company's growth characterized by a founding management team, business plan development, prototype development, and beta testing.

Senior debt: A debt instrument that expressly has a higher priority for repayment than that of general unsecured creditors. Typically used for long-term financing for low-risk companies or for later-stage financing.

Senior securities: Securities that have a preferential claim over common stock on a company's earnings and in the case of liquidation. Generally, preferred stock and bonds are considered senior securities.

Series A preferred stock: Series A preferred stock is the first round of stock offered during the seed or early-stage round by a portfolio company to the venture capitalist. Series A preferred stock is convertible into common stock in certain cases such as an IPO or the sale of the company. Later rounds of preferred stock in a private company are called Series B, Series C, and so on.

Service Corps of Retired Executives (SCORE): They provide counseling advice for small businesses. See www.score.org.

Share capital: The money invested directly in a company by its members. When the shares are first made available by the company, investors can apply to buy them. The company determines and states the price for the shares.

Share certificate: A document that certifies who owns shares in a company. It specifies the type and number of shares owned by the shareholder and lists the serial numbers of the shares.

Share purchase agreement/stock purchase agreement: An agreement in which one or more purchasers buy shares issued by one or more target companies from one or more sellers. The agreement will set out/forth the type and amount of shares sold, representations and warranties, indemnification in the event of misrepresentation, and may also include postclosing covenants (such as the obligation for the sellers not to compete with the purchasers).

Shelf registration: A registration statement that covers securities that are not to be sold in a single offering immediately upon effectiveness, but rather are proposed to be sold over a period of time or on a continuous basis. A similar concept is included in the prospectus directive.

Shell corporation: A corporation with no assets and no business. Typically, shell corporations are designed for the purpose of going public and later acquiring existing businesses. Also known as Specified Purpose Acquisition Companies (SPACs).

Silent partner: A silent partner is an investor who does not have any management responsibilities but provides capital and shares liability for any losses experienced by the entity. Silent partners are liable for any losses up to the amount of their invested capital and participate in any tax and cash flow benefits.

Skimming: Pricing strategy in which price is initially set at a high level to obtain a high profit; is mainly used for new products or services for which there are few alternatives for the customer (typically contrasted with a "penetration" pricing strategy).

Small business: Just what exactly constitutes "small?" There actually is an official definition, but it varies widely from industry to industry.

Small Business Administration (SBA): The United States Government Agency in charge with "providing customer-oriented, full-service programs and accurate, timely information to the entrepreneurial community."

Small Business Investment Company (SBIC): A company licensed by the Small Business Administration to receive government leverage in order to raise capital to use in venture investing.

Small Business Investment Companies (SBICs): Small Business Investment Companies or SBICs are lending and investment firms that are licensed and regulated by the Small Business Administration. The licensing enables them to borrow from the federal government to supplement the private funds of their investors. SBICs prefer investments between $100,000 and $250,000 and have much more generous underwriting guidelines than a venture capital firm.

Sole proprietorship: A business owned and operated by one person.

Sophisticated investor: An investor who is deemed to be sophisticated and sufficiently knowledgeable with respect to financial matters that it can fend for itself in the purchase of securities and does not require the full protection of securities law.

Special resolution: A resolution that must be approved by holders of at least 75% of the shares with voting rights. (Some types of share give their owners the right to vote at shareholder meetings, but there are other types that do not.)

Spinoff: The creation of a new independent company from an existing company by the transfer of the assets of one or more business units or product lines of the company to a new corporation and the distribution of stock of that new corporation to stockholders of the old one.

Spinout: The creation of a new independent company by a university or government agency technology transfer unit whose purpose is to commercialize technology developed at such university or government agency.

Split or stock split: An increase in the number of outstanding shares of a company's stock, such that the proportionate equity of each shareholder remains the same. The market price per share theoretically should drop proportionately. Usually done to make a stock with a very high per share price more accessible to small investors. Requires approval from the board of directors and sometimes shareholders.

Staggered board: This is an antitakeover measure in which the election of the directors is split in separate periods so that only a percentage (e.g., one-third) of the total number of directors come up for election in a given year. It is designed to make taking control of the board of directors more difficult.

Start-up: Start-up is a new business venture in its earliest stage of development.

A company at its initial stages of development—even before setup— that typically has little or no earnings and revenues. Start-up capital is typically provided for product development and initial marketing.

Start-up capital: Start-up capital is the amount of cash that is needed for the new business to go from conception to production. It is sometimes referred to as *seed money*.

Stock options: The right to purchase or sell a stock at a specified price within a stated period. Options are a popular investment medium, offering an opportunity to hedge positions in other securities, to speculate on stocks with relatively little investment, and to capitalize on changes in the market value of options contracts themselves through a variety of options strategies.

A widely used form of employee incentive and compensation. The employee is given an option to purchase its shares at a certain price (at or below the market price at the time the option is granted) for a specified period of years.

Stockholder agreement: An agreement among stockholders, typically in a private company, to ensure maintenance of stable ownership and management of a company for the life of the investment. Venture capital investors will typically require a stockholder agreement that may cover, among other things, a right of first refusal in favor of the issuer or other stockholders on a proposed sale by a stockholder of his or her stock, a right to participate in insider sales (i.e., sales by existing shareholders); an agreement to elect certain directors; and provisions as to buyout.

Strategic alliance: An ongoing relationship between two businesses in which they combine efforts for a specific purpose.

Strategic investors: Corporate or individual investors that add value to investments they make through industry and personal ties that can assist companies in raising additional capital as well as provide assistance in the marketing and sales process.

Street name: A term used to refer to securities beneficially owned by individual investors, but registered in the name of a nominee of a securities or brokerage firm, which are then allocated within that firm to the accounts of individual investors who purchase the securities.

Subscription agreement: An agreement further to which one or more investors undertake to subscribe to, and whereby the competent corporate body (or the members thereof) undertakes to decide (or to vote in favor of), an upcoming issue by one or more target companies of shares, bonds, convertible bonds, warrants, or other financial instruments to such investors. The agreement will set out/forth the type and amount of instruments to be issued, the representations and warranties, the indemnification in the event of misrepresentation and may also include postclosing covenants (such as further investment obligations or restrictions on the transfer of the instruments that will be acquired).

Subsidiary: A company controlled by another company. The control is normally by virtue of having more than 50% of the voting rights.

Sweat equity: The contribution to an innovative project or start-up in the form of effort, knowledge, or toil.

Syndicate: The group of underwriters that will become legally obligated to purchase securities in a firm commitment public offering. Also, the department within the lead underwriter's firm that compiles the book.

Syndication: Syndication is the process whereby a group of venture capitalists will each put in a portion of the amount of money needed to finance a small business.

T

Takeover: Acquiring control of a corporation by stock purchase or exchange, either hostile or friendly.

Tangible asset: An asset that physically exists and can touched.

Tangible property: Property that physically exists and can be touched.

Target company: The company that the offeror is considering investing in. In the context of a public-to-private deal, this company will be the listed company that an offeror is considering investing in with the objective of bringing the company back into private ownership.

Telemarketing: Using the telephone as a means of marketing. This has been virtually the only medium employed in underwritten public offerings, where securities firms have their registered representatives telephone prospects to announce the offering, make a sales presentation, and take an order—preferably all in one call. In a direct public offering, telemarketing is one component of the marketing program. It may be passive (limited to answering incoming responses from prospects to the proposition) or active (initiating follow-up calls to prospects, after the fulfillment for their conversion into a sale).

Tenancy: Type of tenancy agreement under which the landlord has the right to take the property back at the end of the tenancy agreement.

Tender: Offer to perform work for an agreed price.

Term sheet: Term sheet is a nonbinding agreement setting forth the basic terms and conditions under which an investment will be made. The term sheet is a template that is used to develop more detailed legal documents.

Termination for cause: Termination of an employee's employment with justification, typically defined in some detail.

Tiered risk: The level and amount of risk encountered at the various stages of development.

Time value of money: The basic principle that money can earn interest; therefore, something that is worth $1 today will be worth more in the future if invested. This is also referred to as future value.

Trade secret: Information, such as a formula, pattern, device, or process, that is not known to the public and that gives the person possessing the information a competitive advantage. May sometimes include customer lists, marketing, and business plans and suppliers.

Trademark: In intellectual property, a mark that is registered at trademark registries and which is used on products produced by the owner. It is illegal for anyone else to display the mark.

Trust: A financial arrangement under which property is held by named people for someone else's benefit.

Trust corporation: A company that acts as a trustee and holds a trust's assets.

Trust deed: A legal document that is used to

- Create a trust
- Change a trust
- Control a trust

Trustee: A designated person who holds property and looks after it on behalf of someone else.

U

Underwriter: Underwriter is an investment banking firm committing successful distribution of a public issue, failing which the firm would take the securities being offered into its own books. An underwriter may also be a company that backs the issue of a contract, agreeing to accept responsibility for fulfilling the contract in return for a premium.

Underwriter's warrants: Warrants sometimes granted to underwriters as a form of additional compensation in a public offering, typically in a smaller, higher risk offering.

Underwriting agreement: The document pursuant to which the underwriters of a public offering contractually commit to purchase from the issuer the securities that are the subject of the public offering (or, in a best efforts offering, in which they agree to use best efforts to sell the securities). Also called a "placing agreement" in some countries.

Underwriting discount or commission or spread: The difference between the price at which underwriters buy securities from the issuer in a firm commitment public offering and the public offering price.

Unfair dismissal: Firing an employee unfairly. When an employee has been dismissed, it is the employer's responsibility to prove that the dismissal was fair and reasonable.

Uniform commercial code (UCC): Set of laws regulating commercial transactions, especially ones involving the sale of goods and secured transactions.

Unliquidated damages: Monetary damages decided by a court because the parties to a contract had not agreed in advance how much the damages would be for breaking the terms of the contract.

Unsecured creditor: Someone who has lent money without getting any security for the loan.

Unsecured debt: Loans not secured against a company's assets.

V

Valuation: The act or process of determining the value of a business, business ownership interest, security, or intangible asset.

Valuation approach: A general way of determining a value indication of a business, business ownership interest, security, or intangible asset using one or more valuation methods.

Valuation method: Within approaches, a specific way to determine value. The policy guidelines a management team uses to value the holdings in the fund's portfolio. More generally, valuation is an estimate of the price of an item at a given time, based on a model and comparison with the value of similar items.

Valuation procedure: The act, manner, and technique of performing the steps of an appraisal method.

Vendor: A person who sells something.

Venture capital: Original financing provided for new higher-risk ventures such as start-up companies. Over time, the term has expanded to also include investment in management buyouts and other situations in which venture capitalists invest. Venture capital investments are generally characterized by high risk and an expectation of high return.

A form of financing for a company in which the business gives up partial ownership and control of the business in exchange for capital over a limited time frame, usually 3–5 years. Investments typically range from $500,000 to $5 million, although there are occasionally venture capital investments for as low as $50,000 or as high as $20 million.

Venture capital financing: An investment in a start-up business that is perceived to have excellent growth prospects but does not have access to capital markets. Type of financing sought by early-stage companies seeking to grow rapidly.

Venture capitalist: A financial institution specializing in the provision of equity and other forms of long-term capital to enterprises, usually to firms with a limited track record but with the expectation of substantial growth. The venture capitalist may provide both funding and varying degrees of managerial and technical expertise.

Vesting schedules: Timetables for stock grants and options mandating that entrepreneurs earn (vest) their equity stakes over a number of years, rather than upon conversion of the stock options. This guarantees to investors and the market that the entrepreneurs will stick around, rather than converting and cashing in their shares.

Voidable: Able to be cancelled under certain circumstances.

Volatility: The volatility of a stock describes the extent of its variance over time between high and low market prices. High volatility denotes a wide variation and low volatility, a more stable stock. See Beta.

Voluntary arrangement: An agreement between a debtor and the creditors. If a person or a company cannot cover their debts when they are due, they can come to a voluntary arrangement with the creditors to pay the debts over a period. If the creditors agree with the proposals, it avoids bankruptcy of the individual or liquidation of the company.

Voluntary redemption: The right of a company to repurchase some or all of an investor's outstanding shares at a stated price at a given time in the future. The purchase price is usually the issue price, increased by cumulative dividends.

Voting right: The common stockholders' right to vote their stock in the affairs of the company. Preferred stock usually has the right to vote when preferred dividends are in default for a specified amount of time. The right to vote may be delegated by the stockholder to another person.

Vulture capitalist: Negative term for an investor who smells fast money and who is not serious about investing in companies with long-term potential. Compare with Venture capitalist.

W

Waiting period: The period of time between the filing of a registration statement with the SEC and the time when it is declared effective. See Quiet period.

Wall Street: A shorthand description for the US financial community, generally. The term comes from a street in lower Manhattan, New York, on which the American and New York Stock Exchanges, together with many financial professionals, are located.

Warrant: A certificate that gives the person holding it

- The right to buy shares at a given price
- Shares options that are vested

Warranty: In contract law, a warranty generally means a guarantee or promise that provides assurance by one party to the other party that specific facts or conditions are true or will happen.

Weighted average cost of capital (WACC): The cost of capital (discount rate) determined by the weighted average, at market value, of the cost of all financing sources in the business enterprise's capital structure.

Win–win situation: Circumstance in which all parties or companies gain or obtain a fairly distributed benefit.

Worst case: Business scenario based on the assumption that the majority of events affecting the targeted result will be unfavorable.

Write-off: The write-down of a portfolio company's value to zero. The value of the investment is eliminated and the return to investors is zero or negative.

Index

Page numbers followed by f and t indicate figures and tables, respectively.